T0318897

Curbside Consultation in IBD

Third UPDATED Edition

49 Clinical Questions

Curbside Consultation in Gastroenterology
SERIES

SERIES EDITOR, FRANCIS A. FARRAYE, MD, MSc

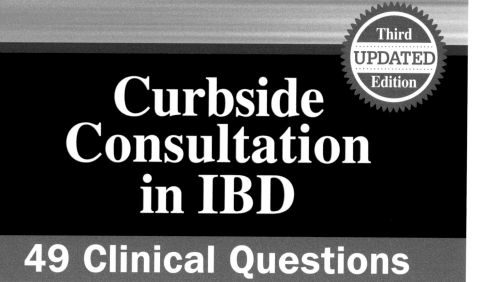

Curbside Consultation in IBD

Third UPDATED Edition

49 Clinical Questions

Editors

David T. Rubin, MD
Joseph B. Kirsner Professor of Medicine
Chief, Section of Gastroenterology, Hepatology, and Nutrition
Co-Director, Digestive Diseases Center
University of Chicago Medicine
Chicago, Illinois

Sonia Friedman, MD
Associate Professor of Medicine
Harvard Medical School
Brigham and Women's Hospital
Boston, Massachusetts

Francis A. Farraye, MD, MSc
Director
Inflammatory Bowel Disease Center
Mayo Clinic
Jacksonville, Florida
Professor of Medicine
Mayo Clinic School of Medicine

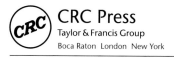
CRC Press
Taylor & Francis Group
Boca Raton London New York

CRC Press is an imprint of the
Taylor & Francis Group, an **informa** business

First Published in 2022 by SLACK Incorporated

Published 2024 by CRC Press
2385 NW Executive Center Drive, Suite 320, Boca Raton FL 33431

and by CRC Press
4 Park Square, Milton Park, Abingdon, Oxon, OX14 4RN

CRC Press is an imprint of Taylor & Francis Group, an informa business

Figures 6-1 and 6-2 are illustrated by Jill K. Gregory, CMI, and are printed with permission from © Mount Sinai Health System.

Cover Artist: Katherine Christie

This book contains information obtained from authentic and highly regarded sources. While all reasonable efforts have been made to publish reliable data and information, neither the author[s] nor the publisher can accept any legal responsibility or liability for any errors or omissions that may be made. The publishers wish to make clear that any views or opinions expressed in this book by individual editors, authors or contributors are personal to them and do not necessarily reflect the views/opinions of the publishers. The information or guidance contained in this book is intended for use by medical, scientific or health-care professionals and is provided strictly as a supplement to the medical or other professional's own judgement, their knowledge of the patient's medical history, relevant manufacturer's instructions and the appropriate best practice guidelines. Because of the rapid advances in medical science, any information or advice on dosages, procedures or diagnoses should be independently verified. The reader is strongly urged to consult the relevant national drug formulary and the drug companies' and device or material manufacturers' printed instructions, and their websites, before administering or utilizing any of the drugs, devices or materials mentioned in this book. This book does not indicate whether a particular treatment is appropriate or suitable for a particular individual. Ultimately it is the sole responsibility of the medical professional to make his or her own professional judgements, so as to advise and treat patients appropriately. The authors and publishers have also attempted to trace the copyright holders of all material reproduced in this publication and apologize to copyright holders if permission to publish in this form has not been obtained. If any copyright material has not been acknowledged please write and let us know so we may rectify in any future reprint.

Library of Congress Control Number: 2021941152

ISBN: 9781630916503 (pbk)
ISBN: 9781003523567 (ebk)

DOI: 10.1201/9781003523567

Dedication

This book is dedicated to my students, whom I teach to always challenge dogma and ask probing questions.

—*David T. Rubin, MD*

This book is dedicated to all my patients who have taught me so much about living with IBD and have inspired me by their courage.

—*Sonia Friedman, MD*

This book is dedicated to my family: my wife, Renee M. Remily, MD; my children, Jennifer Farraye, MSN and Alexis Farraye; and to my parents, who taught me that perseverance and commitment can result in great accomplishments. Finally, I thank my patients and their families for their confidence in allowing me to care for them.

—*Francis A. Farraye, MD, MSc*

Contents

About the Editors

David T. Rubin, MD, is the Joseph B. Kirsner Professor of Medicine; Chief of the Section of Gastroenterology, Hepatology, and Nutrition; and the Co-Director of the Digestive Diseases Center at the University of Chicago Medicine. He earned a medical degree with honors at the University of Chicago Pritzker School of Medicine and completed his residency in internal medicine and fellowships in gastroenterology and clinical medical ethics at the University of Chicago, where he served as Chief Resident and Chief Fellow. He also currently serves as an associate faculty member at the MacLean Center for Clinical Medical Ethics, an associate investigator at the University of Chicago Comprehensive Cancer Center, and is a member of the University of Chicago Committee on Clinical Pharmacology and Pharmacogenomics. He is the chair of the National Scientific Advisory Committee of the Crohn's and Colitis Foundation, where he also serves as a Board of Trustees member. Prior to these appointments, Dr. Rubin served as the Director of the Fellowship in Gastroenterology, Hepatology, and Nutrition at the University of Chicago for 11 years.

Dr. Rubin is a Fellow of the American Gastroenterological Association (AGA), the American College of Gastroenterology (ACG), the American Society for Gastrointestinal Endoscopy (ASGE), the American College of Physicians (ACP), and the Royal College of Physicians (Edinburgh). He is on the Board of Trustees for the ACG. Among numerous awards and honors, Dr. Rubin was chosen by his peers as a member of Best Doctors (recognized for superior clinical ability) and America's Top Physicians (gastroenterology). Additionally, he twice received the ACG's Governor's Award of Excellence in Clinical Research (2003 and 2013), and the UChicago Postgraduate Teaching Award in recognition of significant contributions for fellowship education (2006). In 2012, he received the Crohn's and Colitis Foundation's Rosenthal Award, a national leadership award bestowed upon a volunteer who has contributed in an indisputable way to the quality of life of patients and families. In 2020, Dr. Rubin received the Sherman Prize for Excellence in Crohn's and Colitis. He is an Associate Editor of the journal *Gastroenterology* and Editor-in-Chief of the ACG On-Line Education Universe. In 2018, Dr. Rubin completed the Harvard T.H. Chan School of Public Health Leadership Development Course for Physicians.

In addition to *Curbside Consultation in IBD,* Dr. Rubin is an associate editor of the 11th edition of *Sleisenger and Fordtran's Gastrointestinal and Liver Disease,* and an author or coauthor of more than 450 articles on treatment and management of IBD, cancer in IBD and novel paradigms, as well as the first author of the 2019 ACG Guidelines for ulcerative colitis. His current research is in the area of biosensor monitoring of IBD, prevention of progressive complications from uncontrolled inflammation, and a variety of collaborative studies related to the causes of IBD and its complications. He is also a featured media contact for issues related to IBD, appearing on satellite radio, television, and print media and maintains a popular and verified Twitter feed @IBDMD.

Sonia Friedman, MD, is Associate Professor of Medicine at Harvard Medical School and an Associate Physician at Brigham and Women's Hospital in Boston, Massachusetts. She is an Adjunct Professor of Clinical Epidemiology at the University of Southern Denmark in Odense, Denmark. Dr. Friedman completed her undergraduate degree in biology at Stanford University and her MD at Yale Medical School. She did her medical internship and residency at University of Pennsylvania and her gastroenterology fellowship at Mount Sinai Medical Center in New York City. She specialized in IBD during her fellowship and now has a large IBD practice in the gastroenterology division of Brigham and Women's Hospital. She has been at Brigham and Women's for the past 21 years and is Director of Women's Health at the Center for Crohn's and Colitis.

Dr. Friedman's research interests include reproductive health and the safety of medications taking during conception and/or during pregnancy in patients with IBD. Her clinical interests are the care of patients with Crohn's disease and ulcerative colitis. She specializes in the management of infertility and pregnancy in patients with IBD. Dr. Friedman is a frequent speaker and invited regional and national lecturer on the management of IBD. She has authored or co-authored papers on cancer in Crohn's disease, adherence to surveillance colonoscopy, management of polyps and cancer in IBD, medical management of IBD, fertility, sexual function, pregnancy, and men's health in IBD, as well as the long-term outcomes of children exposed to IBD and IBD medications in utero.

Dr. Friedman is the Deputy Editor of the journal *Inflammatory Bowel Diseases* and is on the *Gastroenterology* and *Digestive Diseases and Sciences* editorial boards. She is a member of the National Academies of Sciences, Engineering, and Medicine Committee on Assessment of NIH Research on Autoimmune Diseases as well as the Crohn's and Colitis Foundation Unbiased Peer Review Task Force. She is a member of the Crohn's and Colitis Foundation Clinical Research Alliance and is a member of the organizing committee of the Crohn's and Colitis Foundation Congress. She has received a recent Crohn's and Colitis Foundation Senior Research Award as well as an American College of Gastroenterology Clinical Research Award to continue her work on reproductive health in IBD.

Francis A. Farraye, MD, MSc, is a Professor of Medicine at the Mayo Clinic School of Medicine and Director of the Inflammatory Bowel Disease Center at the Mayo Clinic in Jacksonville, Florida. After graduating from the State University of New York (SUNY) at Stony Brook, Dr. Farraye earned his medical doctorate from Albert Einstein College of Medicine in New York, New York, and his master's degree in epidemiology from the Harvard School of Public Health in Boston, Massachusetts. He completed an internal medicine residency and gastroenterology fellowship at the Beth Israel Hospital in Boston.

Dr. Farraye is a clinical investigator with an active academic practice managing patients with IBD. A frequent speaker and invited lecturer on topics on the diagnosis and management of IBD, Dr. Farraye has authored or co-authored more than 450 original scientific manuscripts, chapters, reviews, and abstracts. He is the series editor for the text *Curbside Consultation in Gastroenterology* and co-wrote the texts *Curbside Consultation in IBD* and *GI Emergencies: A Quick Reference Guide.* His newest books for patients are *Questions and Answers About Ulcerative Colitis* and *Questions and Answers About Crohn's Disease.* He is the Editor-in-Chief for *IBD Journal Scan,* published weekly by the American Society of Gastrointestinal Endoscopy.

Dr. Farraye is a Fellow of the American College of Physicians, American Society of Gastrointestinal Endoscopy, and American Gastroenterological Association and a Master in the American College of Gastroenterology. He has served on numerous national and international committees and currently is the Chair of the North Florida Chapter Medical Advisory Committee for the Crohn's and Colitis Foundation. The New England Crohn's and Colitis Foundation named Dr. Farraye Humanitarian of the Year in 2003. In 2009, the American College of Gastroenterology awarded Dr. Farraye the William Carey Award for service to the college. In 2020, Dr. Farraye was a recipient of the Life Time Achievement Award from the New England Crohn's and Colitis Foundation.

Contributing Authors

Bincy P. Abraham, MD, MS (Question 25)
Houston Methodist and Weill Cornell
Houston, Texas

Shintaro Akiyama, MD, PhD (Question 41)
Department of Gastroenterology
Faculty of Medicine
University of Tsukuba
Tsukuba, Ibaraki, Japan

Jessica R. Allegretti, MD, MPH (Question 35)
Director of Clinical Research
Director, Fecal Microbiota Transplant Program
Associate Director, Crohn's and Colitis Center
Division of Gastroenterology, Hepatology and
Endoscopy
Brigham and Women's Hospital
Assistant Professor of Medicine
Harvard Medical School
Boston, Massachusetts

Ashwin N. Ananthakrishnan, MD, MPH
(Question 40)
Associate Professor of Medicine
Massachusetts General Hospital
Boston, Massachusetts

Jordan E. Axelrad, MD, MPH (Question 36)
Division of Gastroenterology
Department of Medicine
NYU Grossman School of Medicine
New York, New York

Filip J. Baert, MD, PhD (Question 23)
Department of Gastroenterology
AZ Delta
Roeselare, Belgium

Edward L. Barnes, MD, MPH (Question 12)
Assistant Professor of Medicine
Associate Director
Gastroenterology and Hepatology
Fellowship Program
Division of Gastroenterology and Hepatology
University of North Carolina
Chapel Hill, North Carolina

Alyse Bedell, PhD (Question 46)
Department of Psychiatry and
Behavioral Neuroscience
University of Chicago
Chicago, Illinois

Shomron Ben-Horin, MD (Question 48)
Department of Gastroenterology
Sheba Medical Center
Tel Aviv University
Tel Aviv, Israel

Madeline Bertha, MD (Question 7)
Gastroenterology and Hepatology Fellow
Feinberg School of Medicine
Northwestern University
Chicago, Illinois

David G. Binion, MD (Question 42)
Professor of Medicine
Clinical and Translational Science
University of Pittsburgh School of Medicine
Co-Director, IBD Center
Director of Nutrition Support Service
Medical Director
Small Intestinal Transplantation
UPMC Presbyterian Hospital
Pittsburgh, Pennsylvania

Diana Bolotin, MD, PhD (Question 30)
Associate Professor
Chief
Section of Dermatology
University of Chicago Medicine
Chicago, Illinois

Brian P. Bosworth, MD (Question 9)
Associate Chief Medical Officer
Chief of Medicine
NYU Langone Health Main Campus
Professor of Medicine
NYU Grossman School of Medicine
New York, New York

Michael Buie, BHSc (Question 43)
Department of Community Health Sciences
University of Calgary
Calgary, Alberta, Canada

Anthony Buisson, MD, PhD (Question 5)
IBD Unit
CHU Estaing
Clermont-Ferrand, France

Freddy Caldera, DO, MS (Question 44)
Associate Professor
Division of Gastroenterology and Hepatology
Department of Medicine
School of Medicine and Public Health
University of Wisconsin–Madison
Madison, Wisconsin

Victor G. Chedid, MD, MSc (Question 39)
Division of Gastroenterology and Hepatology
Mayo Clinic
Rochester, Minnesota

Adam Cheifetz, MD (Question 19)
Director
Center for Inflammatory Bowel Disease
Medical Director
Infusion Services
Beth Israel Deaconess Medical Center
Professor of Medicine
Harvard Medical School
Boston, Massachusetts

Britt Christensen, BSc, MBBS (Hons), MPH, PhD (Question 13)
Head of Inflammatory Bowel Disease Unit
Gastroenterology Department
The Royal Melbourne Hospital
Parkville, Victoria, Australia

William T. Clarke, MD, MSc (Question 20)
Division of Gastroenterology
Duke University School of Medicine
Durham, North Carolina

Jennie Clough, MBBS (Question 11)
IBD Research Fellow
Guy's and St Thomas' Hospital
London, United Kingdom

Erica R. Cohen, MD (Question 45)
Director of IBD Program
Capital Digestive Care
Chevy Chase, Maryland

Jean-Frederic Colombel, MD (Question 6)
Professor of Medicine
Co-Director of the
Inflammatory Bowel Disease Center
Icahn School of Medicine at Mount Sinai
New York, New York

Susan Connor, MBBS (Hons 1), B Med Sci, PhD (Question 21)
Department of Gastroenterology and Hepatology
Liverpool Hospital
South Western Sydney Clinical School
University of New South Wales
Sydney, New South Wales, Australia
Ingham Institute of Applied Medical Research
Liverpool, New South Wales, Australia

Ferdinando D'Amico, MD, PhD (Question 17)
IBD Center
Humanitas Research Hospital–IRCCS
Rozzano, Milan, Italy

Silvio Danese, MD, PhD (Question 17)
Department of Biomedical Sciences
Humanitas University
Pieve Emanuele, Milan, Italy
Humanitas Research Hospital-IRCCS
IBD Center
Rozzano, Milan, Italy

Punyanganie S. de Silva, MBBS, MPH (Question 49)
Assistant Professor
Harvard Medical School
Attending Physician
Crohn's & Colitis Centre
Brigham & Women's Hospital
Boston, Massachusetts

Jean A. Donet, MD (Question 2)
Assistant Professor of Medicine
University of California San Francisco
Fresno, California

Iris Dotan, MD (Question 27)
Division of Gastroenterology
Rabin Medical Center
Petah Tikva, Israel
Sackler Faculty of Medicine
Tel Aviv University
Tel Aviv, Israel

David Drobne, MD, PhD (Question 23)
Assistant Professor
Department of Gastroenterology
University Medical Centre Ljubljana
Medical Faculty
University of Ljubljana
Ljubljana, Slovenia

Joseph D. Feuerstein, MD (Question 20)
Associate Professor of Medicine
Center for Inflammatory Bowel Disease
Beth Israel Deaconess Medical Center
Harvard Medical School
Boston, Massachusetts

Kerri Glassner, DO (Question 25)
Assistant Professor Clinical Medicine
Fondren IBD Center
Houston Methodist and Weill Cornell
Houston Methodist Gastroenterology Associates
Houston, Texas

Idan Goren, MD (Question 27)
Division of Gastroenterology
Rabin Medical Center
Petah Tikva, Israel
Sackler Faculty of Medicine
Tel Aviv University
Tel Aviv, Israel

Kay Greveson, BA, MSc (Question 48)
Lead IBD Nurse
Royal Free Hospital
London, United Kingdom

Bilal Hameed, MD (Question 31)
Associate Professor of Medicine
Clinic Chief, Hepatology
University of California, San Francisco
San Francisco, California

Muhammad Bader Hammami, MD (Question 34)
Assistant Professor of Medicine
Loma Linda University
Loma Linda, California
Health Sciences Assistant Clinical Professor
University of California, Riverside
Riverside, California

Stephen B. Hanauer, MD (Question 7)
Clifford Joseph Barborka Professor of Medicine
Northwestern Feinberg School of Medicine
Medical Director
Digestive Health Center
Chicago, Illinois

Jana G. Hashash, MD, MSc (Question 42)
Division of Gastroenterology and Hepatology
American University of Beirut
Beirut, Lebanon
Division of Gastroenterology, Hepatology, and Nutrition
University of Pittsburgh
Pittsburgh, Pennsylvania

Hans Herfarth, MD, PhD (Question 12)
Professor of Medicine
Co-Director
UNC Multidisciplinary
Inflammatory Bowel Diseases Center
Division of Gastroenterology and Hepatology
University of North Carolina
Chapel Hill, North Carolina

Peter M. Irving, MBBS, MA, MD (Question 11)
IBD Unit
Guy's and St Thomas' Hospital
NHS Foundation Trust
London, United Kingdom

Steven H. Itzkowitz, MD (Question 36)
Professor of Medicine
Oncological Sciences
Medical Education Director
Gastroenterology Fellowship Program
The Dr. Henry D. Janowitz
Division of Gastroenterology
The Samuel Bronfman
Department of Medicine
Icahn School of Medicine at Mount Sinai
New York, New York

Sunanda V. Kane, MD, MSPH (Question 39)
Division of Gastroenterology and Hepatology
Mayo Clinic
Rochester, Minnesota

Gilaad G. Kaplan, MD, MPH (Question 43)
Professor of Medicine
Division of Gastroenterology and Hepatology
Departments of Medicine and Community
Health Sciences
Cumming School of Medicine
University of Calgary
Calgary, Alberta, Canada

Seymour Katz, MD (Question 32)
Clinical Professor of Medicine
Director of Outreach IBD Programs
New York University
Grossman School of Medicine
New York, New York

Arthur Kavanaugh, MD (Question 28)
Professor of Medicine
Division of Rheumatology, Allergy, and
Immunology
Department of Medicine
University of California, San Diego
La Jolla, California

Maia Kayal, MD (Question 6)
Assistant Professor
The Susan and Leonard Feinstein IBD Center
Dr. Henry D. Janowitz
Division of Gastroenterology
Icahn School of Medicine at Mount Sinai
New York, New York

Laurie Keefer, PhD (Question 46)
Icahn School of Medicine at Mount Sinai
New York, New York

Jami Kinnucan, MD (Question 26)
Assistant Professor of Medicine
Michigan Medicine
University of Michigan
Ann Arbor, Michigan

Mark Lazarev, MD (Question 2)
Associate Professor of Medicine
Division of Gastroenterology and Hepatology
The Johns Hopkins Hospital
Baltimore, Maryland

Jonathan A. Leighton, MD (Question 4)
Division of Gastroenterology and Hepatology
Mayo Clinic Arizona
Scottsdale, Arizona

Irving Levine, MD (Question 9)
Fellow
Division of Gastroenterology and Hepatology
Department of Medicine
Zucker School of Medicine at
Hofstra/Northwell Health System
New Hyde Park, New York

Alexander N. Levy, MD (Question 35)
Division of Gastroenterology and Hepatology
Tufts Medical Center
Boston, Massachusetts

James D. Lewis, MD, MSCE (Question 47)
Professor of Medicine and Epidemiology
Perelman School of Medicine
University of Pennsylvania
Philadelphia, Pennsylvania

Amy L. Lightner, MD (Question 38)
Director, Center for Regenerative Medicine
and Surgery
Associate Professor of Colorectal Surgery
Digestive Disease Institute
Associate Professor of Inflammation and
Immunity
Lerner Research Institute
Core Member in the Center for Immunotherapy
Cleveland Clinic
Cleveland, Ohio

Jimmy K. Limdi, MBBS (Question 37)
Head
Section of Inflammatory Bowel Disease
Pennine Acute Hospitals NHS Trust
Honorary Clinical Professor of
Gastroenterology
University of Manchester
Manchester, United Kingdom

Uma Mahadevan, MD (Question 34)
Professor of Medicine
University of California, San Francisco
San Francisco, California

Gil Y. Melmed, MD, MS (Question 45)
Co-Director
Clinical Inflammatory Bowel Disease
Professor of Medicine
Division of Digestive Diseases
Department of Medicine
Cedars-Sinai
Los Angeles, California

Oluwakemi Onajin, MD (Question 30)
Section of Dermatology
University of Chicago
Chicago, Illinois

Mark T. Osterman, MD, MSCE (Question 14)
Associate Professor of Medicine
University of Pennsylvania
Perelman School of Medicine
Philadelphia, Pennsylvania

Aoibhlinn O'Toole, MD (Question 33)
Consultant Gastroenterologist
Senior Lecturer
Royal College of Surgeons Ireland
Gastroenterology National Specialty Director
for Training
Royal College of Physicians Ireland
Beaumont Hospital
Dublin, Ireland

Baldeep S. Pabla, MD, MSCI (Question 3)
Assistant Professor
Department of Gastroenterology, Hepatology,
and Nutrition
Vanderbilt University Medical Center
VUMC Inflammatory Bowel Disease Clinic
Nashville, Tennessee

Carolina Palmela, MD (Question 1)
Division of Gastroenterology
Hospital Beatriz Ângelo
Loures, Portugal

Remo Panaccione, MD (Question 10)
Professor of Medicine, University of Calgary
CCC Chair in IBD Research
Director, Inflammatory Bowel Disease Unit
Director, Gastrointestinal Research
Assistant Dean of MD Admissions
Undergraduate Medical Education
Cumming School of Medicine
University of Calgary
Calgary, Canada

Konstantinos Papamichael, MD, PhD (Question 19)
Center for Inflammatory Bowel Disease
Beth Israel Deaconess Medical Center
Instructor in Medicine
Harvard Medical School
Boston, Massachusetts

Shabana F. Pasha, MD (Question 4)
Division of Gastroenterology and Hepatology
Mayo Clinic Arizona
Scottsdale, Arizona

Shivani A. Patel, PharmD, BCPS (Question 24)
Clinical Pharmacy Specialist
University of Chicago Medicine
Chicago, Illinois

Joel Pekow, MD (Question 16)
Associate Professor of Medicine
Section of Gastroenterology, Hepatology, and
Nutrition
University of Chicago
Chicago, Illinois

Tamar Pfeffer Gik, RD, MSc (Question 47)
Inflammatory Bowel Disease Center
Division of Gastroenterology
Beilinson Hospital
Rabin Medical Center
Petah Tikva, Israel

Ralley Prentice, MBBS (Question 13)
Inflammatory Bowel Disease Research Fellow
Monash Health
St Vincent's Hospital
Melbourne, Victoria, Australia

David B. Sachar, MD (Question 8)
Clinical Professor of Medicine and
Emeritus Director of the
Dr. Henry D. Janowitz Division of
Gastroenterology
Icahn School of Medicine at Mount Sinai
New York, New York

Atsushi Sakuraba, MD, PhD (Question 41)
Associate Professor
Section of Gastroenterology, Hepatology and
Nutrition
University of Chicago
Chicago, Illinois

Akriti P. Saxena, MD (Question 14)
Assistant Professor of Clinical Medicine
Division of Gastroenterology and Hepatology
University of Pennsylvania
Philadelphia, Pennsylvania

David A. Schwartz, MD (Question 3)
Director
Inflammatory Bowel Disease Center
Director
McClain Family Directorship in
Gastroenterology
Professor of Medicine
Vanderbilt University Medical Center
Nashville, Tennessee

Seth R. Shaffer, MD, MS (Question 22)
Department of Internal Medicine
Max Rady College of Medicine
Rady Faculty of Medicine
Inflammatory Bowel Disease Clinical and
Research Centre
University of Manitoba
Winnipeg, Manitoba, Canada

Abha G. Singh, MD (Question 28)
Associate Professor of Medicine
Division of Rheumatology, Allergy, and
Immunology
Department of Medicine
University of California, San Diego
La Jolla, California

Arun Swaminath, MD (Question 26)
Chief of Gastroenterology
Lenox Hill Hospital
Northwell Health
New York, New York
Associate Professor of Medicine
Hofstra Northwell School of Medicine
Hempstead, New York

Eva Szigethy, MD, PhD (Question 29)
Professor, Department of Psychiatry,
Pediatrics and Medicine
Co-Director, IBD Total Care Subspecialty
Medical Home
Director, Behavioral Health
UPMC Chief Medical Office
Consultant, UPMC Health Plan
Behavioral Unit of Digitally Delivered Interventions
University of Pittsburgh Medical Center
Pittsburgh, Pennsylvania

Norah Terrault, MD, MPH (Question 31)
Professor of Medicine
University of Southern California
Los Angeles, California

Joana Torres, MD, PhD (Question 1)
Division of Gastroenterology
Hospital Beatriz Ângelo
Loures, Portugal

Andrew R. Watson, MD, MLitt (Question 42)
Department of Surgery
University of Pittsburgh Medical Center
Pittsburgh, Pennsylvania

Emily Weaver, LCSW (Question 29)
University of Pittsburgh Medical Center
Pittsburgh, Pennsylvania

Roni Weisshof, MD (Question 18)
Department of Gastroenterology
Rambam Health Care Campus
Haifa, Israel
Section of Gastroenterology, Hepatology, and
Nutrition
Department of Medicine
University of Chicago
Chicago, Illinois

Rachel W. Winter, MD, MPH (Question 15)
Brigham and Women's Hospital
Harvard Medical School
Boston, Massachusetts

Yang (Clare) Wu, MBChB (Question 21)
South Western Sydney Clinical School
University of New South Wales
Sydney, New South Wales, Australia

Akihiro Yamada, MD, PhD (Question 41)
Division of Gastroenterology
Department of Internal Medicine
Toho University Sakura Medical Center
Sakura City, Chiba, Japan

*Toni M. Zahorian, PharmD, BCACP
(Question 24)*
Trellis Rx
Parkview Health
Fort Wayne, Indiana

Preface

We have been so pleased with the success and positive feedback from our colleagues for the first two editions of *Curbside Consultation in IBD: 49 Clinical Questions*. Writing these prior editions was made successful by the contributions of our expert colleagues from around the world, who shared their experiences and insights in such practical ways. However, what we realized shortly after completing the second edition was that we could easily add many more questions to our list. And so we have, with this updated and excellent third edition.

In keeping with the format of the *Curbside Consultation* series, we created this new edition with 49 questions, but substituted some chapters with entirely new questions and authors. Importantly, we updated the prior questions as well, especially when those topics needed further explanation and distribution.

The field of inflammatory bowel disease continues to expand rapidly, and we are fortunate to live in a time when there are so many more therapies available and improving approaches to the chronic management of these difficult diseases. But keeping pace with the advances in the field, let alone the experience necessary to apply them to practice, is a great challenge. We are hopeful that this edition of *Curbside Consultation in IBD* complements the prior editions nicely, and, if you are a first-time owner of this series of books, you find the format engaging and highly educational.

We welcome your feedback and new questions and hope that through our "curbsides" you are able to provide your patients with a better quality of life.

Introduction

Curbside Consultations in IBD: 49 Clinical Questions, Third Edition has been written for clinicians who care for patients with Crohn's disease and ulcerative colitis. We recognize that these clinicians may be gastroenterologists with a specific interest in inflammatory bowel disease (IBD), academic specialists, general gastroenterologists, and advanced practice providers who work in an office and have their own practice of patients with IBD, all of whom find care for this special population of patients challenging. The structure of the book is based on the best-selling series from SLACK Incorporated and is meant to replicate the casual conversation that occurs in the hallway of a hospital or clinic, or these days by text message, between colleagues who are seeing a difficult patient and are unsure of the best path forward.

The 49 questions included in this edition are based on commonly asked questions, areas that had significant advances in our field and changed the way we practice in the last several years, and additional topics related to dilemmas in our field in which there is little evidence to guide us. This edition is organized by general topic, from diagnosis to treatments, to surgery to chronic care and management otherwise. The book is designed to be a handbook as well as an enjoyable cover-to-cover read. Some may find this book useful from time to time with difficult cases. Others will find that reading it through adds to their body of knowledge and contributes to their plan for their population of patients. We hope that the succinct yet practical description and recommendations translate well to your patients.

SECTION I

DIAGNOSIS AND PROGNOSIS

QUESTION

HOW CAN WE ASSESS PROGNOSIS IN CROHN'S DISEASE?

Carolina Palmela, MD and
Joana Torres, MD, PhD

Crohn's disease (CD) is a chronic disabling disease with a major impact on patients' lives.[1] CD is a destructive disease that can result in progressive bowel damage and ultimately in disability. Only 10% of patients achieve prolonged clinical remission, and more than 50% report either an increase in symptoms intensity or chronic-intermittent/chronic-continuous symptoms over time.[1] Natural history studies coming from population-based cohorts have shown that at diagnosis up to one-third of patients already present with a complicated behavior (strictures, fistula, or abscesses) and that over time most patients will eventually develop a complication, with 50% of patients requiring surgery within 10 years after diagnosis.[1] One-third will need multiple operations and around 10% will require a permanent stoma.[2] Finally, extensive small bowel disease and/or multiple surgeries can potentially result in intestinal failure and short bowel syndrome, one rare but fearful and irreversible complication of the disease.[2]

Therapeutic strategies in CD result from a delicate and difficult balance between benefits and risks. The recognition that chronic and untreated inflammation in CD (even if asymptomatic) ultimately results in poor outcomes has led to a recent paradigm shift in treatment, with the belief that early intervention with immunosuppressant and/or biologic therapy can prevent disease progression and avoid complications. However, treating all patients with biologics and/or combination therapy is probably economically unsustainable and would risk exposing those with an indolent disease course to unnecessary risks or side effects of this potent therapy.[2] The challenge is selecting patients who will benefit the most from early intensive therapy, while sparing those with mild-moderate disease who may experience spontaneous and long-term remission without disease progression and who will derive minimal benefit from such treatment. Therefore, patient profiling

Rubin DT, Friedman S, Farraye FA, eds. *Curbside Consultation in IBD:*
49 Clinical Questions, Third Edition (pp 3-8).
© 2022 Taylor & Francis Group.

using prognostic factors at diagnosis and during follow-up, for the selection of the best candidates for early aggressive therapies and intensive monitoring, is of main importance.

Many studies with different designs and different patient populations have tried to find clinical, endoscopic, serological, and genetic predictors of specific disease complications. So far, none have been demonstrated as accurate when used alone.

Several definitions of poor prognosis in CD have been suggested over the years, such as disabling or complicated disease. Disabling CD has been defined by different authors as the presence of more than two steroid courses and/or steroid dependency, disabling chronic symptoms, the need for immunosuppressive therapy, hospitalization for disease flare or complications of the disease, and intestinal resection or surgery for perianal disease.[3,4] Alternatively, other authors have used complicated CD, defined as the presence of bowel damage (stricture, abscess, and/or fistula) and/or the requirement for surgery and/or the presence of extra-intestinal manifestations[5] as a poor prognosis outcome. Table 1-1 summarizes clinical, endoscopic, molecular, and genetic prognostic predictors in CD and the associated impact on disease course.

Clinical Prognostic Factors

In a recent meta-analysis of 1961 patients with CD, the demographic and clinical characteristics associated with significantly higher risk of developing disabling disease at 5 years after initial diagnosis were young age (< 40 years) at diagnosis, initial requirement of steroids for treating the first flare, and the presence of perianal disease.[6] Several authors have reported clinical factors associated with complicated CD, including young age at diagnosis, small bowel disease (ileal and/or ileocolonic), upper gastrointestinal extent, stricturing or penetrating behavior, perianal disease, and smoking.[5,7-10] Disease located in the small bowel (ileal disease and/or ileocolonic disease), as opposed to colonic disease, has been consistently identified as an independent risk factor for surgery.[11] This may be due to the fact that small bowel involvement is more frequently associated with penetrating and stricturing behavior than colonic disease. The presence of penetrating and stricturing complications, as compared to an inflammatory phenotype, is possibly the most important independent factor associated with the need for surgery, both in adult and pediatric populations. Furthermore, patients who have surgery for penetrating complications have a higher chance of being re-operated on and a short amount of time before a second surgery, which indicates that this is a group of patients with an especially aggressive type of disease.[2]

Endoscopic Prognostic Factors

The presence of extensive and deep ulcerations at colonoscopy has been shown to be associated with an increased rate of penetrating complications and surgery in patients with ileocolonic CD.[12] Such ulcerations predict a more aggressive clinical course and should trigger a more intensive attitude in terms of therapy and monitoring. Endoscopic healing should be the pursued treatment target.

Laboratorial Prognostic Factors

C-reactive protein (CRP) and fecal calprotectin (FCal) are frequently used laboratory biomarkers to evaluate intestinal inflammation. Although these markers have been associated with risk of disease relapse, their utility for long-term prognostication has yet to be proven. A recent systematic review concluded that in asymptomatic patients with inflammatory bowel disease (IBD) the increase of FCal levels measured longitudinally was correlated with increased prob-

Table 1-1

Clinical, Endoscopic, Molecular, and Genetic Prognostic Predictors in Crohn's Disease and the Associated Impact on Disease Course

Prognostic Factor	Impact on Disease Course
Young age (< 40 years) at diagnosis	• Disabling CD[3,8] • Complicated CD (including surgery)[5,8] • Disease recurrence[8]
Complicated behavior (B2 and/or B3)	• Complicated CD (including surgery)[5,8] • Severe CD[4] • Disease recurrence[8] • Hospitalization[9]
Ileal (L1) and ileocolonic (L3) disease	• Complicated CD (including surgery and disease behavior progression)[5,8,10] • Disabling CD[4] • Time to hospitalization[9]
Upper GI extent (L4)	• Complicated CD (including surgery)[5,8]
Perianal disease	• Disabling CD[3,4] • Complicated CD[5,7]
Smoking	• Complicated CD[5,7] • Higher recurrence rate (surgical or nonsurgical)[8] • More frequent perianal disease[10]
Disease duration > 10 years	• Complicated CD[7]
Deep ulcerations at index colonoscopy	• Increased rate of penetrating complications and surgery[12]
Requirement of steroids at diagnosis	• Disabling CD[3,4]
Positive antimicrobial markers	• Complicated phenotype and surgery[16]
NOD2 mutations	• Ileal disease[18] • Surgery[17] • Complicated CD[17]

ability of disease relapse within the next 2 to 3 months.[13] The recently published CALM (effect of tight control management on Crohn's disease) study also showed that timely escalation of therapy on the basis of symptoms combined with CRP and FCal levels was associated with better clinical and endoscopic outcomes at 1 year (as compared to symptom-only driven decisions).[14] Studies assessing the effects of this strategy in long-term outcomes, such as bowel damage, surgeries, hospital admissions, and disability, are still needed.

Several adult and pediatric cohorts have indicated that circulating antibodies against bacterial antigens are associated with complicated CD and progression toward stricturing or penetrating phenotypes. Subsets of patients with differing immune responses to microbial antigens have been described: antibodies to the *Escherichia coli* outer-membrane porin C (OmpC), anti-*Saccharomyces cerevisiae* (ASCA), antiflagellin (anti-CBir1), as well as anti-perinuclear antineutrophil antibody (pANCA).[15] These immune responses have been associated with fibrostenosing, penetrating small bowel disease, and small bowel surgery. It has been suggested that the presence (number of markers) and magnitude (antibody level) of immune responses to microbial antigens are significantly associated with more aggressive disease phenotypes.[16] Nonetheless, serologic factors have a low sensitivity, and most of them are unavailable outside of the United States.

Genetic Prognostic Risk Factors

Genetics have also been shown to predict a more aggressive disease course. The original *nucleotide-binding oligomerization domain-containing protein 2* (NOD2) studies found an association between NOD2 and small bowel fibrostenosing disease. A large meta-analysis of 36 studies showed that the presence of any NOD2 mutation was associated with complicated (stricturing or penetrating) disease (relative risk 1.17) and an increase (58%) in the risk of CD surgery.[17] These findings were not confirmed in the largest genotype-phenotype study conducted so far, where NOD2 mutations did not associate with specific complications but rather with younger age at diagnosis and ileal location.[18] The combination of NOD2 genotype and immune reactivity has also been shown to predict prognosis in a subset of adult patients with CD.[19] Other genetic markers have been studied, including PRDM1 variants, IL23R, JAK2, and TNFS15, which also seem to be associated with complicated CD. However, so far there are insufficient data to support the recommendation to use genetic testing in clinical practice to predict CD course.

Limitations of Current Prognostic Factors and Future Perspectives

The use of prognostic factors to guide CD management is an evolving field. Most of the currently available prognostic factors in CD are clinical and lack precision. For example, while young age at diagnosis is indisputably a poor prognostic factor, the truth is that the majority of patients are younger than 40 years at the time of diagnosis. Furthermore, many of the clinical risk factors have been identified in retrospective studies and have yet to be prospectively validated. The use of serologic and genetic factors in prognostication is also limited by lack of sensitivity and broad availability. Adequately powered prospective studies are necessary to develop appropriate algorithms that can truly predict poor prognosis in the individual patient with CD.

Because it is a complex disease, it is likely that CD prognostication will also be a complex matter and require the integration of clinical, molecular, and endoscopic prognostic factors. The recently developed and validated PROSPECT (Personalized Risk and Outcome Prediction) tool is an example of such a tool, incorporating clinical (gender, duration of disease, and disease location), serologic (ASCA, ANCA, and anti-CBir1), and genetic (NOD2 status) factors to predict an individual patient's risk of developing a CD complication or surgery.[20] The prospective RISK (Risk Stratification and Identification of Immunogenetic and Microbial Markers of Rapid Disease Progression in Children With Crohn's Disease) study also derived and validated a risk-stratification model based on clinical and serological factors in newly diagnosed children with CD.[21] Age at diagnosis, Black race, isolated ileal location, ASCA, anti-CBir1, and a novel extracellular matrix gene signature showed an area under the curve of 0.72 and a negative predictive value of 94% for the development of stricturing or penetrating behavior.

Conclusion

We are currently moving from an era of "one treatment fits all" to an era of personalized medicine. CD is a dynamic disease, and therefore reassessment of disease and of prognosis should likewise be a dynamic and continuous process. Stratifying patients and individualizing therapy are crucial steps to optimize patient management. Briefly, patients presenting with a young age at diagnosis (< 40 years), deep ulcerations at endoscopy, ileal or ileocolonic involvement, perianal disease, severe rectal disease, and penetrating or stenosing behavior should be regarded as having a higher likelihood of progressing to complications and/or surgery and may be candidates for intensive therapy and monitoring. Preliminary findings suggest that immune and genetic markers may be predictive of a more aggressive disease course, but larger prospective studies are needed. Composite scores incorporating clinical information and molecular profiling will hopefully allow us to better personalize CD treatment in the future.

Because of the current limitations of prognostic factors, it is essential to be mindful of the importance of complementing prognostication with a treat-to-target approach. Using this approach, and monitoring disease and the effects of therapy at regular intervals, provides the clinicians with the possibility of adjusting therapy (either escalating, deescalating, or changing therapeutic class) accordingly, therefore increasing the chances to keep disease and inflammation under tight control, which is believed to be key in preventing disease progression and changing disease natural history.

References

1. Torres J, Mehandru S, Colombel JF, Peyrin-Biroulet L. Crohn's disease. *Lancet.* 2017;389(10080):1741-1755.
2. Torres J, Caprioli F, Katsanos KH, et al. Predicting outcomes to optimize disease management in inflammatory bowel diseases. *Journal of Crohn's & Colitis.* 2016;10(12):138-1394.
3. Beaugerie L, Seksik P, Nion-Larmurier I, Gendre JP, Cosnes J. Predictors of Crohn's disease. *Gastroenterology.* 2006;130(3):650-656.
4. Loly C, Belaiche J, Louis E. Predictors of severe Crohn's disease. *Scand J Gastroenterol.* 2008;43(8):948-954.
5. Zallot C, Peyrin-Biroulet L. Clinical risk factors for complicated disease: how reliable are they? *Dig Dis.* 2012;30(3):67-72.
6. Dias CC, Rodrigues PP, da Costa-Pereira A, Magro F. Clinical prognostic factors for disabling Crohn's disease: a systematic review and meta-analysis. *World J Gastroenterol.* 2013;19(24):3866-3871.
7. Lakatos PL, Czegledi Z, Szamosi T, et al. Perianal disease, small bowel disease, smoking, prior steroid or early azathioprine/biological therapy are predictors of disease behavior change in patients with Crohn's disease. *World J Gastroenterol.* 2009;15(28):3504-3510.
8. Romberg-Camps MJ, Dagnelie PC, Kester AD, et al. Influence of phenotype at diagnosis and of other potential prognostic factors on the course of inflammatory bowel disease. *Am J Gastroenterol.* 2009;104(2):371-383.
9. Golovics PA, Mandel MD, Lovasz BD, et al. Is hospitalization predicting the disease course in Crohn's disease? Prevalence and predictors of hospitalization and re-hospitalization in Crohn's disease in a population based inception cohort between 2000-2012. *Gastroenterology;* 2014:S483.
10. Louis E, Mary JY, Vernier-Massouille G, et al. Maintenance of remission among patients with Crohn's disease on antimetabolite therapy after infliximab therapy is stopped. *Gastroenterology.* 2012;142(1):63-70.e65; quiz e31.
11. Solberg IC, Vatn MH, Høie O, et al. Clinical course in Crohn's disease: results of a Norwegian population-based ten-year follow-up study. *Clin Gastroenterol Hepatol.* 2007;5(12):1430-1438.
12. Allez M, Lemann M, Bonnet J, Cattan P, Jian R, Modigliani R. Long-term outcome of patients with active Crohn's disease exhibiting extensive and deep ulcerations at colonoscopy. *Am J Gastroenterol.* 2002;97(4):947-953.
13. Heida A, Park KT, van Rheenen PF. Clinical utility of fecal calprotectin monitoring in asymptomatic patients with inflammatory bowel disease: A systematic review and practical guide. *Inflamm Bowel Dis.* 2017;23(6):894-902.
14. Colombel JF, Panaccione R, Bossuyt P, et al. Effect of tight control management on Crohn's disease (CALM): a multicentre, randomised, controlled phase 3 trial. *Lancet.* 2018;390(10114):2779-2789.
15. Targan SR, Landers CJ, Yang H, et al. Antibodies to CBir1 flagellin define a unique response that is associated independently with complicated Crohn's disease. *Gastroenterology.* 2005;128(7):2020-2028.

16. Dubinsky MC, Lin YC, Dutridge D, et al. Serum immune responses predict rapid disease progression among children with Crohn's disease: immune responses predict disease progression. *Am J Gastroenterol.* 2006;101(2):360-367.

17. Adler J, Rangwalla SC, Dwamena BA, Higgins PD. The prognostic power of the NOD2 genotype for complicated Crohn's disease: a meta-analysis. *Am J Gastroenterol.* 2011;106(4):699-712.

18. Cleynen I, Boucher G, Jostins L, et al. Inherited determinants of Crohn's disease and ulcerative colitis phenotypes: a genetic association study. *Lancet.* 2016;387(10014):156-167.

19. Lichtenstein GR, Targan SR, Dubinsky MC, et al. Combination of genetic and quantitative serological immune markers are associated with complicated Crohn's disease behavior. *Inflamm Bowel Dis.* 2011;17(12):2488-2496.

20. Siegel CA, Horton H, Siegel LS, et al. A validated web-based tool to display individualized Crohn's disease predicted outcomes based on clinical, serologic and genetic variables. *Aliment Pharmacol Ther.* 2015;43(2):262-271.

21. Kugathasan S, Denson LA, Walters TD, et al. Prediction of complicated disease course for children newly diagnosed with Crohn's disease: a multicenter inception cohort study. *Lancet.* 2017;389(10080):1710-1718.

HOW DO YOU EVALUATE AND TREAT MID-PROXIMAL SMALL BOWEL CROHN'S DISEASE?

Jean A. Donet, MD and Mark Lazarev, MD

The Montreal classification defines L4 Crohn's disease (CD) as any disease location proximal to the terminal ileum, which anatomically includes L4-esophagogastroduodenal (EGD), L4-jejunal, and L4-proximal ileal involvement. This chapter will focus on L4-jejunal and L4-proximal ileal disease. L4 disease prevalence is about 15%—it is more common to have L4-EGD disease than L4-jejunal or proximal ileal disease.[1] The vast majority of patients with L4 disease have evidence of CD in other locations, mostly in the terminal ileum.

L4-jejunal disease has a worse prognosis compared to non-L4 disease in Western and Eastern populations.[1,2,3] Data from the National Institute of Diabetes and Digestive and Kidney Diseases (NIDDK) IBD Genetics Consortium have shown that L4-jejunal disease is a significantly greater risk factor for stricturing behavior and multiple abdominal surgeries compared to either L4-EGD or isolated terminal ileal (without proximal) disease.[1] In a multivariable analysis, jejunal disease was found to be an independent risk factor for possessing a stricturing phenotype (OR-2.9 [1.89–4.45]), and for requiring multiple surgeries (OR-2.39 [1.36 4.20])[1]. Groups in Korea and China have recently reported similar findings.[2,3,20] Kim et al identified 222 patients with proximal small bowel involvement among 1329 patients with CD. Patients with proximal small bowel disease were more likely to have stricturing disease (19.8% vs 12.7%) and more likely to require surgery. Population-based studies have also suggested a slight increased risk of small bowel adenocarcinomas and neuroendocrine tumors in patients with small bowel CD; only a minority of patients with this condition are diagnosed preoperatively.[4]

Rubin DT, Friedman S, Farraye FA, eds. *Curbside Consultation in IBD:*
49 Clinical Questions, Third Edition (pp 9-14).
© 2022 Taylor & Francis Group.

Diagnosis

Jejunal and proximal ileal CD can represent a diagnostic challenge that is specific to its location, since this portion of the small bowel is beyond the reach of standard upper endoscopy and ileocolonoscopy. This could lead to a delay in the diagnosis and also makes disease reassessment more difficult. In these circumstances, radiological imaging, video-capsule endoscopy (VCE), and enteroscopy should be recognized as complementary investigations for the diagnosis and monitoring of disease in this subgroup of patients.

Cross-Sectional Imaging

Computed tomography enterography (CTE) and magnetic resonance enterography (MRE) have emerged as the most used and effective methods for imaging the small bowel in CD. They can detect intramural, extramural, or proximal and mid small bowel inflammation in approximately 50% of patients with CD who have normal routine endoscopic examinations.[5]

The Society of Abdominal Radiology Crohn's Disease focused panel, the Society of Pediatric Radiology, and the American Gastroenterological Association have published joint recommendations for use of CTE and MRE in small bowel CD.[5] Findings associated with **inflammation** include (1) segmental mural hyperenhancement, more specific of CD when asymmetric; (2) wall thickening, categorized as mild (3 to 5 mm), moderate (5 to 10 mm), and severe (> 10 mm); (3) intramural edema; and (4) ulcerations. Strictures are defined as luminal narrowing with unequivocal upstream dilation > 3 cm. Fixed luminal narrowing without upstream dilation cannot be reliably diagnosed as a stricture on a single image and can lead to false positives. It should be highlighted that the majority of CD strictures will have both an inflammatory and a fibrotic component, and currently there are no robust radiologic means to accurately assess the degree of fibrosis within a stricture. The presence of inflammation might suggest a possibility, although not guaranteed, that the stricture may respond to medical therapy. CTE and MRE can also detect features of **penetrating disease** and **mesenteric inflammation**, including fistulas, sinus tracts, inflammatory mass (the term *phlegmon* is discouraged), abscess, perienteric edema/inflammation, engorged vasa recta (*comb sign*), fibrofatty proliferation (*creeping fat*), mesenteric venous thrombosis, and adenopathy. In addition, CTE and MRE could reveal **extra-intestinal** pathology, including sacroiliitis, primary sclerosing cholangitis, avascular necrosis, pancreatitis, nephrolithiasis, and cholelithiasis.

Both CTE and MRE have a comparable diagnostic yield. According to the most recent meta-analysis, CTE and MRE have similar sensitivity and specificity for the diagnosis of small bowel inflammation in CD (CTE sensitivity 87%, specificity 91%; MRE sensitivity 86%, specificity 93%).[6] However, MRE avoids exposure to ionizing radiation, a significant disadvantage with CTE. The selection of CTE vs MRE will be based on patient characteristics and institution availability/expertise.

Cross-sectional imaging is also useful for monitoring the response to therapy in patients with small bowel CD. Radiological transmural response (TR), indicated by improvement of imaging findings of inflammation, is associated with a reduced probability of CD-related surgeries, hospitalizations, and rescue corticosteroid therapy.[7] A recent retrospective study has also shown that sustained radiological response can be a powerful treatment target to avoid small bowel surgery on long-term follow-up.[8]

Video-Capsule Endoscopy and Enteroscopy

The diagnostic yield of VCE is superior to MRE for patients who are suspected of having CD.[9] This is due to its higher capability to detect early/subtle and proximal disease. VCE has high sensitivity and low specificity. There is a broad differential diagnosis when lesions are found on CE, and even healthy people may have minor mucosal breaks on VCE. Therefore, unless the patient has confirmed CD in other parts of the gastrointestinal tract, diagnosing small bowel CD solely on the basis of VCE is discouraged, and enteroscopy with biopsies is generally recommended. In cases of established CD, VCE and cross-sectional imaging are comparable. VCE has a high negative predictive value of 96%.[10] The quantification of inflammation in the small bowel using the Lewis score (LS) at the time of diagnosis has prognostic value in patients with isolated small bowel CD. A retrospective study from Portugal showed that patients with moderate to severe inflammatory activity (LS ≥ 790) presented higher rates of corticosteroid use and hospitalizations when compared to patients with mild inflammatory activity (135 ≤ LS < 790).[11] VCE has also proven valid for longitudinal monitoring of small bowel CD.[12,13] Caution should be exercised in patients with suspected small bowel strictures, and a patency capsule should be employed prior to the study. Deep enteroscopy is not usually part of routine diagnostic testing in patients with suspected CD. However, it may be needed in patients with isolated small bowel findings on cross-sectional imaging or VCE, who require biopsy of small bowel tissue to make an accurate diagnosis.

Barium Studies (Small Bowel Follow-Through and Enteroclysis)

The rise of CTE and MRE has led to a dramatic reduction in the use of barium studies. However, barium examinations remain useful for patients who have a suspected stricture not visualized on cross-sectional imaging and where radiologic expertise exists in performing/interpreting these studies. It may also be useful in patients with complex postoperative anatomy or those with intravenous contrast allergies.

Contrast-Enhanced Small Bowel Ultrasound

Contrast-enhanced small bowel ultrasound has emerged as a technique comparable to cross-sectional imaging for the evaluation of CD. However, it is operator dependent and not widely available. Its role has not been discussed in the recent American College of Gastroenterology guidelines for CD management.[14]

Fecal Calprotectin

It has been long believed that the accuracy of fecal calprotectin (FCal) in reflecting the inflammatory activity of CD diminishes with the proximate disease location. The utility of FCal for patients with small bowel CD remains controversial. A recent prospective study from Canada did not find a correlation between FCal levels and disease activity in the small bowel assessed by imaging or ileocolonoscopy.[15] Another recent study from Japan found good correlation between FCal and endoscopic activity assessed by double-balloon endoscopy in small bowel CD.[16] Other studies have found different degrees of correlation between FCal and VCE according to the cut-off value used.[17,18] FCal ≥ 100 μg/g has a sensitivity, specificity, positive predictive value, and negative predictive value of 78.6%, 87.9%, 89.2%, and 76.3%, respectively, for the detection of significant inflammatory activity defined as LS ≥ 135.[18]

Treatment

Patients with jejunal and proximal ileal CD have a worse prognosis. Efforts should be made for early identification of these patients, with the goal of instituting early and aggressive treatment that could potentially decrease or delay the development of complications (Figure 2-1). Only selected patients with very limited and mild small bowel disease can potentially be observed closely, receiving only sporadic short courses of budesonide if needed, and rapidly escalating therapy if there are any signs of ongoing inflammation. Mesalamines, in particular Pentasa, have been commonly used for these patients; however, these likely have limited value. Patients with moderate to severe disease should be managed aggressively by a multidisciplinary team. Different biologics are currently approved—anti–tumor necrosis factor agents (infliximab, adalimumab, certolizumab pegol), agents targeting leukocyte trafficking (natalizumab, vedolizumab), and agents targeting interleukin (IL) 12/IL-23 (ustekinumab). The landmark randomized trials that led to the approval of these biologics for CD did not consistently separate jejunal/proximal ileal locations and did not report on efficacy based on disease location. Additionally, no head-to-head studies have directly compared the efficacy between these drugs.

If a stricture is found, the relative proportion of active inflammation and fibrosis may help to determine whether the disease is likely to respond to medical therapy, although this can be difficult to determine radiologically. The location, length, and number of strictures will influence the choice between surgical resection, strictureplasty, or endoscopic dilation. Bowel-length preservation is an important principle in these patients, and despite the advent of newer therapies and refined endoscopic therapies, loss of functional bowel is almost inevitable once stricturing has occurred. In general, balloon dilation through device-assisted enteroscopy can be attempted for short (< 4 cm) and fibrotic strictures. However, surgery will be required for longer strictures and strictures associated with significant upstream bowel dilation or fistulizing disease. A recent Italian study reported that the most frequent surgery for patients with jejunal CD is a combined surgery (46.3%), consisting of resection of the most affected tract and strictureplasty of the residual strictures. There was no difference in the rates of surgical complications or stricture recurrence based on the type of surgery performed.[19]

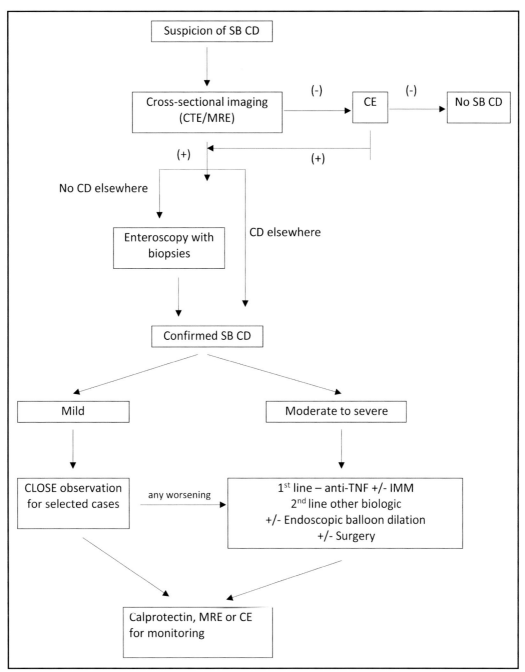

Figure 2-1. Diagnostic and therapeutic algorithm for small bowel CD. (CE = capsule endoscopy; CTE = computed tomography enterography; IMM = immunomodulator; MRE = magnetic resonance enterography; SB CD = small bowel Crohn's disease; TNF = tumor necrosis factor.)

References

1. Lazarev M, Huang C, Bitton A, et al. Relationship between Crohn's disease location and disease behavior and surgery: a cross-sectional study of the IBD Genetics Consortium. *Am J Gastroenterol*. 2013;108(1):106-112.
2. Kim Oz, Han DS, Park CH. The clinical characteristics and prognosis of Crohn's disease in Korean patients showing proximal small bowel involvement: results from the CONNECT study. *Gut Liver*. 2018;12(1):67-72.
3. Mao R, Tang RH, Qiu Y. Different clinical outcomes in Crohn's disease patients with esophagogastroduodenal, jejunal, and proximal ileal disease involvement: is L4 truly a single phenotype? *Therap Adv Gastroenterol*. 2018, 11:1-9.
4. Bojesen RD, Riis LB, Hogdall E, et al. Inflammatory bowel disease and small bowel cancer risk, clinical characteristics, and histopathology: a population-based study. *Clin Gastroenterol Hepatol*. 2017;15(12):1900-1907.e2.
5. Bruining DH, Zimmermann EM, Loftus EV Jr, et al. Consensus recommendations for evaluation, interpretation and utilization of computed tomography and magnetic resonance enterography in patients with small bowel Crohn's disease. *Gastroenterology*. 2018;154:1172-1194.
6. Park SH. Ye BD, Lee TY, et al. Computed tomography and magnetic resonance small bowel enterography: current status and future trends focusing on Crohn's disease. *Gastroenterol Clin North Am*. 2018;47(3):475-499.
7. Deepak P, Fletcher JG, Fidler JL, et al. Radiological response is associated with better long-term outcomes and is a potential treatment target in patients with small bowel Crohn's disease. *Am J Gastroenterol*. 2016;111:997-1006.
8. Deepak P, Fletcher J, Fidler J, et al. Predictors of durability of radiological response in patients with small bowel Crohn's disease. *Inflamm Bowel Disease*. 2018;24(8):1815-1825.
9. Gonzalez-Suarez B, Rodriguez S, Ricart E. Comparison of capsule endoscopy and magnetic resonance enterography for the assessment of small bowel lesions in Crohn's disease. *Inflamm Bowel Dis*. 2018;24(4):775-780.
10. Hall B, Holleran G, Costigan D, et al. Capsule endoscopy: high negative predictive value in the long term despite a low diagnostic yield in patients with suspected Crohn's disease. *United European Gastroenterology J*. 2013;1: 461-468.
11. Dias de Castro F, Boal P, Monteiro S, et al. Lewis score—prognostic value in patients with isolated small bowel Crohn's Disease. *Journal of Crohn's and Colitis*. 2015;9(12):1146-1151.
12. Melmed GY, Dubinsky MC, Rubin DT, et al. Utility of videocapsule endoscopy for longitudinal monitoring of Crohn's disease activity in the small bowel: a prospective study. *Gastrointest Endosc*. 2018;88(6):947-955.e2.
13. Park S, Ye B, Kim K, et al. Guidelines for video capsule endoscopy: emphasis on Crohn's disease. *Clin Endosc*. 2015;48:128-135.
14. Lichtenstein GR, Loftus EV, Isaacs KL. ACG clinical guideline: management of Crohn's disease in adults. *Am J Gastroenterol*. 2018;113:481-517.
15. Zittan E, Kelly OB, Gralnek IM. Fecal calprotectin correlated with active colonic inflammatory bowel disease but not with small intestinal Crohn's disease activity. *JGH Open*. 2018;2(5):201-206.
16. Matsuura R, Watanabe O, Nakamura M, et al. Fecal calprotectin reflects endoscopic activity in patients with small-bowel Crohn's disease according to double-balloon endoscopy findings. *Nagoya J Med Sci*. 2018;80(2):257-266.
17. Yousuf H, Aleem U, Egan R, et al. Elevated fecal calprotectin levels are a reliable non-invasive screening tool for small bowel Crohn's disease in patients undergoing capsule endoscopy. *Dig Dis*. 2018;36(3):202-208.
18. Monteiro S, Barbosa M, Colcalves C, et al. Fecal calprotectin as a selection tool for small bowel capsule endoscopy in suspected Crohn's disease. *Inflamm Bowel Dis*. 2018;24(9):2033-2038.
19. Tonelli F, Alemanno G, Di Martino C. Results of surgical treatment for jejunal Crohn's disease: choice between resection, strictureplasty, and combined treatment. *Langnbecks Arch Surg*. 2017;402(7):1071-1078.
20. Sun XW, Wei J, Yang Z, et al. Clinical features and prognosis of Crohn's disease with upper gastrointestinal tract phenotype in Chinese patients. *Dig Dis Sci*. 2019 Nov;64(11):3291-3299. https://doi.org/10.1007/s10620-019-05651-1.

QUESTION

3

What Is Your First-Line Approach to the Diagnosis and Treatment of Patients With Perianal Crohn's Disease?

Baldeep S. Pabla, MD, MSCI and David A. Schwartz, MD

Perianal fistulizing Crohn's disease (CD) is one of the more dreaded complications for patients with this disease. If not treated appropriately from the onset, it can often negatively affect the patient's quality of life in a dramatic way, secondary to pain or incontinence. In the worst cases, severe disease requires definitive surgical management with a proctectomy. To prevent these potential outcomes, we approach patients with CD with perianal disease using a modified top-down approach, employing a multimodality (radiology, surgery, and medicine) treatment strategy (Figure 3-1).

When a patient presents with a possible perianal fistula, we start by reassessing their perianal disease. Fistulas should be divided into complex and simple fistulas to help plan treatment. A simple fistula is a superficial, intersphincteric, or low transsphincteric fistula with only one opening. It is neither associated with an abscess nor connected to an adjacent structure. A complex fistula is one that involves more of the anal sphincter (ie, high transsphincteric, extrasphincteric, or suprasphincteric), has multiple openings, horseshoes (crosses the midline either anteriorly or posteriorly), is associated with a perianal abscess, and/or connects to an adjacent structure, such as the vagina or bladder.

Delineation of the fistulizing process is done first with a thorough physical examination, but it is important to also image the patient with either magnetic resonance imaging (MRI) or endorectal ultrasound (EUS). Physical examination is not accurate in this setting because of the pain, induration, and scarring associated with perianal CD. Studies have shown that MRI and EUS are highly accurate in assessing perianal CD.[1] Creating this virtual roadmap of the patient's perianal disease is important prior to starting treatment because several studies have demonstrated that failure to fully recognize and treat all of the perianal process (ie, abscess and fistula's branches)

Rubin DT, Friedman S, Farraye FA, eds. *Curbside Consultation in IBD:*
49 Clinical Questions, Third Edition (pp 15-19).
© 2022 Taylor & Francis Group.

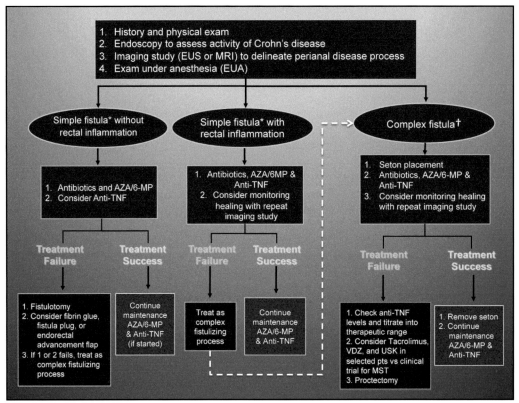

Figure 3-1. Treatment algorithm. *Simple fistula: a superficial, intersphincteric, or low transsphincteric fistula with only one opening; it is neither associated with an abscess nor connected to an adjacent structure. †Complex fistula: involves more of the anal sphincter (ie, high transsphincteric, extrasphincteric, or suprasphincteric), has multiple openings, horseshoes (crosses the midline either anteriorly or posteriorly), is associated with a perianal abscess, and/or connects to an adjacent structure, such as the vagina or bladder. (6-MP = 6-mercaptopurine; Anti-TNF = anti-tumor necrosis factor; AZA = azathioprine; MST = mesenchymal stem cell therapy; USK = ustekinumab; VDZ = vedolizumab.)

can result in a simple fistula becoming complex and/or recurrent fistulas or abscesses.[2] Once a fistula becomes complex, the chance for complete closure of the fistula is dramatically reduced,[2] so the goal of treatment becomes primarily one of symptom control (ie, cessation of drainage) and not complete closure or fibrosis of the tract. So, in essence, there may be only a limited opportunity to achieve fistula closure. Imaging with EUS or MRI increases the odds of accomplishing this goal.

At this point, we send the patient to a surgeon for an examination under anesthesia. By using the imaging roadmap, the surgeon can make sure all abscesses are drained and setons are placed in all of the fistulas prior to starting treatment. Retrospective studies have shown that seton placement prior to starting infliximab reduces the rate of fistula recurrence dramatically (44% vs 79%).[3] Seton placement prior to biologic therapy has also been shown to result in fewer hospitalizations and lower health care costs.[4] Setons work by preventing the premature closure of the cutaneous opening of the fistula tract (ie, prior to the time when fistula inactivity occurs; Figure 3-2).

Once drainage has been established, it is time to institute medical therapy. Because of the potential negative outcomes associated with perianal CD, we use anti–tumor necrosis factor-α (anti-TNF-α) antibodies at the onset, along with immunomodulators (azathioprine or 6-mercaptopurine) and an antibiotic (ciprofloxacin or metronidazole) in patients with a simple fistula who have concomitant rectal luminal disease or those with a complex fistula (see Figure 3-1).

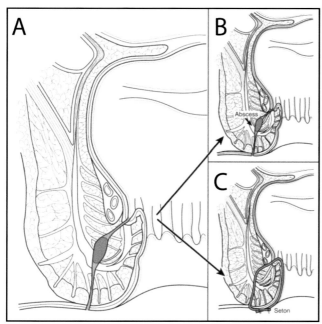

Figure 3-2. (A) Typical transsphincteric fistulas prior to treatment. (B) Without seton placement prior to anti-TNF therapy, one gets premature closure of cutaneous openings and abscess formation. (C) Seton placement prior to initiation of medical treatment prevents abscess formation by allowing the fistula to drain until inflammation is absent.

Similar to the rationale for the top-down approach (using anti-TNF-α therapy before steroids or proven failure of oral thiopurines) for luminal CD, this modified top-down approach aims to aggressively treat the fistulizing disease from the onset with the most effective treatment currently available to achieve healing and prevent the complications that can occur with perianal CD. Studies have shown that anti-TNF-α treatment with infliximab, adalimumab, or certolizumab pegol results in complete cessation of drainage in about 50% to 60% of patients treated.[5–8] Of the initial responders, 30% to 40% of patients maintain cessation of fistula drainage through 6 months with certolizumab pegol and for more than 1 year with infliximab and adalimumab.[5–8]

In ACCENT II (a CD clinical trial evaluating infliximab in a new long-term treatment regimen), the infliximab fistula maintenance trial, infliximab was used to maintain fistula closure over the course of 1 year.[6] In this trial, the 195 patients who were considered responders (≥ 50% reduction in draining fistulas) at week 14 to the initial induction sequence of 5 mg/kg of infliximab at 0, 2, and 6 weeks were randomized to receive either 5 mg/kg or placebo every 8 weeks. At week 54, 36% of patients who were on maintenance infliximab had complete cessation of drainage of all of their fistulas, compared with only 19% of patients in the placebo cohort (P = .009).[6] Fistula healing was studied as a secondary endpoint in the adalimumab maintenance trial, CHARM (Crohn's Trial of the Fully Human Antibody Adalimumab for Remission Maintenance).[7] Complete fistula closure at week 56 was seen in 33% of the treated group (combined 40 mg weekly and every other week adalimumab dosing arms), compared with 13% in the placebo arm (P = .016). The response was durable. In the patients who demonstrated fistula closure at week 26, all maintained fistula closure at week 56.[7] Finally, a randomized clinical trial assessed certolizumab pegol's effect on fistula closure.[8] Participants with draining fistulas received an induction dose of certolizumab pegol at 0, 2, and 4 weeks. Responders at week 6 were randomized to receive additional maintenance therapy with certolizumab pegol or to receive placebo. At week 26, the certolizumab pegol arm showed a 36% response with 100% fistula closure, compared with a 17% response in the placebo arm (P = .038). The results of these studies suggest that infliximab, adalimumab, and certolizumab pegol have a similar benefit in perianal CD (36% infliximab vs 19% placebo, 33% adalimumab vs 13% placebo, and 36% certolizumab pegol vs 17% placebo), although the certolizumab pegol study was half as long as the other 2 studies.

Several novel agents have been recently approved for the treatment of CD, though data regarding their efficacy in management of perianal disease are lacking, and as such these agents are not used as first-line therapies to manage this condition. Vedolizumab, an $\alpha_4\beta_7$ integrin antibody, was approved for the treatment of CD and ulcerative colitis by the US Food and Drug Administration (FDA) in 2014. While there are limited data regarding perianal disease, data from Gemini 2, an integrated induction and maintenance trial in patients with active CD, did demonstrate that 41.2% of patients on every 8-week dosing vs 11.1% of patients on placebo had fistula closure ($P = .03$).[9] A recent paper reporting further exploratory analysis from this trial demonstrated that this improvement was also seen for those patients with isolated perianal disease, though this result did not meet statistical significance.[10] Ustekinumab, a monoclonal antibody against the p40 subunit of interleukin (IL) 12 and IL-23, is another new biologic agent that was approved by the FDA for the treatment of CD in 2016. Observational data with ustekinumab suggest this agent may be effective with 61% to 67% of patients with perianal disease.[11,12] The phase 2 and 3 trials that lead to its approval did include a small number of patients with fistulas. A subanalysis of these patients showed that fistula response and resolution at 8 weeks approached significance, with the authors suggesting that longer follow-up would be necessary to determine if this signal represents true response.[13]

For patients with simple fistulas who do not have concomitant luminal disease, the use of antibiotics (ciprofloxacin or metronidazole) as a bridge to immunomodulator treatment is reasonable.[14] A prospective open-label trial of 52 patients with CD perianal fistulas compared those patients treated only with ciprofloxacin or metronidazole for 8 weeks to those patients who transitioned or were already on azathioprine at a dose of 2.0 to 2.5 mg/kg per day. Although the results at week 8 were similar between the 2 groups, those who were maintained on azathioprine had a greater response by week 20 than those who were not (48% vs 15%, respectively; $P = .03$). Patients who fail this therapy should start therapy with anti-TNF-α antibodies. Surgical fistulotomy, fibrin glue or fibrin plug therapy, or an endorectal advancement flap can be considered in these patients as well. If these therapies fail these patients should be treated as having complex fistulas (see Figure 3-1).

A new therapy that has garnered much excitement is the use of mesenchymal stem cell therapy. Though local intralesional injection of stem cell therapy for the management of perianal fistulae has been studied in the management of CD since 2005, the use of allogenic stem cells was first reported in 2011.[15] A recently published randomized placebo-controlled trial demonstrated combined remission, defined as fistula closure of all tracts draining at time of randomization with an absence of fluid collections > 2 cm as assessed by MRI, to be 56.3% in patients with refractory perianal disease treated with Cx601 allogenic expanded adipose derived stem cells vs 38.6% in controls at 52 weeks ($P = .01$).[16] This trial led to the approval of this drug in Europe, and trials in the United States are ongoing.

Usually, fistulas will stop draining after 2 to 6 weeks of treatment if anti-TNF-α therapy is used. However, inflammation and purulence with the fistula persists long after this time. EUS and MRI studies have shown that the internal portion of the fistula remains active long after the fistula stops draining, so it is our practice to rely on imaging rather than physical exam to determine when the inflammation has largely resolved in order to guide us on when to remove the setons. Further support for this approach is shown in a recent prospective study characterizing the usefulness of MRI in determining fistula healing for patients on anti-TNF treatment.[17] This study demonstrated that the deep fistula healing takes longer than needed to achieve cessation of drainage. Furthermore, the study showed that significant variability exists in fistula healing among patients receiving this therapy. MRI was used in this study to determine which patients needed their therapy increased (adalimumab increased from every other week to weekly if inflammation was seen on MRI) to improve fistula healing.[17] We have shown in a retrospective study[18] and in 2 small randomized prospective trials[19,20] that using EUS to guide therapy in this way improves the long-term treatment success rate with a combination of medical and surgical therapy.

References

1. Schwartz DA, Wiersema MJ, Dudiak KM, et al. A comparison of endoscopic ultrasound, magnetic resonance imaging, and exam under anesthesia for evaluation of Crohn's perianal fistulas. *Gastroenterology*. 2001;121(5): 1064-1072.
2. Williamson PR, Hellinger MD, Larach SW, Ferrara A. Twenty-year review of the surgical management of perianal Crohn's disease. *Dis Colon Rectum*. 1995;38(4):389-392.
3. Regueiro M, Mardini H. Treatment of perianal fistulizing Crohn's disease with infliximab alone or as an adjunct to exam under anesthesia with seton placement. *Inflamm Bowel Dis*. 2003;9(2):98-103.
4. Schwartz DA, Wang A, Ozbay B, et al. Comparison of health care utilization and costs between patients with perianal fistulizing Crohn's disease treated with biologics with or without previous seton placement. *Inflamm Bowel Dis*. 2017;23(10):1860-1866.
5. Present DH, Rutgeerts P, Targan S, et al. Infliximab for the treatment of fistulas in patients with Crohn's disease. *N Engl J Med*. 1999;340(18):1398-1405.
6. Sands BE, Anderson FH, Bernstein CN, et al. Infliximab maintenance therapy for fistulizing Crohn's disease. *N Engl J Med*. 2004;350(9):876-885.
7. Colombel JF, Sandborn WJ, Rutgeerts P, et al. Adalimumab for maintenance of clinical response and remission in patients with Crohn's disease: the CHARM trial. *Gastroenterology*. 2007;132(1):52-65.
8. Schreiber S, Lawrance IC, Thomsen OØ, Hanauer SB, Bloomfield R, Sandborn WJ. Randomised clinical trial: certolizumab pegol for fistulas in Crohn's disease—subgroup results from a placebo-controlled study. *Aliment Pharmacol Ther*. 2011;33(2):185-193.
9. Sandborn WJ, Feagan BG, Rutgeerts P, et al. Vedolizumab as induction and maintenance therapy for Crohn's disease. *N Engl J Med*. 2013;369(8):711-721.
10. Feagan BG, Schwartz D, Danese S, et al. Efficacy of Vedolizumab in fistulising Crohn's disease: exploratory analyses of data from GEMINI 2. *J Crohns Colitis*. 2018;12(5):621-626.
11. Wils P, Bouhnik Y, Michetti P, et al. Subcutaneous ustekinumab provides clinical benefit for two-thirds of patients with Crohn's disease refractory to anti-tumor necrosis factor agents. *Clin Gastroenterol Hepatol*. 2016;14(2):242-250.e2.
12. Khorrami S, Ginard D, Marín-Jiménez I, et al. Ustekinumab for the treatment of refractory Crohn's disease: the Spanish experience in a large multicenter open-label cohort. *Inflamm Bowel Dis*. 2016;22(7):1662-1669.
13. Sands BE, Gasink C, Jacobstein D, et al. Fistula healing in pivotal studies of ustekinumab in Chron's disease. *Gastroenterology*. 2017;152(5):S185.
14. Dejaco C, Harrer M, Waldhoer T, Miehsler W, Vogelsang H, Reinisch W. Antibiotics and azathioprine for the treatment of perianal fistulas in Crohn's disease. *Aliment Pharmacol Ther*. 2003;18(11-12):1113-1120.
15. Garcia-Olmo D, Schwartz DA. Cumulative evidence that mesenchymal stem cells promote healing of perianal fistulas of patients with Crohn's disease: going from bench to bedside. *Gastroenterology*. 2015;149(4):853-857.
16. Panés J, García-Olmo D, Van Assche G, et al. Long-term efficacy and safety of stem cell therapy (Cx601) for complex perianal fistulas in patients with Crohn's disease. *Gastroenterology*. 2018;154(5):1334-1342.e4.
17. Ng SC, Plamondon S, Gupta A, et al. Prospective evaluation of anti-tumor necrosis factor therapy guided by magnetic resonance imaging for Crohn's perineal fistulas. *Am J Gastroenterol*. 2009;104(12):2973-2986.
18. Schwartz DA, White CM, Wise PE, Herline AJ. Use of endoscopic ultrasound to guide combination medical and surgical therapy for patients with Crohn's perianal fistulas. *Inflamm Bowel Dis*. 2005;11(8):727-732.
19. Spradlin NM, Wise PE, Herline AJ, Muldoon RL, Rosen M, Schwartz DA. A randomized prospective trial of endoscopic ultrasound to guide combination medical and surgical treatment for Crohn's perianal fistulas. *Am J Gastroenterol*. 2008;103(10):2527-2535.
20. Wiese DM, Beaulieu D, Slaughter JC, et al. Use of endoscopic ultrasound to guide adalimumab treatment in perianal Crohn's disease results in faster fistula healing. *Inflamm Bowel Dis*. 2015;21(7):1594-1599.

QUESTION

WHAT IS THE UPDATED ROLE OF CAPSULE ENDOSCOPY IN IBD?

Shabana F. Pasha, MD and Jonathan A. Leighton, MD

The role of capsule endoscopy (CE) has expanded considerably in the evaluation and management of patients with inflammatory bowel disease (IBD). In conjunction with ileocolonoscopy (IC) and cross-sectional imaging (CTE/MRE), CE is a complementary tool for detecting and monitoring small bowel inflammation associated with Crohn disease (CD). It also has a potential role in the future, for colon evaluation in CD and ulcerative colitis (UC; Table 4-1).

Capsule Endoscopy in Suspected Crohn Disease

While cross-sectional imaging is useful to assess transmural inflammation and penetrating and fibrostenotic CD complications, CE is superior to both CTE and MRE for detection of early and mild mucosal inflammation in CD (Figure 4-1). A large meta-analysis demonstrated an incremental yield with CE of 47% (95% CI, 31% to 63%) over CTE and 22% (95% CI, 5% to 39%) over ileocolonoscopy in patients with non-stricturing CD.[1] Another study that compared cross-sectional imaging and CE also found that CE had a higher sensitivity (100%) compared with both CTE (85%) and MRE (81%) for small bowel inflammation.[2] Due to its high negative predictive value (> 96%), CE is the most useful of all currently available tests to rule out a diagnosis of small bowel CD.[3] It is therefore recommended after negative IC to evaluate patients with suspected CD, in the absence of obstructive symptoms.

The main disadvantage of CE lies in the low specificity of small bowel findings. Mucosal inflammation, similar to CD, can be seen in patients with nonsteroidal anti-inflammatory drug (NSAID) use, underlying infectious enteritis, and autoimmune and other inflammatory disor-

Rubin DT, Friedman S, Farraye FA, eds. *Curbside Consultation in IBD:*
49 Clinical Questions, Third Edition (pp 21-26).
© 2022 Taylor & Francis Group.

Table 4-1

Current and Future Indications for Capsule Endoscopy in IBD

Suspected Crohn Disease
Diagnosis of early or mild small bowel CD after negative ileocolonoscopy
Established Crohn Disease
Assessment of small bowel disease extent and severity
Evaluation for post-operative CD recurrence
Classification of IBD undefined
Future Roles
Monitoring response to therapy and assessment of mucosal healing in small bowel CD
Evaluating and monitoring UC and Crohn colitis
Single noninvasive test for evaluating and monitoring small bowel and colonic CD

ders. For this reason, the Lewis score and Capsule Endoscopy Crohn Disease Activity Index (CECDAI), both validated indices for assessment of disease severity and extent of involvement in established CD, are not useful as diagnostic tools in suspected CD. A careful selection of patients based on clinical symptoms and laboratory markers, including fecal calprotectin, has been shown to improve the positive predictive value of CE. In a recent meta-analysis, an elevated fecal calprotectin > 50 mg/kg had a sensitivity of 89%, specificity of 55%, and negative predictive value of 91.8% for diagnosis of small bowel CD with CE.[4]

Capsule Endoscopy in Established Crohn Disease

CE has several potential roles in established CD, including assessment of disease extent and activity (Figure 4-2), monitoring response to therapy, documentation of mucosal healing, and evaluation for postoperative recurrence, as well as in the classification of IBD undefined (IBD-U).

ASSESSMENT OF DISEASE EXTENT AND ACTIVITY

CE findings can guide management of patients toward escalation or change in medical therapy and surgical management. A meta-analysis found that CE was superior to CTE, but not MRE, for detection of active small bowel inflammation in established CD, with an incremental yield of 32% (95% CI, 16% to 47%).[1] Subsequent studies have shown that CE is superior to both CTE and

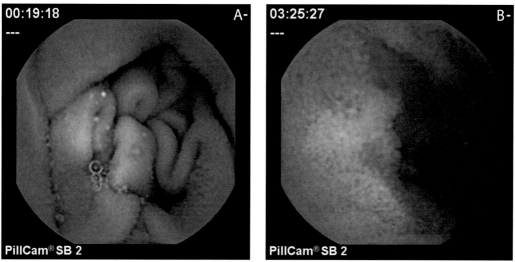

Figure 4-1. Aphthous ulcers seen on capsule endoscopy.

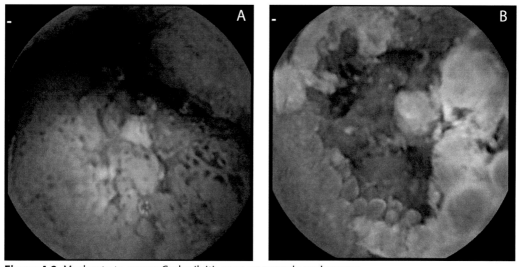

Figure 4-2. Moderate to severe Crohn ileitis seen on capsule endoscopy.

MRE for detection of proximal small bowel inflammation. In a study by Jensen et al, proximal CD was detected in a significantly higher number of patients with CE, as compared with CTE/MRE ($P < .05$).[2] Another study demonstrated jejunal inflammation on CE in 56% of patients with established CD, with isolated jejunal involvement in 17%.[5] The presence of proximal small bowel involvement was found to be an independent predictor of CD relapse, although this needs to be confirmed in prospective studies. In a retrospective study by Dussault et al, CE findings resulted in a change in management in over 50% of patients within 3 months of undergoing the test.[6]

Monitoring Response to Therapy and Mucosal Healing

Mucosal healing is now recognized as an important treatment goal in CD, with increasing evidence to support improved outcomes in patients who achieve deep remission. A prospective longitudinal study demonstrated that use of serial CEs for monitoring small bowel inflammation in nonstricturing CD is both safe and feasible.[7] A recent meta-analysis of 5 observational studies also confirmed that mucosal healing on CE was associated with improved outcomes after a follow-up of 3 to 24 months (OR 11.06; 95% CI, 3.74 to 32.73; $P < .001$).[8]

However, several questions still need to be addressed before CE can be approved for this indication, including which patients might benefit from and safely undergo CE monitoring, appropriate timing of repeat CE examinations, how CE findings compare with ileoscopy and cross-sectional imaging, and how CE findings might influence management decisions.

Detection of Postoperative Recurrence

IC is currently the test of choice to assess for postoperative CD recurrence. CE may have a role in patients with either suspected or known proximal small bowel involvement inaccessible with IC and in those patients who wish to pursue noninvasive testing. In a small study, postoperative recurrence was detected in the neoterminal ileum in fewer patients with CE, but a significantly higher number of patients had proximal small bowel inflammation not detected with IC. In addition, CE was preferred over IC by all patients.[9] Another recent study found a higher recurrence rate with a panenteric examination using the Pillcam colon capsule, as compared with IC.[10]

Classification of IBD-U

CE can detect small bowel inflammation in 30% to 40% of patients with IBD-U.[11] However, the clinical relevance of CE findings remains unclear due to lack of data on long-term follow-up. CE should ideally be performed after confirming that patients have been abstinent of NSAIDs for at least 8 to 12 weeks prior to the test. While the presence of small bowel inflammation on CE can be helpful to confirm a diagnosis of CD, a negative CE also does not rule out possibility of a future diagnosis of CD in these patients.

Colon Evaluation in Crohn's Disease and Ulcerative Colitis

Preliminary studies have evaluated the role of colon capsule endoscopy (CCE) in both CD and UC.

Crohn's Disease

A prospective study of 40 patients with CD reported significant agreement between CCE and IC for active colitis using the Crohn's Disease Endoscopic Index of Severity (CDEIS) score (intraclass correlation coefficient or ICC 0.65; 95% CI, 0.43 to 0.80). While the highest agreement between the tests was observed in the terminal ileum (ICC 0.73; 95% CI, 0.54 to 0.85), there was a trend toward lower agreement in the distal colon, with an underestimation of severity of disease on CCE.[12]

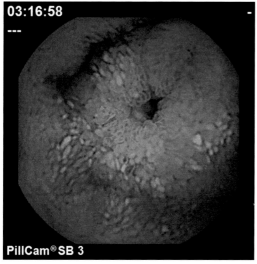

Figure 4-3. Severe ulcerated stenosis in a patient with CD resulting in capsule retention.

ULCERATIVE COLITIS

A study of 100 patients with UC found that CCE had a sensitivity and specificity of 89% and 75%, respectively, for detection of active colitis.[13] Similarly, another study of 150 patients found excellent interobserver agreement for inflammation scores (ICC > .80) and a sensitivity of 97% and 94% for mucosal inflammation.[14] A small study of 25 patients with UC found a significant correlation between CCE and IC for both extent of involvement (K 0.522, *P* < .001) and disease severity (K 0.751, *P* < .001).[15]

Additional studies are necessary to define the utility of capsule endoscopy for evaluation of colonic inflammation. The main limitations of the test are an intensive preparation coupled with an inability to obtain biopsies, especially in patients who require high-risk colorectal cancer surveillance.

HOW TO MINIMIZE RISK AND MANAGE CAPSULE RETENTION

Capsule retention is defined as presence of the capsule endoscope in the gastrointestinal tract for a minimum of 2 weeks, or any duration, if it results in obstructive symptoms that necessitate endoscopic and/or surgical retrieval (Figure 4-3). According to a recent meta-analysis, CE retention in suspected CD was 2.35% (95% CI, 1.31% to 4.19%) and 4.63% (95% CI, 3.42% to 6.25%) in established CD.[16] Retention rates in established CD were decreased to 2.88% (95% CI, 1.74% to 4.74%) after patency capsule and 2.32% (95% CI, 0.87% to 6.03%) after CTE/MRE. It is therefore important to confirm luminal patency prior to CE in all patients with established CD, as well as patients with suspected CD who are at increased retention risk due to NSAID use, prior surgery, or obstructive symptoms.

In the absence of an acute obstruction that would necessitate emergent surgical intervention, most patients with CE retention can be managed conservatively with the administration of steroids or biologics to reduce inflammation and facilitate spontaneous passage of the capsule. Endoscopic retrieval is an alternative approach to elective surgery in those patients who fail conservative management.

FUTURE DEVELOPMENTS

A panenteric (Pillcam Crohn or SBC) capsule endoscope has recently been developed. This is a 2-headed capsule similar to the Pillcam colon capsule, with a 172-degree field of view and a frame rate up to 35 per second. In a feasibility study by Leighton et al, the per-subject diagnostic yield for active inflammation with SBC capsule was significantly higher than ileocolonoscopy (83.3% vs 69.7%; 95% CI, 2.6% to 24.7%).[17] This capsule could potentially serve as a single non-invasive test for evaluation of both small bowel and colonic CD in the future.

References

1. Dionisio PM, Gurudu SR, Leighton JA, et al. Capsule endoscopy has a significantly higher diagnostic yield in patients with suspected and established small-bowel Crohn's disease: a meta-analysis. *Am J Gastroenterol.* 2010;105(6):1240-1248; quiz 1249.
2. Jensen MD, Nathan T, Rafaelsen SR, Kjeldsen J. Diagnostic accuracy of capsule endoscopy for small bowel Crohn's disease is superior to that of MR enterography or CTE. *Clin Gastroenterol Hepatol.* 2011;9(2):124-129.
3. Tukey M, Pleskow D, Legnani P, Cheifetz AS, Moss AC. The utility of capsule endoscopy in patients with suspected Crohn's disease. *Am J Gastroenterology.* 2009;104(11):2734-2739.
4. Kopylov U, Yung DE, Engel T, et al. Fecal calprotectin for the prediction of small bowel Crohn disease by capsule endoscopy: a systematic review and meta-analysis. *Eur J Gastroenterol Hepatol.* 2016;28(10):1137-1144.
5. Flamant M, Trang C, Maillard O, et al. The prevalence and outcome of jejunal lesions visualized by small bowel capsule endoscopy in Crohn's disease. *Inflamm Bowel Dis.* 2013;19(7):1390-1396.
6. Dussault C, Gower-Rousseau C, Salleron J, et al. Small bowel capsule endoscopy for management of Crohn's disease: a retrospective tertiary care center experience. *Digestive and Liver Disease.* 2013;45(7):558-561.
7. Melmed GY, Dubinsky MC, Rubin DT. Utility of video capsule endoscopy for longitudinal monitoring of Crohn's disease activity in the small bowel: a prospective study. *Gastrointes Endosc.* 2018;88(6):947-955.
8. Niv Y. Small-bowel mucosal healing assessment by capsule endoscopy as a predictor of long-term clinical remission in patients with Crohn's disease: a systematic review and meta-analysis. *Eur J Gastroenterol Hepatol.* 2017;29(7):844-848.
9. Pons BV, Nos P, Bastida G, et al. Evaluation of postsurgical recurrence in Crohn's disease: a new indication for capsule endoscopy? *Gastrointes Endosc.* 2007;66(3):533-540.
10. Haussman J, Schmelz R, Walldorf J, et al. Pan-intestinal capsule endoscopy in patients with postoperative Crohn's disease: a pilot study. *Scandinavian J of Gastroenterol.* 2017;52(8):840–845.
11. Manoury V, Savoye G, Bourreille A. Value of wireless capsule endoscopy in patients with indeterminate colitis (inflammatory bowel disease type unclassified). *Inflamm Bowel Dis.* 2007;13(2):152-155.
12. D'Haens G, Lowenberg M, Samaan MA, et al. Safety and feasibility of using the second generation Pillcam colon capsule to assess active colonic Crohn disease. *Clin Gastroenterol Hepatol.* 2015;13(8):1480-1486.
13. Sung J, Ho KY, Chiu HM, Ching J, Travis S, Peled R. The use of Pillcam colon in assessing mucosal inflammation in ulcerative colitis: a multicenter study. *Endoscopy.* 2012;44(8):754-758.
14. Shi HY, Chan FKL, Higashimori A, et al. A prospective study on second-generation colon capsule endoscopy to detect mucosal lesions and disease activity in ulcerative colitis (with video). *Gastrointest Endoscop.* 2017;86(6):1139-1146.
15. Ye CA, Gao YJ, Ge ZZ, et al. PillCam colon capsule endoscopy versus conventional colonoscopy for the detection of severity and extent of ulcerative colitis. *J Dig Dis.* 2013;14(3):117-124.
16. Pasha SF, Pennazio M, Rondonotti E, et al. Capsule retention in Crohn disease: a meta-analysis. *Inflamm Bowel Dis.* 2020;26(1):33-42.
17. Leighton JA, Helper DJ, Gralnek I, et al. Comparing diagnostic yield of a novel pan-enteric video capsule endoscope with ileocolonoscopy in patients with active Crohn's disease: a feasibility study. *Gastrointest Endosc.* 2017;85(1):196-205.

HOW SHOULD WE BE USING FECAL MARKERS IN OUR PATIENTS?

Anthony Buisson, MD, PhD and David T. Rubin, MD

In the last decade, the management of patients with inflammatory bowel diseases (IBD) has dramatically evolved. A treat-to-target approach with endoscopic mucosal healing is currently the reference. In addition, a tight monitoring of inflammatory activity using objective tools is recommended. In this context, fecal biomarkers, which are more accepted by patients than repeated colonoscopies, could be promising alternatives.[1] Among them, calprotectin is the fecal marker that demonstrates the strongest performances in patients with IBD. It belongs to the family of S100 proteins and is secreted by neutrophils in the stool. We focused this chapter on fecal calprotectin (FCal).

The first situation where FCal can be used is to differentiate patients with IBD from patients with irritable bowel syndrome (IBS). Meta-analyses reported a very high negative predictive value that can lead to avoiding two-thirds of colonoscopies. The consensual cut-off value of 50 µg/g is well accepted, with a sensitivity of 96% and specificity of 93%.[2]

FCal is a surrogate marker of endoscopic activity both in Crohn's disease (CD) and ulcerative colitis (UC). FCal values are significantly higher in patients with endoscopic activity compared to those with mucosal healing.[3] In addition, the level of FCal is nicely correlated with endoscopic scores such as Crohn's Disease Endoscopic Index of Severity (CDEIS; correlation coefficient ρ = from 0.42 to 0.83) or simplified endoscopic score for CD (SES-CD; ρ = from 0.49 to 0.75) in patients with CD and Rachmilewitz index (ρ = from 0.55 to 0.83), or endoscopic Mayo score (ρ = from 0.61 to 0.76) in those with UC.[3] In UC, FCal is also correlated with histological activity and could detect histological healing. Many studies attempted to define the best threshold to detect endoscopic activity in IBD. However, IBD physicians have to keep in mind the factors influencing the level of FCal. The values of FCal can vary with up to 5-fold quantitative differ-

Rubin DT, Friedman S, Farraye FA, eds. *Curbside Consultation in IBD: 49 Clinical Questions, Third Edition* (pp 27-30).
© 2022 Taylor & Francis Group.

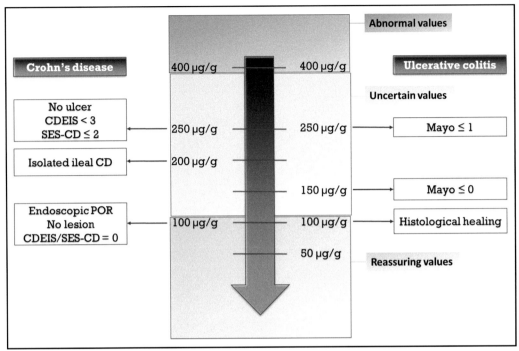

Figure 5-1. Using benchmarks to interpret FC values.

ences between assays.[4] Thus, all comparisons between FCal values should be performed using the same assay. The other key point is that the more stringent the definition of remission, the lower the best threshold. Finally, the most impactful factor influencing the level of FCal is the extent of the inflammatory disease. It may explain why patients with short-segment ileitis or limited proctitis have low FCal values despite the presence of significant lesions.[5] For clinical practice, regardless of the type of assay, we can retain that FCal < 100 μg/g is reassuring and should not modify the therapeutic management. In contrast, FCal > 400 μg/g should lead to confirm persistent inflammation by endoscopy or to intensify the treatment. Between 100 and 400 μg/g, the interpretation should be more cautious and consider initial disease extent, the type of assay and the therapeutic target. We propose benchmark values according to clinical situation in Figure 5-1.

FCal is predictive of relapse in patients in clinical remission, as shown by a meta-analysis (pooled sensitivity = 0.78 [0.72–0.83] and pooled specificity = 0.73 [0.68–0.76]) with cut-off values ranging from 50 to 300 μg/g.[6] FCal level is highly accurate to predict and monitor the risk of relapse after therapeutic deescalation in patients with IBD.[7] FCal > 100 μg/g was predictive of clinical relapse (HR = 3.96 [2.47–6.35]; P < .0001) regardless of the type of deescalation.[7] Serial monitoring with FCal could be performed 3 months after therapeutic deescalation and then every 6 months.[7] A value of FCal < 200 μg/g during the surveillance was highly predictive of no clinical relapse, whereas FCal > 400 μg/g should lead to therapeutic intensification due to the high risk of clinical relapse.[7]

FCal could be helpful after ileocolonic resection in patients with CD. The level of FCal increased with the grade of Rutgeerts index. Patients with endoscopic postoperative recurrence at 6 months had higher values of FCal than those without recurrence. In 2 different studies, cut-off values of 100 μg/g demonstrated a high negative predictive value (91% and 93%) but moderate positive predictive value (53% and 69%), suggesting that FCal could avoid most postoperative endoscopies.[8,9] However, it means that measuring FCal alone will miss 1 in 10 patients with endoscopic postoperative recurrence. Consequently, we consider that FCal may replace colonoscopy in patients refusing to undergo colonoscopy at 6 months post-surgery but remains necessary in the other patients owing to the high prediction of CD course (using Rutgeerts index as the reference). Recent preliminary data suggest that the kinetics of FCal within the first 3 months after surgery could predict earlier endoscopic postoperative recurrence. Additional data are needed to confirm its utility in this specific situation.

Evidence is growing that FCal could be a noninvasive tool to evaluate therapeutic efficacy in patients with IBD. Recently, the CALM (Effect of Tight Control Management on Crohn's Disease) trial compared 2 ways of monitoring patients with CD treated with adalimumab.[10] In the first arm (conventional care), the patients had a therapeutic intensification if the Crohn's Disease Activity Index (CDAI) did not decrease by at least 70 points. In the second group, called the "tight control group," the therapies were upgraded in cases of CDAI > 150 or C-reactive protein (CRP) > 5 mg/L or FCal > 250 μg/g.[10] The authors reported that the tight control group achieved better endoscopic and clinical outcomes than the conventional care group.[10] In a post hoc analysis of this study, the authors reported that most of the therapeutic intensification was related to increased level of FCal in the tight control group.[10] A recent meta-analysis on individual data reported that patients achieving clinical remission, normal CRP, and a FCal decrease > 50% after 3 months of anti-TNF therapy had a likelihood > 90% to maintain clinical remission 1 year later compared to clinical remission alone (53%) and clinical remission and normal CRP (60%). These data illustrate the potential of FCal to assess therapeutic efficacy and that it could be used as therapeutic target in patients with IBD, but also that the value of relative FCal changes in an individual patient.

Conclusion

In clinical practice, we should use FCal to distinguish IBD and IBS patients, to assess disease activity, to predict symptomatic relapse in patients with clinical remission or after therapeutic deescalation, to detect CD endoscopic postoperative recurrence, or to assess therapeutic efficacy. FCal cut-off values have to be cautiously interpreted, taking into account type of assay, initial disease extent, and therapeutic target.

References

1. Buisson A, Gonzalez F, Poullenot F, et al. Comparative acceptability and perceived clinical utility of monitoring tools: a nationwide survey of patients with inflammatory bowel disease. *Inflamm Bowel Dis*. 2017;23(8):1425-1433.
2. van Rheenen PF, Van de Vijver E, Fidler V. Fecal calprotectin for screening of patients with suspected inflammatory bowel disease: diagnostic meta-analysis. *BMJ*. 2010;341:c3369.
3. D'Haens G, Ferrante M, Vermeire S, et al. Fecal calprotectin is a surrogate marker for endoscopic lesions in inflammatory bowel disease. *Inflamm Bowel Dis*. 2012;18(12):2218-2224.
4. Labaere D, Smismans A, Van Olmen A, et al. Comparison of six different calprotectin assays for the assessment of inflammatory bowel disease. *United Eur Gastroenterol J*. 2014;2(1):30-37.
5. Goutorbe F, Goutte M, Minet-Quinard R, et al. Endoscopic factors influencing fecal calprotectin value in Crohn's disease. *J Crohns Colitis*. 2015;9(12):1113-1119.
6. Mao R, Xiao Y, Gao X, et al. Fecal calprotectin in predicting relapse of inflammatory bowel diseases: a meta-analysis of prospective studies. *Inflamm Bowel Dis*. 2012;18(10):1894-1899.
7. Buisson A, Mak WY, Andersen MJ, et al. Fecal calprotectin is a very reliable tool to predict and monitor the risk of relapse after therapeutic de-escalation in patients with inflammatory bowel diseases. *J Crohns Colitis*. 2019;13(8):1012-1024.
8. Boschetti G, Laidet M, Moussata D, et al. Levels of fecal calprotectin are associated with the severity of postoperative endoscopic recurrence in asymptomatic patients With Crohn's disease. *Am J Gastroenterol*. 2015;110(6):865-872.

9. Wright EK, Kamm MA, De Cruz P, et al. Measurement of fecal calprotectin improves monitoring and detection of recurrence of Crohn's disease after surgery. *Gastroenterology*. 2015;148(5):938-947.e1.

10. Colombel J-F, Panaccione R, Bossuyt P, et al. Effect of tight control management on Crohn's disease (CALM): a multicenter, randomised, controlled phase 3 trial. *Lancet Lond Engl*. 2018;390(10114):2779-2789.

QUESTION

WHAT ENDPOINTS SHOULD WE AIM FOR IN IBD MEDICAL THERAPY?

Maia Kayal, MD and Jean-Frederic Colombel, MD

New Therapeutic Strategies in IBD

The conventional approach to the treatment of Crohn's disease (CD) and ulcerative colitis (UC) has focused on symptom control using a step-up pharmacological intervention strategy with progressive intensification of therapy. It is now recognized that CD and UC are chronic progressive diseases and that treatment strategies should not only aim for symptom control, but also for blocking disease progression, bowel damage, and disability.[1,2] The 3 pillars of modern care in CD and UC are early intervention, treat to target, and tight control (Figure 6-1).

Treat to Target

Treat to target is a proactive therapeutic approach that involves baseline disease assessment and risk stratification, identification of an appropriate target, selection of therapy, regular assessment of disease activity (tight control) with composite measures, and adjustment of therapy until the predefined target is achieved (Figure 6-2).

In 2015, the International Organization for the Study of Inflammatory Bowel Disease (IOIBD) established the Selecting Targets of Remission in Inflammatory Bowel Disease (STRIDE) committee, whose objective was to achieve international expert consensus on evidence-based treatment targets that could be used in treat-to-target strategies and applied in routine clinical practice.

Rubin DT, Friedman S, Farraye FA, eds. *Curbside Consultation in IBD:*
49 Clinical Questions, Third Edition (pp 31-34).
© 2022 Taylor & Francis Group.

Figure 6-1. The pillars of modern IBD care. (Illustrated by Jill K. Gregory, CMI. Printed with permission from © Mount Sinai Health System.)

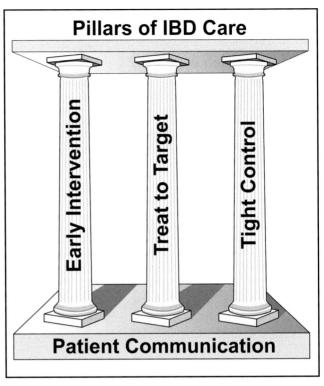

Pillars of IBD Care

Early Intervention
Treat to Target
Tight Control

Patient Communication

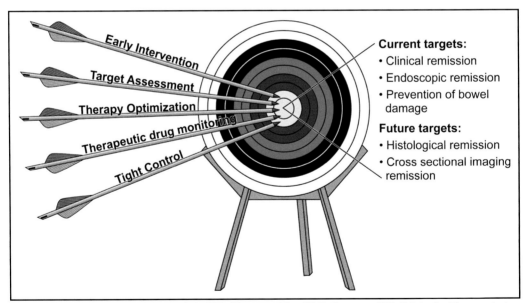

Early Intervention
Target Assessment
Therapy Optimization
Therapeutic drug monitoring
Tight Control

Current targets:
- Clinical remission
- Endoscopic remission
- Prevention of bowel damage

Future targets:
- Histological remission
- Cross sectional imaging remission

Figure 6-2. Treat-to-target approach in IBD. (Illustrated by Jill K. Gregory, CMI. Printed with permission from © Mount Sinai Health System.)

Table 6-1
Crohn's Disease Targets

Crohn's Disease Composite Endpoint	
Clinical/PRO remission	Endoscopic remission
• Resolution of abdominal pain and normalization of bowel habits ◦ Assess every 3 months	• Resolution of ulceration on ileocolonoscopy or imaging ◦ Assess 6 months after treatment

Table 6-2
Ulcerative Colitis Targets

Ulcerative Colitis Composite Endpoint	
Clinical/PRO remission	Endoscopic remission
• Resolution of rectal bleeding and normalization of bowel habits ◦ Assess every 3 months	• Resolution of friability and ulceration on colonoscopy (Mayo 0-1) ◦ Assess 3 months after treatment

The STRIDE committee recommended a composite endpoint of clinical/patient-reported outcome (PRO) remission and endoscopic remission as the primary therapeutic target for both CD and UC.[3] For CD, clinical/PRO remission is defined as resolution of abdominal pain and normalization of bowel habits with eventual normalization of quality of life, formally assessed via the Crohn's Disease Activity Index (CDAI score < 150 defines remission, score decrease by 70 defines response). CD endoscopic remission is defined as resolution of ulceration on ileocolonoscopy or resolution of inflammation on cross-sectional imaging in those patients who cannot be adequately assessed with ileocolonoscopy (Table 6-1). For UC, clinical/PRO remission is defined as resolution of rectal bleeding and normalization of bowel habits, with eventual normalization of quality of life. Endoscopic remission is defined as resolution of friability and ulceration on flexible sigmoidoscopy or colonoscopy formally assessed via the Mayo Score (Mayo 0 indicates remission; Mayo 1 indicates response). For clinical/PRO remission in both CD and UC, assessment is recommended at 3-month intervals during active disease (Table 6-2). For endoscopic remission, assessment is recommended at 3-month intervals during active UC and 6-month intervals during active CD.

The target of endoscopic remission is supported by indirect evidence of its association with improved outcomes such as sustained clinical remission, fewer hospitalizations, and fewer surgeries in post hoc analysis of randomized controlled trials. The ongoing REACT2 (Randomized Evaluation of an Algorithm for Crohn's Treatment) trial will compare an intervention approach based on clinical symptoms with an intervention approach based on endoscopy. The REACT2 trial will provide insight into the efficacy and feasibility of the treat-to-target approach with the current recommended targets.

Adjunctive targets for CD and UC are histological remission and biomarker remission (normal C-reactive protein (CRP), normal calprotectin); however, these have not been formally recommended as targets due to insufficient evidence.

Tight Control

The STRIDE committee did not recommend biomarkers as targets but did suggest their use to facilitate noninvasive disease monitoring. The tight control management algorithm involves close serial monitoring of patients with objective markers and continued adjustment of therapies toward predefined target end points. The tight control strategy is integral to the treat-to-target approach, and its application is thought to block disease progression and prevent bowel damage.

The tight control approach was first validated in the CALM (Effect of Tight Control Management on Crohn's Disease) trial, a randomized controlled trial that evaluated immunomodulator and biologic naïve adult patients with moderate-severe CD, active endoscopic disease, and elevated CRP and/or calprotectin. The clinical management group had treatment escalation driven by CDAI and prednisone use, while the tight control group had treatment escalation driven by CDAI, prednisone use, fecal calprotectin, and CRP. The primary outcome was the proportion of patients with mucosal healing defined as Crohn's Disease Endoscopic Index of Severity (CDEIS) score < 4 and lack of deep ulcerations at 48 weeks. There were higher rates of endoscopic remission observed in the tight control group as compared with the clinical management group, indicating symptom drive management did not adequately control underlying inflammation.

The CALM trial established that a tight control algorithm with regular assessment of objective markers results in improved clinical and endoscopic outcomes compared with symptom-driven care.[4]

It is not yet established if treat to target with tight control will improve long-term outcomes in IBD.

Future Targets

Future potential targets include histological remission and cross-sectional imaging remission in conjunction with endoscopic remission.[5] Many studies have already used histological remission as a target in UC with promising results. Treatment targets will continue to evolve as supporting evidence is collected.

References

1. Colombel JF, Narula N, Peyrin-Biroulet L. Management strategies to improve outcomes of patients with IBD. *Gastroenterology.* 2017:152(2):351-361.
2. Bouguen G, Levesque BG, Feagan BG, et al. Treat to target: a proposed new paradigm for the management of Crohn's disease. *Clin Gastroenterol Hepatol.* 2015;13(6):1042-1050.
3. Peyrin-Biroulet L, Sandborn W, Sands BE, et al. Selecting therapeutic targets in inflammatory bowel disease (STRIDE): determining therapeutic goals for treat-to-target. *Am J Gastroenterol.* 2015;110(9):1324-1338.
4. Colombel JF, Panaccione R, Bossuyt P, et al. Effect of tight control management on Crohn's disease (CALM): a multicenter, randomized, controlled phase 3 trial. *Lancet.* 2018:390(10114):2279-2789.
5. Pouillon L, Peyrin-Biroulet L. It is time to revise the STRIDE guidelines determining therapeutic goals for treat-to-target in inflammatory bowel disease. *J Crohns Colitis.* 2018:12(4):509.

SECTION II

MEDICAL TREATMENT

WHEN SHOULD WE BE USING 5-AMINOSALICYLIC ACIDS IN IBD? HOW DO YOU OPTIMIZE THEIR USE?

Stephen B. Hanauer, MD and Madeline Bertha, MD

5-aminosalicylic acids (5-ASAs) are one of the oldest therapies available for the treatment of inflammatory bowel disease (IBD) and are the main "foundational" therapy for induction and maintenance of mild to moderately active ulcerative colitis (UC). Although once widely used for the treatment of Crohn's disease (CD), evidence suggests that there is a limited (if any) role for their use in CD. 5-ASA is a very safe drug with a wide dosing range and relatively few adverse effects; given their frequent use, it is necessary to understand the different delivery systems, dosing, indications, and potential side effects of these medications.

5-ASA is a hydrophilic small molecule that is readily absorbed in the small intestine, where it is converted in the liver to its inactive form, N-acetyl-5-ASA, and then excreted by the kidneys. In the large intestine 5-ASA can be acetylated either within the epithelium or in the lumen by gut bacteria. Acetylated-5-ASA does not cross into the epithelium and is therefore minimally absorbed from the lumen. Consequently, oral formulations of 5-ASAs have been pharmacologically manufactured to allow for maximized delivery to the distal small bowel and colon. This is accomplished by either the encapsulation of 5-ASA to prevent small bowel absorption or via linkage to an azo bond that is then broken down by luminal bacteria (primarily colonic) for delivery into the colon. The azo bond, or pro drug, formulations include sulfasalazine, olsalazine, and balsalazide. Each drug contains 5-ASA bound by an azo bond to either sulfapyridine, 5-ASA, or N-(4-Aminobenzoyl)-beta-alanine, respectively. Other formulations are composed of 5-ASA alone, with variable delivery mechanisms (delayed release, controlled release, delayed and sustained release) that allow for targeted release of 5-ASA in different parts of the distal small and large bowel.[1] In addition, 5-ASAs have been formulated in rectal preparations (suppositories, foams, or suspensions) and can be utilized either alone or in combination with their oral counterpart.[2]

Rubin DT, Friedman S, Farraye FA, eds. *Curbside Consultation in IBD: 49 Clinical Questions, Third Edition* (pp 37-39).
© 2022 Taylor & Francis Group.

5-ASAs are very forgiving molecules with a wide therapeutic range and relatively few adverse effects at cumulative daily doses up to 8.8 g (4.8 g orally and 4 g rectally). The oral mesalamine formulations are well tolerated with few dose-related side effects. Relatively common adverse effects that are associated with all of the 5-ASAs include headache and gastrointestinal discomfort. Uncommon idiosyncratic reactions include myocarditis, pancreatitis, pleuritis, and hepatitis. Nephrotoxicity is a very rare but serious side effect that has led to the US Food and Drug Administration's recommendation for regular monitoring of renal function. Sulfasalazine, the original 5-ASA compound, has additional risks due to the sulfa moiety that include "intolerances" such as nausea and headache (improved when administered with food and in divided doses) as well as risks of sulfa allergy, hemolytic anemia, and azoospermia.[3]

5-ASAs are the first-line therapy for induction and maintenance of mild to moderately active UC. The primary consideration when initiating a 5-ASA for the treatment of UC is the extent of the disease involved, as this determines the ideal route of delivery. For individuals with proctitis or proctosigmoiditis, topical (rectal) mesalamine suppositories or retention enemas have proven to be the most efficacious. Clinical studies have shown clear superiority for topical mesalamine alone or in combination with oral 5-ASAs for the treatment of distal disease. More recently, topical mesalamine, in combination with oral mesalamine, has also been shown to be more effective than oral mesalamine alone in extensive UC (disease that extends beyond the splenic flexure). There is no role for 5-ASAs in severe disease. Once remission is obtained, patients are continued on the induction dose of 5-ASA indefinitely.[4,5]

With regard to 5-ASA dosing and frequency in mild to moderately active UC, it is generally accepted to start with 2.4 g/day for the induction of remission (unless the patient has a history of difficult-to-treat UC). If the patient has not achieved clinical remission by 6 to 8 weeks, the dose can be increased up to 4.8 g/day.[4,5] Recent studies have shown that continuing treatment for an additional 8 weeks allows for the recruitment of an additional 60% of responders. A subgroup of patients with a history of difficult-to-treat UC may benefit from initiating oral therapy at 4.8 g/day or in combination with rectal mesalamine.[5] Once remission is obtained, the patient should be continued, indefinitely, on maintenance therapy at the same dose required to induce remission.[6]

In the setting of CD, the role of 5-ASA has been less consistent and more controversial. The National and European Cooperative Crohn's Disease Study from 1979 to 1984 found sulfasalazine therapy effective in treatment of CD when the colon was involved (ileocolitis or colitis).[7] These findings were explained by the need for bacteria azo-reductase activity to liberate 5-ASA into the colon. Subsequently, with the development of oral mesalamine compounds, a number of controlled trials demonstrated inconsistent clinical benefits. Overall, meta-analyses of numerous inductive and maintenance studies have failed to demonstrate superiority over placebo in either induction or clinical remission or maintenance of steroid-induced remission.[8] Of note, trials performed in the 1980s to 2000 evaluated symptoms without assessing biomarkers or endoscopy. As such, while the use of sulfasalazine continues to be recommended in guidelines for the treatment of colonic disease, there is no defined role of the use of other 5-ASAs in the induction and maintenance of CD.[8] Nevertheless, many clinicians continue to use mesalamine for mild CD based on safety more than efficacy.

In contrast to sulfasalazine, which requires administration with food and divided doses to prevent common intolerances, mesalamine formulations can be administered once daily to improve compliance.[9] While oral therapy is effective for distal UC, either topical therapy alone, or in combination, can improve responses.[10] Once remission is achieved, the rectal formulations, while usually well tolerated, are often tapered to allow improved compliance with oral (mono) therapy. Nevertheless, we have found that many patients who require rectal therapy to achieve remission may require some maintenance with topical therapy to maintain remissions. In these situations, the rectal administration can often be reduced to an alternate-day or multiple-day weekly schedule. As stated, the specific formulation appears to be less important than the cumulative daily dose of 5-ASA from whichever delivery system. Hence, when changing formulations, the ultimate dose of 5-ASA needs to be considered to either enhance an effect or maintain responses/remissions.

References

1. Sandborn WJ, Hanauer SB. Systematic review: the pharmacokinetic profiles of oral mesalazine formulations and mesalazine pro-drugs used in the management of ulcerative colitis. *Aliment Pharmacol Ther.* 2003;17(1):29-42.
2. Marteau P, Probert CS, Lindgren S, et al. Combined oral and enema treatment with Pentasa (mesalazine) is superior to oral therapy alone in patients with extensive mild/moderate active ulcerative colitis: a randomized, double blind, placebo controlled study. *Gut.* 2005;54(7):960-965.
3. Sonu I, Lin MV, Blonski W, Lichtenstein GR. Clinical pharmacology of 5-ASA compounds in inflammatory bowel disease. *Gastroenterol Clin North Am.* 2010;39(3):559-599.
4. Hanauer SB, Sandborn WJ, Dallaire C, et al. Delayed-release oral mesalamine 4.8 g/day (800 mg tablets) compared to 2.4 g/day (400 mg tablets) for the treatment of mildly to moderately active ulcerative colitis: the ASCEND I trial. *Can J Gastroenterol.* 2007;21:827-834.
5. Hanauer SB, Sandborn WJ, Kornbluth A, et al. Delayed-release oral mesalamine at 4.8 g/day (800 mg tablet) for the treatment of moderately active ulcerative colitis: the ASCEND II trial. *Am J Gastroenterol.* 2005;100:2478-2485.
6. Hanauer SB, Sninsky CA, Robinson M, et al. An oral preparation of mesalamine as long-term maintenance therapy for ulcerative colitis: a randomized, placebo- controlled trial. *Ann Intern Med.* 1996;124(2):204-211.
7. Summers RW, Switz DM, Sessions JT, et al. National Cooperative Crohn's Disease Study: results of drug treatment. *Gastroenterology.* 1979;77(4):847-869.
8. Akobeng AK, Gardener E. Oral 5-aminosalicylic acid for maintenance of medically-induced remission in Crohn's disease. *Cochrane Database Syst Rev.* 2005;1:CD003715.
9. Ford AC, Khan KJ, Sandborn WJ, Kane SV, Moayyedi P. Once-daily dosing vs. conventional dosing schedule of mesalamine and relapse of quiescent ulcerative colitis: systematic review and meta-analysis. *Am J Gastroenterol.* 2011;106(12):2070-2077.
10. Ford AC, Khan KJ, Achkar JP, Moayyedi P. Efficacy of oral vs. topical, or combined oral and topical 5-aminosalicylates, in ulcerative colitis: systematic review and meta-analysis. *Am J Gastroenterol.* 2012;107(2):167-176.

WHAT IS STEROID DEPENDENCE AND HOW IS IT MANAGED?

David B. Sachar, MD

The vast majority of patients with inflammatory bowel disease (IBD; 75% to 90%) will respond acutely to a course of treatment with steroids, with half or more achieving complete remission within 30 days.[1] Many of these responders, however, will ultimately prove to be steroid dependent, a classification clearly defined by a European Crohn's and Colitis Organization (ECCO) consensus group in 2006 and reprised in 2008:

> [inability] to reduce corticosteroids below the equivalent of prednisolone 10 mg/day (or budesonide below 3 mg/day) within 3 months of starting corticosteroids, without recurrent active disease or [occurrence of] a relapse within 3 months of stopping corticosteroids.[2]

The only logical treatment for steroid dependence, therefore, is by definition steroid-sparing therapy. The quickest and most immediately effective steroid-sparing therapy is, of course, *surgery*. But here we are discussing medical management of steroid dependency, which can be described in 2 categories.

First, there is the scenario in which the high acute remission rate on steroids is exploited while it lasts, with prompt transition to a maintenance drug. The second approach is to eschew steroid use altogether by using a different agent to induce remission acutely, and then subsequently to maintain the remission either with the same medication or a different one.

We will consider these 2 avenues of therapy individually and consider both in Crohn's disease (CD) and ulcerative colitis (UC) separately.

Rubin DT, Friedman S, Farraye FA, eds. *Curbside Consultation in IBD: 49 Clinical Questions, Third Edition* (pp 41-44).
© 2022 Taylor & Francis Group.

Crohn's Disease

The strategy of transitioning to another steroid-sparing regimen directly from steroids, during a period of remission, is time-honored. Two decades ago, a landmark multicenter study in children with CD showed that early addition of 6-mercaptopurine to a regimen of corticosteroids significantly lessened the need for prednisone and improved maintenance of remission. The early introduction of 6-mercaptopurine in treatment of children in steroid-induced remission of CD reduced the 18-month relapse rate from 47% on placebo to only 9% (*P* = .007).[3]

This finding of the steroid-sparing effect of thiopurine maintenance has been frequently confirmed in subsequent years.[4] Indeed, a 2016 Cochrane systematic review of 4 studies (1971-1995) calculated that "there was a statistically significant difference in steroid sparing . . . between azathioprine and placebo [64% vs 46%, RR 1.34]."[5] With respect to methotrexate, the data supporting a possible steroid-sparing effect are similar but less robust or consistent. The most recent Cochrane review on the subject[6] found only one large, randomized trial that demonstrated a significant steroid-sparing benefit of this antimetabolite.

Other than transferring from a steroid-dependent remission to a steroid-free maintenance regimen, a second strategy to prevent steroid dependency is to avoid steroids altogether and use an alternative regimen to induce and maintain remission. This approach is becoming increasingly favored among IBD specialists, especially lately in the era of biologics. While there is some evidence that thiopurines or methotrexate alone may have a modest benefit over placebo in the induction of remission in CD, the overwhelming trend of the past 2 decades has been to turn directly to biologic agents for this purpose.[7]

Anti–tumor necrosis factor (TNF) agents in particular have a well-established track record for inducing steroid-free remission in both children and adults. Infliximab has been clearly shown to have this effect, and similar observations hold true for adalimumab. The 2 agents do not appear to be dramatically different in steroid-sparing ability.[8]

Additionally, the anti-integrin vedolizumab has shown a considerable steroid-sparing effect. In one recent uncontrolled retrospective study, which included 15 steroid-dependent patients with CD, 9 (60%) were eventually weaned off steroids.[9] A more comprehensive review of the literature, comprising both randomized clinical trials and real-world experience has also suggested a role for vedolizumab in long-term steroid-sparing maintenance, albeit not so much in acute induction of remission.[10,11] It is encouraging that vedolizumab seems to have efficacy even in patients who have failed prior treatment with anti-TNFs.[12]

More recently, the promising approach of initial *combination* therapy has been introduced. Christensen et al have demonstrated the safety and efficacy of cyclosporine or tacrolimus in combination with vedolizumab for refractory IBD.[13] Likewise, vedolizumab in combination with steroids can improve induction of remission and thus expedite corticosteroid-free maintenance.[14]

Similarly, the landmark CERTIFI trial of ustekinumab reported that more patients in the ustekinumab group than in the placebo group were in glucocorticoid-free remission at week 22, regardless of whether glucocorticoids had been used at baseline (30.6% vs 17.8%, *P* = .048).[15]

Ulcerative Colitis

In acute, severe cases, the surgical alternatives to medical therapy can be even more compelling in UC than in CD. Nonetheless, systemic steroid treatment has long been the mainstay of urgently quelling a flareup of UC. Yet the same arguments against the use of steroids for long-term maintenance apply in UC as they do in CD. Hence, we must turn our attention in the remainder of this chapter to the management of steroid dependence in UC.

The ECCO definition of steroid dependence in UC is the same as in CD.[2]

The value of both azathioprine and 5-aminosalicylate in maintaining steroid-free remissions of UC has long been recognized, with the former demonstrably more efficacious than the latter.[16] But even with evidence supporting the superiority of azathioprine over placebo, the strategy of relying on thiopurines alone for maintaining steroid-free remission in UC, as in CD, has been more recently supplanted by the introduction of biologics.

Again, as with CD, the experience with infliximab treatment in UC has been the most extensive among the biologic agents. Both infliximab and adalimumab have firmly established themselves as first-line therapy in maintaining remission in UC, at least after aminosalicylates have exhausted their definite but limited benefit.[17] It is of interest, as with the SONIC (Study of Biologic and Immunomodulator Naive Patients in Crohn's Disease) study for CD,[18] that combination therapy for UC with thiopurine plus anti-TNF again seems more effective than the use of either alone.[19]

Perhaps even more solidly than in CD, vedolizumab has achieved a firm niche in the maintenance of steroid-free remissions in UC. Indeed, having already established itself as a second-line drug of choice after anti-TNFs, vedolizumab is currently receiving serious consideration as the first-line biologic for both induction and maintenance in this disease.[20]

Ustekinumab, an inhibitor of interleukin (IL) 12/IL-23, already approved by the US Food and Drug Administration (FDA) for CD, is still under investigation for its role in UC. But the newest entry to the IBD field to be approved by the FDA (as of this writing) is tofacitinib, an oral Janus kinase inhibitor, which is already in the marketplace for UC. In the OCTAVE (Omapatrilat Cardiovascular Treatment Assessment vs Enalapril) Sustain trial, remission at 52 weeks occurred in 34.3% of the patients (68 of 198) in the 5 mg tofacitinib group and in 40.6% (80 of 197) of the 10 mg tofacitinib group, as compared with 11.1% (22 of 198) in the placebo group ($P < .001$ for both comparisons with placebo)—an impressive number needed to treat of only 3.4 for the higher dose.[21]

Finally, we should acknowledge the unique role of exclusive enteral nutrition as an important steroid-sparing treatment in pediatric IBD.[22]

Conclusion

Steroid therapy in IBD might be considered analogous to putting out a fire by calling the fire department with hoses, axes, boots, and ladders. This may be an effective system for extinguishing the blaze acutely, but not for maintaining a long-term fire-prevention program. In certain forms of IBD, without generalized sepsis, peritonitis, abscess, fistulization, or perforation, systemic steroids might be used temporarily as an acute salvage treatment, but once the fire has been controlled, an effective preventive maintenance regimen can be introduced with various regimens of antimetabolites and especially biologic agents, with infliximab or adalimumab as first-line and vedolizumab or ustekinumab as second-line (or perhaps in some cases first-line) medications. None of these promising options, however, should totally blind us to the potential benefits of surgery.

References

1. Faubion WA Jr, Loftus EV Jr, Harmsen WF, Zinsmeister AR, Sandborn WJ. The natural history of corticosteroid therapy for inflammatory bowel disease: a population-based study. *Gastroenterology.* 2001;121(2):255-260.
2. Stange EF, Travis SPL, Vermeire S, et al. European evidence-based consensus on the management of Crohn's disease: definitions and diagnosis. *J Crohn Colitis.* 2008;2:1-23.
3. Markowitz J, Grancher K, Kohn N, Lesser M, Daum F. A multicenter trial of 6-mercaptopurine and prednisone in children with newly diagnosed Crohn's disease. *Gastroenterology.* 2000;119(4):895-902.

4. Bermejo F, Aguas M, Chaparro M, et al. Recommendations of the Spanish working group on Crohn's disease and ulcerative colitis (GETECCU) on the use of thiopurines in inflammatory bowel disease. *Gastroenterol Hepatol.* 2018;41(3):205-221.

5. Chande N, Townsend CM, Parker CE, MacDonald JK. Azathioprine or 6-mercatopurine for induction of remission in Crohn's disease. *Cochrana Database Syst Rev.* 2016;16(6):CD000545.

6. McDonald JW, Wang Y, Tsoulis DJ, MacDonald JK, Feagan BG. Methotrexate for induction of remission in refractory Crohn's disease. *Cochrane Database Syst Rev.* 2014;(10):CD003459.

7. Ford AC, Sandborn WJ, Khan KJ, Hanauer SB, Talley NJ, Moayyedi P. Efficacy of biological therapies in inflammatory bowel disease: systematic review and meta-analysis. *Am J Gastroenterol.* 2011;106:644-659.

8. Benmassaoud A, Al-Taweel T, Sasson MS, et al. Comparative effectiveness of infliximab versus adalimumab in patients with biologic-naive Crohn's disease. *Dig Dis Sci.* 2018;63(5):1302-1310.

9. Crowell KT, Tinsley A, Williams ED, et al. Vedolizumab as a rescue therapy for patients with medically refractory Crohn's disease. *Colorectal Dis.* 2018;20(10):905-912.

10. Scribano ML. Vedolizumab for inflammatory bowel disease: from randomized control trials to real-life evidence. *World J Gastroenterol.* 2018;24(23):2457-2467.

11. Christensen B, Colman RJ, Micic D, et al. Vedolizumab as induction and maintenance for inflammatory bowel disease: 12-month effectiveness and safety. *Inflamm Bowel Dis.* 2018;24(4):849-860.

12. Sands BE, Feagan BG, Rutgeerts P, et al. Effects of vedolizumab induction therapy for patients with Crohn's disease in whom tumor necrosis factor antagonist treatment failed. *Gastroenterology.* 2014;147(3):618-627.

13. Christensen B, Gibson PR, Micic D, et al. Safety and efficacy of combination treatment with calcineurin inhibitors and vedolizumab in patients with refractory inflammatory bowel disease. *Clin Gastroenterol Hepatol.* 2019;17(3):486-493.

14. Sands BE, Van Assche G, Tudor D, Akhundova-Unadkat G, Curtis RI, Tan T. Vedolizumab in combination with corticosteroids for induction therapy in Crohn's disease: a post hoc analysis of GEMINI 2 and 3. *Inflamm Bowel Dis.* 2019;25:1375-1382.

15. Sandborn WJ, Gasink C, Gao LL, et al. Ustekinumab induction and maintenance therapy in refractory Crohn's disease. *N Engl J Med.* 2012;367:1519-1528.

16. Ardizzone S, Maconi G, Russo A, Imbesi V, Colombo E, Bianchi Porro G. Randomized controlled trial of azathioprine and 5-aminosalicylic acid for treatment of steroid dependent ulcerative colitis. *Gut.* 2006;55(1):47-53.

17. Wang Y, MacDonald JK, Vandermeer B, Griffiths AM, El-Matary W. Methotrexate for maintenance of remission in ulcerative colitis. *Cochrane Database Syst Rev.* 2015;11(8):CD007560.

18. Colombel JF, Sandborn WJ, Reinisch W, et al. Infliximab, azathioprine, or combination therapy for Crohn's disease. *N Engl J Med.* 2010;362:1383-1395. https://doi.org/10.1056/NEJMoa0904492

19. Panaccione R, Ghosh S, Middleton S, et al. Combination therapy with infliximab and azathioprine is superior to monotherapy with either agent in ulcerative colitis. *Gastroenterology.* 2014;146(2):392-400.

20. Scott FI, Shah Y, Lasch K, Luo M, Lewis JD. Assessing the optimal position for vedolizumab in the treatment of ulcerative colitis: a simulation model. *Inflamm Bowel Dis.* 2018;24(2):286-295.

21. Sandborn WJ, Su C, Sands BE, et al. Tofacitinib as induction and maintenance therapy for ulcerative colitis. *N Engl J Med.* 2017;376(18):1723-1736.

22. Harris RE, Sim W, Garrick V, et al. Using a steroid-sparing tool in pediatric inflammatory bowel disease to evaluate steroid use and dependency. *J Pediatric Gastroenterol Nutr.* 2019;69(5):557-563.

WHAT ARE THE NEW APPROACHES TO USING AND MINIMIZING STEROIDS?

Irving Levine, MD and Brian P. Bosworth, MD

For nearly half a century, corticosteroids have been the hallmark of therapy in inflammatory bowel disease (IBD). Initially introduced in the 1950s, and formally studied in the 1970s, systemic corticosteroids have demonstrated efficacy at inducing remission in both ulcerative colitis (UC) and Crohn's disease (CD). Through their anti-inflammatory effect of downregulating tumor necrosis factor-α (TNF-α), interleukin (IL) 1, and IL-6, corticosteroids play an important role in interrupting the inflammatory pathway. However, the utility of systemic steroids is limited by their side effect profile. Additionally, as the current goal in IBD therapy shifts to long-term safety and prevention of disease complications, with a renewed focus on mucosal healing as a marker of successful treatment, the efficacy of corticosteroids has come in to question given their inability to induce and maintain mucosal healing. Therefore, identifying appropriate steroid use remains a challenge.

The Importance of Limiting Systemic Corticosteroids

Systemic corticosteroids, while effective, carry a severe side effect profile. Side effects from corticosteroids are correlated with the combination of the average daily dose, as well as duration of therapy. The most serious side effect of corticosteroids is an increased risk of infection, with some studies demonstrating increased mortality with steroid usage.[1] Other systemic side effects include fluid retention, fat redistribution, hypertension, hyperglycemia, cataracts, adrenal suppression, cardiovascular disease, renal dysfunction, osteonecrosis, and avascular necrosis, among others.

Rubin DT, Friedman S, Farraye FA, eds. *Curbside Consultation in IBD:*
49 Clinical Questions, Third Edition (pp 45-50).
© 2022 Taylor & Francis Group.

Gastrointestinal specific side effects include gastritis, peptic ulcer disease (if used in conjunction with nonsteroidal anti-inflammatory drugs), hemorrhage, and acute pancreatitis.

Separate from adverse side effects, systemic corticosteroids are ineffective at accomplishing long-term treatment goals in IBD. The current approach to IBD treatment focuses on mucosal healing and the prevention of long-term complications. In CD, corticosteroids are ineffective at inducing mucosal healing.[2] In UC, by contrast, corticosteroids may be effective at inducing mucosal healing but are unable to maintain remission.[3] The combination of ineffectiveness and adverse effects necessitates a critical analysis of appropriate corticosteroid usage.

Indications for Systemic Corticosteroids

Indications for systemic corticosteroids vary between CD and UC. For CD, the American College of Gastroenterology (ACG) 2018 guidelines[4] recommend a short course of oral corticosteroids for moderate to severely active disease. For severe/fulminant disease, intravenous steroids should be used.

In UC, oral prednisone is recommended for induction of mild disease refractory to 5-aminosalicylic acid (ASA; oral or rectal) and budesonide MMX (for left-sided or extensive colitis). For moderate to severe disease, oral prednisone is an option for initial induction, along with several other options, including biologic therapy and small molecules.[3]

For acute severe UC requiring hospitalization, intravenous steroids should be used, with a daily dose equivalent of 60 mg methylprednisolone. Patients who do not respond within 3 to 5 days of intravenous steroids require colectomy, infliximab, or cyclosporine. Corticosteroids should not be used for maintenance therapy.

Limiting the Side Effects of Systemic Corticosteroids

One approach to limiting side effects of systemic corticosteroids is limiting the duration of therapy, with a focus on tapering regiments. By decreasing the duration of therapy, and thereby decreasing the cumulative dose, side effects can be lessened. Studies demonstrate that among severely active patients with CD, quicker tapers of steroids (7 weeks compared to 15 weeks) provide similar rates of remission (85% and 87%, respectively) and 6-month relapse (53% and 37%, respectively).[6]

In addition to the rapidity of steroid taper, frequency of dosing during a steroid taper can also be adjusted. Conventional tapering regimens include daily steroid administration, with a decrease of the daily steroid dose every few days. Several studies, however, have noted improved side effect profiles by intermittent steroid boluses as a tapering method. For example, every other day or a once-weekly dose of the combined cumulative dose that one would be administered through daily administration provides fewer side effects and less decrease in serum cortisol (a marker of adrenal suppression).[7]

Alternatives to Systemic Corticosteroids

Budesonide, a second-generation synthetic nonsystemic corticosteroid related to 16-alpha-hydroxyprednisolone, has a stronger affinity for the glucocorticoid receptor than dexamethasone, prednisolone, or hydrocortisone. Though initially developed for respiratory diseases, budesonide is now routinely used for treatment of IBD. Budesonide provides topical anti-inflammatory effect with minimal systemic symptoms, as 90% of the drug undergoes first-pass metabolism by the liver.

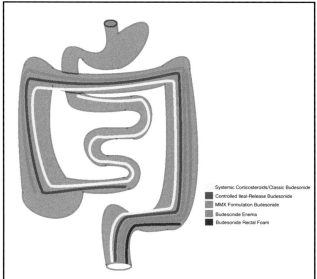

Figure 9-1. Distribution of pharmacologic activity of budesonide. (Yellow = Systemic corticosteroids/classic budesonide; red = controlled ileal-release budesonide; green = MMX formulation budesonide; blue = budesonide edema; purple = budesonide rectal foam. Adapted from Johns Hopkins Medicine https://www.hopkinsmedicine.org/gastroenterology_hepatology/_pdfs/small_large_intestine/crohns_disease.pdf.)

In order to deliver budesonide to the specific region of diseased bowel, several different formulations exist (see Figure 9-1 for location of pharmacologic activity). *Classic oral budesonide*, taken as an oral tablet, has activity throughout the small and large bowel. *Controlled ileal-release budesonide* consists of a coated capsule that prevents dissolution in the acidic gastric environment. Once intestinal pH approaches 5.5, the external capsule decomposes. This allows delivery of the medication to the terminal ileum and right-sided colon.

MMX extended release budesonide consists of a pH-resistant coating as well, yet also has a lipophilic and hydrophilic coating. Upon reaching the terminal ileum, where the pH approaches 7, the resistant coating dissolves. Fluid then accumulates within the hydrophilic layer, allowing the capsule to swell, thereby slowing transit time throughout the colon. Additionally, the lipophilic layer slows the penetration of aqueous fluid into the tablet core. This allows delivery of budesonide to the ileum, ascending, and transverse colon. The MMX budesonide is well tolerated, with a side effect profile including headache and nausea. Gastrointestinal complaints include abdominal pain, diarrhea, and flatulence.

While the previous preparations are oral medications, several rectal preparations of budesonide exist. Liquid budesonide enemas contain approximately 100 mL of liquid enema with budesonide. Budesonide enemas can reach the splenic flexure, yet their utility is limited by patient difficulty in retaining the solution. Rectal foam preparations of budesonide reach approximately 40 cm from the anal verge and are not hindered by the same administration limitations.

Budesonide in Crohn's Disease

In CD, classic oral budesonide is effective at inducing remission compared to placebo. The standard dose is 9 mg per day, yet data in pediatric patients suggest improved responses with higher doses (12 mg/d). However, in severe disease (Crohn's Disease Activity Index > 300), budesonide is inferior compared to conventional corticosteroids, despite being better tolerated. As for maintenance therapy, budesonide is US Food and Drug Administration–approved for mild-moderate CD; however, its effectiveness is not well studied.

Controlled ileal-release budesonide is effective in CD, specifically in disease of the terminal ileum and right-sided colon. Updated ACG guidelines (2018) recommend controlled ileal-release budesonide (9 mg/d) for induction of mild-moderate ileocecal CD.

MMX budesonide has not been studied in CD.

Budesonide in Ulcerative Colitis

In UC, both classic oral budesonide and controlled ileal-release budesonide are minimally effective, as only small quantities reach the left-sided colon.

MMX budesonide is effective at inducing remission compared to placebo in UC. The Core I and Core II trials[8] demonstrated that MMX budesonide induces remission, improves mucosal healing, and decreases C-reactive protein in patients with UC. These results were most apparent in patients with left-sided disease. It remains unclear whether MMX budesonide is effective for maintenance therapy, and current ACG guidelines do not recommend MMX budesonide for maintenance therapy.

For left-sided disease and proctosigmoiditis, rectal formulations of liquid enemas and rectal foam are effective. Liquid budesonide enemas (100 mL) are limited by administration difficulty and may not be effective in patients with severe disease (clinical activity index [CAI] > 8, or patients who have failed 5-ASA formulations). For budesonide rectal foam, studies have demonstrated significantly higher rates of remission, mucosal healing, and decreased rectal bleeding compared to placebo in patients with mild-to-moderate ulcerative proctitis and proctosigmoiditis. The foam is administered as a twice-daily dosing of 2 mg for 2 weeks, followed by a once-daily dosing for 4 weeks.[9]

It should be noted that hydrocortisone enemas and rectal foam also exist, and are effective acute therapy of distal disease, but have not been proven efficacious in maintaining remission.

Other Steroid-Sparing Medications

Alternative medications can be used in place of steroids in active disease. Thiopurines (azathioprine, 6-mercaptopurine) are effective steroid-sparing medications for maintenance therapy in steroid-dependent patients. They can be used in conjunction with steroids in steroid-dependent patients in an attempt to facilitate steroid tapering. However, thiopurines are not useful for inducing symptomatic remission in either UC or CD, given delayed time to action. Alternatively, methotrexate, up to 25 mg weekly, can be used in steroid-dependent CD for maintenance therapy.

Biologic medications, including anti–TNF-α monoclonal antibodies such as infliximab, are effective at inducing response and remission in both moderate-to-severe UC as well as active CD. In CD, concomitant use of thiopurines and infliximab reduces rates of antibody formation to infliximab.

Nonpharmacologic Options to Remain Steroid-Free

Nutritional supplementation and dietary therapy are nonpharmacologic options to improve outcomes in IBD and remain steroid-free. Dietary therapy, specifically elemental diet, is effective therapy at inducing remission in moderately active CD, with some studies demonstrating superiority of elemental diet to corticosteroids.[10] Controversy remains regarding the utility of vitamin D supplementation in patients with IBD. Curcumin, a substance in turmeric, may reduce inflammation and improve symptoms in UC,[11] but larger trials are necessary.

Table 9-1

Various Formulations of Budesonide and Indicated Uses

Corticosteroid	Location of Action	Advantages	When to Use
Controlled ileal release budesonide	Terminal Ileum-right colon	Well tolerated	Ileocolonic CD
MMX formulation	Right colon-left colon	Well tolerated Delivers medication throughout colon	UC with left- or right-sided disease
Budesonide enema	Rectum-splenic flexure	Minimal systemic absorption	UC with left-sided disease
Budesonide foam	Rectum 40 cm above anal verge	Easily administered Minimal systemic absorption	Mild-moderate UC proctitis and proctosigmoiditis

In active moderate-to-severe CD, recent studies have demonstrated clinical and endoscopic improvement with low dose naltrexone (4.5 mg daily).[12] Naltrexone, as a mu-opiod receptor antagonist, blocks endogenous opioid effects, leading to decreased inflammation and wound healing of the epithelial barrier cells.

Conclusion

For nearly half a century, systemic corticosteroids have been the hallmark of IBD therapy. However, given the side effect profile, and inability to induce and maintain mucosal healing, steroid use must be minimized. When systemic corticosteroids are necessary, different tapering regiments help decrease side effects. Several formulations of nonsystemic corticosteroids are available, including oral controlled release, as well as rectal preparations, with specific indications given disease location (Table 9-1). Other steroid-sparing medications and nutritional supplementation can further help the steroid-dependent patient with IBD. With this armamentarium of options, physicians must critically analyze all steroid use in IBD.

References

1. Lichtenstein GR, Feagan BG, Cohen RD, et al. Serious infections and mortality in association with therapies for Crohn's disease: TREAT registry. *Clin Gastroenterol Hepatol.* 2006;4(5):621-630.
2. Atreya R, Neurath MF. Current and future targets for mucosal healing in inflammatory bowel disease. *Visc Med.* 2017;33(1):82-88.
3. Rubin DT, Ananthakrishnan AN, Siegel CA, Sauer BG, Long MD. ACG clinical guideline: ulcerative colitis in adults. *Am J Gastroenterol.* 2019;114(3):384-413.
4. Lichtenstein GR, Loftus EV, Isaacs KL, Regueiro MD, Gerson LB, Sands BE. ACG clinical guideline: management of Crohn's disease in adults. *Am J Gastroenterol.* 2018;113(4):481-517.

5. Kornbluth A, Sachar DB, Practice Parameters Committee of the American College of Gastroenterology. Ulcerative colitis practice guidelines in adults: American College of Gastroenterology, Practice Parameters Committee. *Am J Gastroenterol.* 2010;105(3):501-523; quiz 524.

6. Brignola C, De Simone G, Belloli C, et al. Steroid treatment in active Crohn's disease: a comparison between two regimens of different duration. *Aliment Pharmacol Ther.* 1994;8(4):465-468.

7. Farkas K, Balint A, Valkusz Z, et al. Bolus administration of steroid therapy is more favorable than the conventional use in preventing decrease of bone density and the increase of body fat percentage in patients with inflammatory bowel disease. *J Crohns Colitis.* 2014;8(9):992-997.

8. Sandborn WJ, Travis S, Moro L, et al. Once-daily budesonide MMX(R) extended-release tablets induce remission in patients with mild to moderate ulcerative colitis: results from the CORE I study. *Gastroenterology.* 2012;143(5): 1218-1226.e2.

9. Sandborn WJ, Bosworth B, Zakko S, et al. Budesonide foam induces remission in patients with mild to moderate ulcerative proctitis and ulcerative proctosigmoiditis. *Gastroenterology.* 2015;148(4):740-750.e2.

10. Narula N, Dhillon A, Zhang D, Sherlock ME, Tondeur M, Zachos M. Enteral nutritional therapy for induction of remission in Crohn's disease. *Cochrane Database Syst Rev.* 2018;4(4):CD000542.

11. Taylor RA, Leonard MC. Curcumin for inflammatory bowel disease: a review of human studies. *Altern Med Rev.* 2011;16(2):152-156.

12. Smith JP, Bingaman SI, Ruggiero F, et al. Therapy with the opioid antagonist naltrexone promotes mucosal healing in active Crohn's disease: a randomized placebo-controlled trial. *Dig Dis Sci.* 2011;56(7):2088-2097.

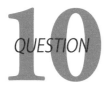

Should You Use Concomitant Immunomodulators With Biological Therapies in IBD?

Remo Panaccione, MD

Biologic therapies—including anti–tumor necrosis factor (TNF) antibodies (infliximab [IFX], adalimumab [ADA], certolizumab [CZP], golimumab [GOL]), integrin inhibitors (vedolizumab [VDZ], natalizumab), and anti–interleukin (IL) 12/IL-23 antibodies (ustekinumab [UST])—have been valuable additions to the therapeutic armamentarium for the treatment for inflammatory bowel disease (IBD). Whether to use biologic therapies for IBD as monotherapy or in combination with immunomodulators such as the thiopurine anti-metabolites (azathioprine [AZA]/6-mercaptopurine [6-MP]) or methotrexate (MTX) has been a matter of debate for the last 2 decades. There are 4 main reasons to consider using concomitant immunomodulators in IBD: (1) to improve overall efficacy, (2) to decrease immunogenicity, (3) to alter pharmacokinetics (decrease drug clearance/increase drug levels), and (4) to treat extraintestinal manifestations or other immune-mediated diseases associated with IBD (eg, psoriasis, rheumatoid arthritis, ankylosing spondylitis). The decision to use or not use a concomitant immunomodulator needs to be balanced with safety concerns for the individual patient. In addition, the practice and rationale for using a combination approach may vary with the individual classes. A combination of the available evidence and practical recommendations is discussed in the sections that follow.

The Case to Improve Overall Efficacy

Combination therapy was not superior in any of the registration trials for Crohn's disease (CD) and ulcerative colitis (UC) for TNF antagonists, VDZ, natalizumab, or UST.[1-11] However, none of these trials were powered to detect these differences, and many patients entering these

Rubin DT, Friedman S, Farraye FA, eds. *Curbside Consultation in IBD: 49 Clinical Questions, Third Edition* (pp 51-58).

trials had failed conventional immunomodulators. Despite this, there is good evidence supporting the use of AZA and IFX in combination with AZA in patients who are bio-naive and immuno-modulatory naive in both moderate to severe CD and UC.[12,13] The SONIC (Study of Biologic and Immunomodulator Naive Patients in Crohn's Disease) trial demonstrated that the combination of IFX and AZA resulted in higher rates of corticosteroid-free clinical remission and mucosal heal-ing (absence of ulcers) after 26 weeks of treatment in patients with CD (56.8% vs 44.4%; P = .02 and 43.9% vs 30.1%; P = .06, respectively) than either treatment alone[12] (Figure 10-1). A recent post hoc analysis of this trial showed significantly higher rates of antidrug antibodies in the mono-therapy patients (36% vs 8%).[14] The benefit of combination therapy seemed mainly driven by the effect of AZA on the pharmacokinetics and immunogenicity of IFX in those on combination therapy.[14] Likewise, the UC-SUCCESS (Infliximab, Azathioprine, or Infliximab + Azathioprine for Treatment of Moderate to Severe Ulcerative Colitis) trial showed increased corticosteroid-free remission in patients with UC on combination therapy after 16 weeks of treatment (39.7% vs 22.1%, P = .017; Figure 10-2), although in this trial the mucosal healing rates (assessed by local investigators) were not higher with combination than with monotherapy (62.8% vs 54.6%, P = .295 in combina-tion vs monotherapy).[13] The superiority of IFX combination therapy in patients with UC also was shown in a systematic review and meta-analysis.[15] In contrast, the only prospective study with ADA did not show a difference of adding an immunomodulator to ADA. Despite some study limitations, the DIAMOND study by Matsumoto et al showed no difference in clinical efficacy in patients with CD on combination therapy vs monotherapy in a 52-week prospective trial (remission rates 68% vs 72%).[16] However, endoscopic improvement (the secondary outcome defined as a decrease of the Simple Endoscopic Score for Crohn's Disease (SES-CD) of at least 8 points from the baseline, or SES-CD ≤ 4) was more frequently attained in patients after 26 weeks of combination treatment (84.2%, n = 5 vs 63.8%, n = 58 [P = .019]). Nevertheless, this endoscopic difference was not sus-tained after 52 weeks of treatment. More recently, there is suggestion that adding AZA to recently diagnosed patients who have not achieved clinical or biomarker remission with ADA is associated with some benefit.[17] There are no dedicated prospective data similar to SONIC, UC-SUCCESS, or DIAMOND with the newer agents VDZ or UST. These studies are certainly needed.

What does this all mean? In clinical practice if the goal is to optimize efficacy, IFX should be used in combination therapy with AZA from the start, weighing the benefits and risks. In bio-naive patients initiating all other agents, monotherapy is preferred given the present data.

The Case to Decrease Immunogenicity

It is well known that all biologics are immunogenic regardless of whether they are a murine chi-mera, humanized, or fully human. In general, the addition of an immunomodulatory, either AZA/6-MP or MTX, reduces the rate of antibody formation by at least 50% regardless of the biologic, as was seen in the registration trials.[1-11] In the anti-TNF era, the best argument for using concomitant immunomodulators was to reduce the risk of immunogenicity (ie, antidrug antibody formation). This has been demonstrated with both the thiopurines and MTX. The extent of reduction in antidrug antibodies appears similar for the thiopurines and MTX.[18,19] Furthermore, in the IFX clinical trials patients on concurrent immunomodulators experienced fewer infusion-related reactions.[1,2] The rate of anti-drug antibody formation is lower with ADA than IFX, so the effect of suppression of anti-drug antibodies with immunomodulators may be less pronounced with ADL combination therapy.[3,4] This has been recently demonstrated in the largest anti-TNF observational cohort study performed in the United Kingdom: the PANTS study.[20] Combination immunosuppressive therapy, however, leads to less immunogenicity and higher ADA serum concentrations.[20] Antidrug antibody forma-tion has been documented early after commencing therapy with anti-TNF, and therefore if starting immunomodulators for this reason, it should be done at the same time as starting the anti-TNF.[21]

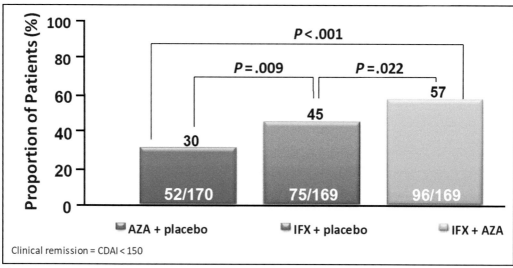

Figure 10-1. Primary endpoint SONIC study: corticosteroid-free remission.

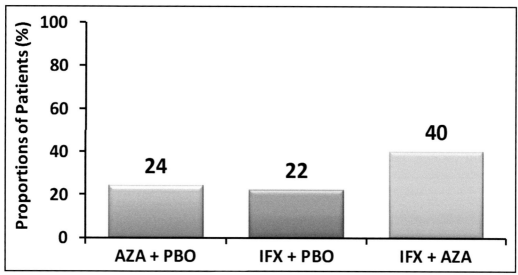

Figure 10-2. Primary endpoint UC-SUCCESS study: corticosteroid-free remission.

The question of how long to continue the combination was addressed in a small underpowered study. Van Assche et al[22] from Belgium reported on a group of 80 patients with CD with disease controlled on combination therapy for a minimum of 6 months. Patients were randomized to maintenance with IFX and placebo vs continued immunomodulator and followed for 104 weeks. The primary outcome was the need to decrease the IFX dosing interval or discontinue IFX. Secondary outcomes included IFX trough levels and safety. While those patients discontinuing their immunomodulator showed significantly lower IFX trough levels at 54 weeks, 1.65 µg/mL vs 2.87 µg/mL ($P < .0001$), and a trend toward higher C-reactive protein levels, there was no difference at 104 weeks with regard to the need for altering the IFX dose or discontinuation. The authors concluded that there was no benefit to immunomodulator beyond 6 months in patients achieving remission with combination IFX and immunomodulator. This has led to the clinical practice of discontinuing immunomodulators at 6 to 12 months, a practice the author does not endorse.

In addition to preventing immunogenicity, introduction of an immunomodulator also has a high chance of reversing antidrug antibody formation, in particular when the antibodies are of low titer and in most cases within 12 months.[23,24]

With the newer agents, VDZ and UST, the rate of immunogenicity is lower than the anti-TNFs.[9-11] For this reason, the absolute benefit of adding an immunomodulatory is much less and the value is less pronounced. Therefore, in bio-naive patients these agents are often used as monotherapy.

What does this all mean? A high-risk bio-naive patient combination therapy should be used with IFX and considered with the other anti-TNFs. In bio-naive patients starting VDZ or UST, beginning with monotherapy is reasonable. However, in patients starting a second biologic, in particular if they have developed antibodies to the first, combination immunomodulators are recommended to prevent immunogenicity. In addition, in those patients who develop low titer antibodies the addition of an immunomodulatory is recommended to attempt to overcome these antidrug antibodies.

The Case to Alter Pharmacokinetics

Altering pharmacokinetics of biologic therapy when using a concomitant immunomodulatory is in part due to reduction in immunogenicity but is likely also due to other independent mechanisms. Presence of antidrug antibodies against IFX has been associated with a 4-fold increase in drug clearance, most likely due to enhanced clearance of drug/antidrug antibody immune complexes.[21] Rapid drug clearance results in low or undetectable circulating drug concentrations, which are associated with lower success rates for induction of remission and loss of response. Indeed, in the SONIC study patients who were on the combination of IFX and AZA had higher trough levels than those on monotherapy[14] (Figure 10-3). Combination therapy may be particularly relevant in complex disease such as perianal fistulizing disease, where higher drug concentrations are desirable. In a cross-sectional study of 117 patients with CD with active fistulas on infliximab for more than 24 weeks, higher trough infliximab levels (> 10 µg/mL) were associated with higher rates of fistula healing compared to lower levels.[25] Rates of mucosal healing and fistula closure were also higher among patients with higher infliximab levels in that study.[25] Whether full doses are needed to achieve these effects is debatable, but a recent study by Roblin et al showed that lower doses of AZA were equally effective in maintaining adequate IFX concentrations and preventing antibody formation as full AZA doses.[26] This has also been shown in other independent studies.[27] The effect of concomitant immunomodulators is not as pronounced with ADA and has not been demonstrated in other studies.[27] It remains a puzzle as to why ADA combination therapy is not as effective as IFX combination therapy. Factors that need to be considered include mode of delivery, absolute drug amount delivered, tissue concentrations, or simply the effects of immunogenicity, as described. A summary of the clinical and pharmacokinetic benefits of concomitant immunomodulators is provided in Table 10-1.

The Case to Treat Extraintestinal Manifestations or Other Immune-Mediated Diseases Associated With IBD

There are cases where concomitant immunomodulators may be used to treat extraintestinal manifestations of IBD and or other immune-mediated diseases. This may become more relevant with some of the newer biologics that may not have the same systemic effects as the anti-TNF

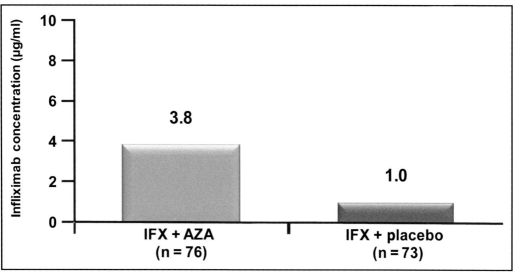

Figure 10-3. Effect of immunomodulator on IFX pharmacokinetics: an analysis of the SONIC study.

Table 10-1

Summary of Clinical and Pharmacokinetic Benefits With Concomitant Immunomodulators

	Crohn's Disease		Ulcerative Colitis	
	Clinical Benefit	Pharmacokinetic/ Immunogenic Benefit	Clinical Benefit	Pharmacokinetic/ Immunogenic Benefit
IFX + AZA/6-MP (treatment naive)	+	+	+	+
IFX + AZA/6-MP (step-up from immunomodulator monotherapy)	–	NA	NA	NA
IFX + MTX	+/–	+	NA	NA
ADA + IMM	+/–	+/–	NA	NA
VDZ + IMM	NA	+	NA	NA
Ustekinumab + IMM	NA	NA	NA	NA

6-MP = 6-mercaptopurine; ADA = adalimumab; AZA = azathioprine; IFX = infliximab; IMM = immunomodulatory; MTX = methotrexate; NA = no adequate data available VDZ = vedolizumab; + = beneficial; +/– = possible benefit; – = no benefit.

therapies. Particular examples may include the treatment of patients with psoriasis or rheumatoid arthritis with VDZ and perhaps MTX when the VDZ is performing well in treating the intestine. This area will be of particular importance in the next several years as more clinical experience with newer agents is established. It also puts an emphasis on individual clinicians to be cognizant of the history of extraintestinal manifestations and other immune-mediated diseases when choosing the biologic itself.

Safety and the Use of Use of Concomitant Immunomodulators in IBD

A common question arises regarding the safety of using concomitant immunomodulators with biologics in IBD. Combination therapy is associated with a different safety profile than biologic monotherapy, regardless of class, which warrants review and discussion with patients. The 2 most concerning safety signals are malignancy (including lymphoma) and serious infections.

Long-term retrospective and prospective series have shown that adding AZA to anti-TNF agents is associated with higher relative risks of opportunistic infection, lymphoma, and nonmelanoma skin cancer.[28-31] With respect to other malignancies, a large global, multicenter prospective cohort study (DEVELOP, n = 5402) examined rates of malignancies among pediatric patients with IBD treated with biologics.[32] Comparing the rates to the general population using the SEER database as the comparator, the authors did not observe any overall risk of malignancy with the biologics alone, but there was a 2.7-fold increased risk of malignancy in thiopurine-exposed patients irrespective of biologic exposure.[32] To date monotherapy with newer agents such as VDZ or UST appear to be safe as monotherapies.[33,34] The impact of adding an immunomodulator remains in question.

A systematic review published in 2011 compiled data on the association between hepatosplenic T-cell lymphoma (HSTCL) and combination therapy for IBD from published reports and the MedWatch reporting system of the US Food and Drug Administration.[35] There was a substantial increase in risk associated with thiopurines, either as monotherapy or combined with anti-TNF therapy, when compared with anti-TNF monotherapy. The overall risk increases dramatically among men younger than 35 years old. This needs to always be taken into consideration when combining anti-TNF with a thiopurine.

Conclusion

Analysis of the currently available evidence for combination therapy in IBD shows that data obtained for one biologic agent may not apply to others. Combination therapy is more effective for IFX, especially in those without prior immunomodulator or IFX use. Combination may be less important for other anti-TNFs and newer agents. The main benefit of combination therapy is likely through favorable effects on immunogenicity and pharmacokinetics. In general, one might consider combination therapy patients with risk factors for disabling disease, complications, or surgery, and in those who are starting a second-line biologic. As safety always plays an important role it is important to evaluate the benefits and risks of combination vs monotherapy on a patient-by-patient basis.

References

1. Hanauer SB, Feagan BG, Lichtenstein GR, et al. Maintenance infliximab for Crohn's disease: the ACCENTI randomized trial. *Lancet*.2002;359(9317):1541-1549.
2. Rutgeerts P, Sandborn WJ, Feagan BG, et al. Infliximab for induction and maintenance therapy for ulcerative colitis. *N Engl J Med*. 2005;353(23):2462-2476.
3. Sandborn WJ, Hanauer SB, Rutgeerts P, et al. Adalimumab for maintenance treatment of Crohn's disease: results of the CLASSIC II trial. *Gut*. 2007;56(9):1232-1239.
4. Colombel JF, Sandborn WJ, Rutgeerts P, et al. Adalimumab for maintenance of clinical response and remission in patients with Crohn's disease: the CHARM trial. *Gastroenterology*. 2007;132(1):52-65.
5. Schreiber S, Khaliq-Kareemi M, Lawrance IC, et al. Maintenance therapy with certolizumab pegol for Crohn's disease. *N Engl J Med*. 2007; 357:239-250.
6. Sandborn WJ, Feagan BG, Stoinov S, et al. Certolizumab pegol for the treatment of Crohn's disease. *N Engl J Med*.2007;357(3):228-238.
7. Sandborn WJ, Feagan BG, Marano C, et al. Subcutaneous golimumab maintains clinical response in patients with moderate-to-severe ulcerative colitis. *Gastroenterology*. 2014;146(1):96-109.e1.
8. Sandborn WJ, Feagan BG, Marano C, et al. Subcutaneous golimumab induces clinical response and remission in patients with moderate-to-severe ulcerative colitis. *Gastroenterology*. 2014;146(1):85-95; quiz e14-5.
9. Feagan BG, Rutgeerts P, Sands BE, et al. Vedolizumabas induction and maintenance therapy for ulcerative colitis. *N Engl J Med*. 2013;369:699-710.
10. Sandborn WJ, Feagan BG, Rutgeerts P, et al. Vedolizumab as induction and maintenance therapy for Crohn's disease. *N Engl J Med*. 2013;369:711-721.
11. Feagan BG, Sandborn WJ, Gasink C, et al. Ustekinumab as induction and maintenance therapy for Crohn's disease. *N Engl J Med*. 2016;375:1946-1960.
12. Colombel JF, Sandborn WJ, Reinisch W, et al. Infliximab, azathioprine, or combination therapy for Crohn's disease. *N Engl J Med*. 2010;362:1383-1395.
13. Panaccione R, Ghosh S, Middleton S, et al. Combination therapy with infliximab and azathioprine is superior to monotherapy with either agent in ulcerative colitis. *Gastroenterology*. 2014;146(2):392-400.e3.
14. Colombel JF, Adedokun OJ, Gasink C, et al. Combination therapy with infliximab and azathioprine improves infliximab pharmacokinetic features and efficacy: a post hoc analysis. *Clin Gastroenterol Hepatol*. 2019 Jul;17(8): 1525-1532.e1.
15. Christophorou D, Funakoshi N, Duny Y, et al. Systematic review with meta-analysis: infliximab and immunosuppressant therapy vs Infliximab alone for active ulcerative colitis. *Aliment Pharmacol Ther*. 2015;41(7):603-612.
16. Matsumoto T, Motoya S, Watanabe K, et al. Adalimumab monotherapy and a combination with azathioprine for Crohn's disease: a prospective, randomized trial. *J Crohns Colitis*. 2016;10(11):1259-1266.
17. Colombel JF, Panaccione R, Bossuyt P, et al. Effect of tight control management on Crohn's disease (CALM): a multicenter, randomized, controlled phase 3 trial. *Lancet*. 2018;390(10114):2779-2789.
18. Feagan BG, McDonald JW, Panaccione R, et al. Methotrexate in combination with infliximab is no more effective than infliximab alone in patients with Crohn's disease. *Gastroenterology*. 2014;146(3):681-688.e1.
19. Vermeire S, Noman M, Van Assche G, et al. Effectiveness of concomitant immunosuppressive therapy in suppressing the formation of antibodies to infliximab in Crohn's disease. *Gut*. 2007;56(9):1226-1231.
20. Kennedy NA, Heap GA, Green HD, et al. Predictors of anti-TNF treatment failure in anti-TNF-naive patients with active luminal Crohn's disease: a prospective, multicenter, cohort study. *Lancet Gastroenterol Hepatol*. 201;4(5):341-353. https://doi.org/10.1016/S2468-1253(19)30012-3
21. Brandse JF, Mathôt RA, van der Kleij D, et al. Pharmacokinetic features and presence of antidrug antibodies associate with response to infliximab induction therapy In patients with moderate to severe ulcerative colitis. *Clin Gastroenterol Hepatol*. 2016;14(2):251-258.e1.
22. Van Assche G, Magdelaine-Beuzelin C, D'Haens G, et al. Withdrawal of immunosuppression in Crohn's disease treated with scheduled infliximab maintenance: a randomized trial. *Gastroenterology*. 2008;134(7):1861-1868.
23. Ben-Horin S, Waterman M, Kopylov U, et al. Addition of an immunomodulatory to infliximab therapy eliminates antidrug antibodies in serum and restores clinical response of patients with inflammatory bowel disease. *Clin Gastroenterol Hepatol*. 2013;11(4):444-447.
24. Strik AS, van den Brink GR, Ponsioen C, et al. Suppression of anti-drug antibodies to infliximab or adalimumab with the addition of an immunomodulatory in patients with inflammatory bowel disease. *Aliment Pharmacol Ther*. 2017;45(8):1128-1134.
25. Yarur AJ, Kanagala V, Stein DJ, et al. Higher infliximab trough levels are associated with perianal fistula healing in patients with Crohn's disease. *Aliment Pharmacol Ther*. 2017;45(7):933-940.

26. Roblin X, Boschetti G, Williet N, et al. Azathioprine dose reduction in inflammatory bowel disease patients on combination therapy: an open-label, prospective and randomized clinical trial. *Aliment Pharmacol Ther.* 2017;46(2):142-149.

27. van Schaik T, Maljaars JP, Roopram RK, et al. Influence of combination therapy with immune modulators on anti-TNF trough levels and antibodies in patients with IBD. *Inflamm Bowel Dis.* 2014;20(12):2292-2298.

28. Lichtenstein GR, Feagan BG, Cohen RD, et al. Drug therapies and the risk of malignancy in Crohn's disease: results from the TREAT registry. *Am J Gastroenterol.* 2014;109(2):212-223.

29. D'Haens G, Reinisch W, Colombel JF, et al. Five-year safety data from ENCORE, a European observational safety registry for adults with Crohn's disease treated with infliximab [Remicade] or conventional therapy. *J Crohns Colitis.* 2017;11(6):680-689.

30. Osterman MT, Sandborn WJ, Colombel JF, et al. Increased risk of malignancy with adalimumab combination therapy, compared with monotherapy, for Crohn's disease. *Gastroenterology.* 2014;146(4):941–949.

31. D'Haens GR, Reinisch W, Satsangi J, et al. Long-term safety of adalimumab in patients with Crohn's disease: final data from PYRAMID registry. *Gastroenterology.* 2017;152(5):S137.

32. Hyams JS, Dubinsky MC, Baldassano RN, et al. Infliximab is not associated with increased risk of malignancy or hemophagocytic lymphohistiocytosis in pediatric patients with inflammatory bowel disease. *Gastroenterology.* 2017:152(8):1901-1914.

33. Colombel JF, Sands BE, Rutgeerts P, et al. The safety of vedolizumab for ulcerativecolitis and Crohn's disease. *Gut.* 2017;66(5):839-851.

34. Ghosh S, Gensler LS, Yang Z, Gasink C, et al. Ustekinumab safety in psoriasis, psoriatic arthritis, and Crohn's disease: an integrated analysis of phase II/III clinical development programs. *Drug Saf.* 2019;42(6):751-768.

35. Kotlyar DS, Osterman MT, Diamond RH, et al. A systematic review of factors that contribute to hepatosplenic T-cell lymphoma in patients with inflammatory bowel disease. *Clin Gastroenterol Hepatol.* 2011;9(1):36-41.e1.

If, When, and How Should Thiopurines Be Used in IBD?

Jennie Clough, MBBS and Peter M. Irving, MBBS, MA, MD

The Role of Thiopurines in IBD

As biologic therapy in inflammatory bowel disease (IBD) becomes increasingly affordable with the advent of biosimilars, the role of thiopurines may be becoming less clear. There is good evidence, however, that optimized thiopurines remain effective as monotherapy for selected patients, and that as immunomodulators they prevent the formation of antibodies to biologic therapies, decreasing the chance of loss of response.

THIOPURINE MONOTHERAPY

Around 60% of patients with IBD will receive thiopurines,[1] of which azathioprine (AZT) and mercaptopurine (MP) are the most commonly prescribed. While the evidence for their use as induction agents is weak, their slow onset of action makes this debate academic, thiopurines having no role in this situation. Thiopurine monotherapy is, however, effective as a maintenance and steroid-sparing strategy in both ulcerative colitis (UC)[2] and Crohn's disease (CD).[3] Studies also support the long-term disease-modifying effects of thiopurines, with an observed 40% reduction in the need for surgery in CD.[4] In addition, rates of clinical and endoscopic postoperative recurrence are significantly lower at 1 year for patients receiving thiopurine therapy,[5] and early azathioprine is associated with a reduction in perianal fistula formation.[6]

Escalation to a thiopurine is recommended in patients with UC who experience 2 disease flares requiring steroids over the course of a year or who are steroid dependent. Their use should

Rubin DT, Friedman S, Farraye FA, eds. *Curbside Consultation in IBD:*
49 Clinical Questions, Third Edition (pp 59-64).
© 2022 Taylor & Francis Group.

be considered earlier in CD, and while 2 trials questioned the role of thiopurines in patients with new onset CD (AZTEC and RAPID), there remains a role for these drugs in patients with early steroid-dependent disease.

Key, however, to the use of thiopurines as monotherapy, as with all drugs, is an understanding of the importance of assessing their effectiveness; if the desired treatment goal is not reached, a change in therapy is indicated. Given that thiopurine tissue levels stabilize at 12 to 16 weeks, due to the time taken for thioguanine nucleotides (TGNs) to be incorporated into DNA, an interval of at least 3 to 4 months is likely to be needed to assess response. For some outcomes, such as mucosal healing in CD, longer intervals may need to be considered.

THIOPURINES IN COMBINATION WITH ANTI–TUMOR NECROSIS FACTOR

The SONIC (Study of Biologic and Immunomodulator Naive Patients in Crohn's Disease) trial demonstrated convincingly that CD infliximab (IFX) therapy, in combination with AZT, was more effective than either drug alone,[7] a finding subsequently mirrored in UC in the UC-SUCCESS (Infliximab, Azathioprine, or Infliximab + Azathioprine for Treatment of Moderate to Severe Ulcerative Colitis) trial.[8] Whether this also holds true for adalimumab (ADA) is less clear, with conflicting results having been reported across both studies and outcome measures.[9]

By way of contrast, thiopurines clearly decrease immunogenicity of both IFX and ADA. For example, data from the recently reported PANTS cohort of more than 1600 new starters on anti–tumor necrosis factor (TNF) demonstrated that 31% of patients on IFX monotherapy had negative drug levels and positive antibodies at 1 year, as did 12% on ADA monotherapy.[10] Thiopurines reduced immunogenicity to both IFX and ADA in a dose-dependent manner, with the lowest rates of antibody formation seen in patients treated with higher thiopurine doses. The role of thiopurines in combination with other biologics is unclear, although early data suggest that vedolizumab and ustekinumab are less immunogenic than anti-TNF drugs, suggesting that there is likely to be less benefit when they are used in combination with thiopurines, at least in terms of immunogenicity.

SCREENING

AZT and MP are metabolized by thiopurine methyltransferase (TPMT), leading to the formation of methylmercaptopurine (MeMP). Accumulation of this metabolite is associated with the development of hepatotoxicity. The activity of TPMT varies in the population, with around 1 in 300 White persons showing complete deficiency, and 1 in 10 being heterozygote carriers of an allele, resulting in around 50% enzyme activity.[1] TPMT activity should, therefore, be checked prior to starting thiopurine therapy.

Nudix hydrolase 15 (NUDT15) variants have also been identified as risk factors for thiopurine-induced myelosuppression in European and Asian populations, with 59% patients with defective expression developing TIM.[11] Defective NUDT15 alleles have been found in approximately 2% of patients with IBD, though screening for defects in NUDT15 is not yet widely available.

If TPMT levels are very low or absent, thiopurines given at standard doses can cause severe myelosuppression. Thiopurine use should be avoided in these populations. If TPMT activity is moderate, it is recommended to halve the usual dose of AZT/MP. Coexistent mutations in both NUDT15 and TPMT are associated with an increased risk of myelotoxicity; dosing alteration is unexplored such that, currently, avoidance of thiopurine therapy is probably reasonable in this situation.

Table 11-1
Screening Prior to Thiopurine Treatment

Investigation	*Action*
Hepatitis C antibody	Requires treatment under specialist hepatology guidance if positive
Hepatitis B surface antigen (HbsAg)	Requires treatment under specialist hepatology guidance if positive
Hepatitis B core antibody (HbcAb)	Vaccinate if negative
HIV	Requires treatment under specialist guidance if positive
Varicella zoster IgG	Vaccinate at least 3 weeks prior to treatment if negative
Epstein Barr virus IgG	Consider antivirals (ganciclovir or foscarnet) in acute infection
	If negative in young men (< 35 years), consider alternative immunosuppressive agent
IFNγ release assay Chest X-ray	Requires treatment under specialist respiratory guidance if positive

Screening for preexisting hepatitis B/C infection, HIV infection, and varicella exposure should be undertaken prior to commencing thiopurine therapy. Unexposed patients should receive varicella vaccination before commencing thiopurines when this is feasible. A chest X-ray and interferon gamma (IFNγ) release assay should be performed to identify latent tuberculosis. Epstein-Barr virus (EBV) status screening allows consideration of avoidance of azathioprine in young EBV-naive patients, as primary EBV infection in this situation can result in fatal lymphoproliferative disorders, which occur due to loss of immune control of EBV-infected B lymphocyte proliferation.[12] The required screening is summarized in Table 11-1.

The pneumococcal vaccine should be administered, preferably prior to treatment, and the influenza vaccine should be given annually. Vaccination for human papilloma virus is also recommended, and women receiving thiopurines should be advised to take part in national cervical cancer screening programs. Live vaccines, such as yellow fever, measles, mumps, and rubella, should not be given during thiopurine treatment.

Recommended starting doses for thiopurines (assuming normal TPMT) are weight-based (2.0 mg/kg to 2.5 mg/kg AZT, 1.0 mg/kg to 1.5 mg/kg MP). Routine blood monitoring should be undertaken for all patients receiving thiopurines to identify early signs of myelosuppression or hepatotoxicity. Full blood count and liver function tests should be checked regularly during initiation (eg, every 2 weeks for the first 2 months), followed by every 3 months for the duration of therapy.

SIDE EFFECTS

Up to one-third of patients cease thiopurine therapy due to side effects,[1] and TPMT polymorphisms account for only around 10% of thiopurine toxicity. Leukopenia occurs in 1.3.% to 12.6% of patients, and 50% to 75% is not predicted by TPMT level.

Hepatotoxicity occurs in 4% of patients and has no relationship to TPMT level[1] but can be associated with a TGN:MeMP ratio of > 11 or MeMP levels > 5700 pmol/8×10^8 RBCs. In patients who develop hepatotoxicity, reducing the dose of AZT to 25% to 33% of the standard dose, with the addition of allopurinol, corrects the shunt. This strategy can also be useful in bypassing gastrointestinal upset, flu-like symptoms, and myalgia.

Pancreatitis occurs in 3% of patients and is an idiosyncratic reaction.[1] An association has been demonstrated with an HLA variant (HLA-DQ1-HLA-DRB1).[13] It is not appropriate to rechallenge with AZT/MP if there is a high suspicion of pancreatitis. Thioguanine (TG) can be considered an alternative agent, which is usually given at a dose of 20 to 40 mg daily.

Up to 6.5% of patients experience idiosyncratic reactions, including flu-like symptoms, arthralgia, rash, or headache. Patients who are intolerant to AZT may benefit from a switch to a metabolic descendent, such as MP or TG.

Thiopurine use is associated with an increased susceptibility to viral infections.[1] In the setting of an acute infection thiopurines should be withheld and restarted once the infection has cleared. Studies suggest that when thiopurines are given in combination with an anti-TNF there is no significantly increased infection risk compared to either agent used alone.[7]

There is a 4- to 5-fold increased risk of malignancy with thiopurine use compared to the general population, particularly lymphoproliferative disease. However, the absolute risk remains low[14] and returns to population levels on cessation of thiopurine therapy. The risk of development of nonmelanoma skin cancer (NMSC) was first identified in transplant recipients. Thiopurines confer a 4- to 6-fold increased risk of NMSC in patients with IBD, and this risk persists even after stopping.[15] Use of a high-factor sunscreen should be advised, and some units advocate annual outpatient screening of skin lesions.[14] Recent evidence suggests that the increase in risk of lymphoma for thiopurine and anti-TNF therapy is probably similar and also additive.

Patients undergoing surgery on thiopurines do not appear to have any increased risk of postoperative complications.[14]

DRUG MONITORING

Thioguanine nucleotides (TGNs) are the primary mediators of therapeutic response, and there is good clinical evidence that TGN monitoring is associated with improved disease outcomes in IBD.[16] Recent data have demonstrated improved rates of mucosal healing in patients with CD with higher TGN levels.[17] Although it takes 12 to 16 weeks for a clinical response to thiopurines to be established, TGN blood monitoring can be initiated from 4 weeks, as steady state blood levels are achieved from 4 to 6 weeks.[1] Lower TGNs may be acceptable in patients taking AZT as CIM rather than monotherapy, although recent data from the PANTS cohort challenge this belief.

In addition to measuring TGN, MMP levels can also be measured. This allows interpretation of reasons for inadequate response. Table 11-2 describes recommended interventions based on TGN/MMP results.

TG is not widely used but has a role in patients who have experienced pancreatitis with AZT/MP, with clinical remission rates of 79% at 12 months. Nodular regenerative hyperplasia has been reported in patients taking TG, but the incidence remains uncertain. The ability of regular screening to monitor for nodular regenerative hyperplasia with, for example, annual MRI scanning is unproven. However, the development of thrombocytopenia or abnormal liver function tests should prompt investigation.[14] TGN levels are typically higher for patients receiving TG than AZT/MP.

Table 11-2
Interpretation of Thioguanine Nucleotides Results

Result	Interpretation	Action
Negligible/undetectable 6-TGN Negligible/undetectable 6-MMP	Nonadherence	Patient education
Low 6-TGN MeMP:TGN <11	Inadequate dosing	Increase AZT dose Recheck in 4 weeks
Low 6-TGN MeMP:TGN >/=11	Hypermethylator	Reduce AZT dose to 25% to 33% Add allopurinol (100 mg)
Normal 6-TGN MeMP:TGN <11	Therapeutic	If in clinical remission, no change advised If symptomatic, consider change of therapy
High 6-TGN	Overdosing	Consider reducing AZT dose by 25 mg to 50 mg, especially if 6-TGN > 550 Recheck in 4 weeks. If symptomatic, consider change of therapy

Good safety data exist for the use of thiopurines in men and women around conception and pregnancy. However, there are no safety data on the use of allopurinol in pregnancy, and it would therefore be advisable to avoid allopurinol during pregnancy.

THIOPURINE WITHDRAWAL

It is suggested that thiopurine withdrawal can be considered after 5 years of treatment if the patient remains in clinical remission. Treatment for longer than 4 years has been shown to increase the rates of NMSC and lymphoma, with a greater risk in patients over the age of 50 years. When thiopurines are withdrawn, 1-year clinical relapse rates are 23% in CD and 12% in UC.[18] A raised C-reactive protein prior to withdrawal was found to be highly predictive of relapse.[14]

Conclusion

Thiopurines continue to have a role in IBD both as a monotherapy and in combination with anti-TNF therapy. Pharmacogenetic markers are able to identify patients at higher risk of side effects, and optimization using thiopurine metabolite monitoring improves response rates. Special consideration needs to be taken for older cohorts of patients, for whom the risks of infection and lymphoproliferative disease are higher. Most importantly, as with all treatments, if reassessment shows a lack of or incomplete response to thiopurines, changes in therapeutic strategies are required.

References

1. Warner B, Johnston E, Arenas-Hernandez M, Marinaki A, Irving P, Sanderson J. A practical guide to thiopurine prescribing and monitoring in IBD. *Frontline Gastroenterol*. 2018;9(1):10-15
2. Timmer A, Patton PH, Chande N, McDonald JW, MacDonald JK. Azathioprine and 6-mercaptopurine for maintenance of remission in ulcerative colitis. *Cochrane Database Syst Rev*. 2016;(5):CD000478.
3. Sandborn WJ, Sutherland LR, Pearson D, May G, Modigliani R, Prantera C. Azathioprine or 6-mercaptopurine for induction of remission in Crohn's disease. In: Sandborn WJ, ed. *Cochrane Database of Systematic Reviews*. Chichester, UK: John Wiley & Sons; 1998:1465-1858.
4. Chatu S, Subramanian V, Saxena S, Pollok RC. The role of thiopurines in reducing the need for surgical resection in Crohn's disease: a systematic review and meta-analysis. *Am J Gastroenterol*. 2014;109(1):23-34.
5. Peyrin-Biroulet L, Deltenre P, Ardizzone S, et al. Azathioprine and 6-mercaptopurine for the prevention of postoperative recurrence in Crohn's disease: a meta-analysis. *Am J Gastroenterol*. 2009;104(8):2089-2096.
6. Cosnes J, Bourrier A, Laharie D, et al. Early administration of azathioprine vs conventional management of Crohn's disease: a randomized controlled trial. *Gastroenterology*. 2013;145(4):758-765.e2.
7. Colombel JF, Sandborn WJ, Reinisch W, et al. Infliximab, azathioprine, or combination therapy for Crohn's disease. *N Engl J Med*. 2010;362(15):1383-1395.
8. Panaccione R, Ghosh S, Middleton S, et al. Combination therapy with infliximab and azathioprine is superior to monotherapy with either agent in ulcerative colitis. *Gastroenterology*. 2014;146(2):392-400.e3.
9. Matsumoto T, Motoya S, Watanabe K, et al. Adalimumab monotherapy and a combination with azathioprine for Crohn's disease: a prospective, randomized trial. *J Crohns Colitis*. 2016;10(11):1259-1266.
10. Kennedy NA, Heap GA, Green HD, et al. Predictors of anti-TNF treatment failure in anti-TNF-naive patients with active luminal Crohn's disease: a prospective, multicentre, cohort study. *Lancet Gastroenterol Hepatol*. 2019;4(5):341-353.
11. Walker GJ, Harrison JW, Heap GA, et al. Association of genetic variants in NUDT15 with thiopurine-induced myelosuppression in patients with inflammatory bowel disease. *JAMA—J Am Med Assoc*. 2019;321(8):753-761.
12. Louis E, Irving P, Beaugerie L. Use of azathioprine in IBD: modern aspects of an old drug. *Gut*. 2014;63(11):1695-1699.
13. Heap GA, Weedon MN, Bewshea CM, et al. HLA-DQA1–HLA-DRB1 variants confer susceptibility to pancreatitis induced by thiopurine immunosuppressants. *Nat Genet*. 2014;46(10):1131-1134.
14. Goel RM, Blaker P, Mentzer A, Fong SCM, Marinaki AM, Sanderson JD. Optimizing the use of thiopurines in inflammatory bowel disease. *Ther Adv Chronic Dis*. 2015;6(3):138-146.
15. Peyrin–Biroulet L, Khosrotehrani K, Carrat F, et al. Increased risk for nonmelanoma skin cancers in patients who receive thiopurines for inflammatory bowel disease. *Gastroenterology*. 2011;141(5):1621-1628.e5.
16. Smith M, Blaker P, Patel C, et al. The impact of introducing thioguanine nucleotide monitoring into an inflammatory bowel disease clinic. *Int J Clin Pract*. 2013;67(2):161-169.
17. Mao R, Guo J, Luber R, et al. 6-thioguanine nucleotide levels are associated with mucosal healing in patients with Crohn's disease. *Inflamm Bowel Dis*. 2018;24(12):2621-2627.
18. Kennedy NA, Kalla R, Warner B, et al. Thiopurine withdrawal during sustained clinical remission in inflammatory bowel disease: relapse and recapture rates, with predictive factors in 237 patients. *Aliment Pharmacol Ther*. 2014;40(11-12):1313-1323.

HOW SHOULD METHOTREXATE BE USED IN IBD?

Hans Herfarth, MD, PhD and Edward L. Barnes, MD, MPH

Methotrexate (MTX) is a folate antagonist, initially developed in 1948 for the treatment of leukemia. In the setting of lymphoma or solid cancer therapy, this drug is used at high doses (in the range of grams). In contrast to its usage in cancer therapy, lower doses of MTX, in the range of 10 to 30 mg, are typically used for the treatment of autoimmune diseases such as psoriasis, rheumatoid arthritis, and Crohn's disease (CD; Table 12-1).

Methotrexate Administration

MTX is administered once weekly, either orally, subcutaneously (SC), or intramuscularly (IM). MTX SC application has the same bioavailability as MTX IM and is preferred since the IM administration is more painful compared to SC injections. Oral administration achieves the same bioavailability as SC administration at doses up to 15 mg weekly.[1] Above 15 mg the small bowel absorption of MTX is more variable. Thus, it is recommended to apply MTX subcutaneously at doses above 15 mg/week or if there is suspicion of impaired small bowel absorption (eg, jejunal CD).[1] MTX has a relatively short serum half-life of 6 to 8 hours, and more than 80% of the drug in its intact form is excreted in the urine by glomerular and tubular secretion. The remaining 20% are converted to MTX polyglutamates, which are retained for some time in tissues such as the liver and kidney. In the setting of a decreased glomerular or tubular filtration rate, MTX toxicity increases, and the dose needs to be adapted. Given the delayed onset of therapeutic efficacy of MTX (around 6 to 8 weeks), one should consider an additional induction therapy such as steroids.

Rubin DT, Friedman S, Farraye FA, eds. *Curbside Consultation in IBD:*
49 Clinical Questions, Third Edition (pp 65-69).
© 2022 Taylor & Francis Group.

Table 12-1
Dosing of Methotrexate for Different IBD Indications

Disease	*MTX Dose Adult*	*MTX Pediatric Dose*
Crohn's disease	25 mg SC once weekly (in stable remission may be reduced to 15 mg SC or oral once weekly)	15 mg/m² (body surface area) once weekly to a maximum dose of 25 mg (in stable remission may be reduced to dose of 10 mg/m² once a week to a maximum dose of 15 mg)
Crohn's disease or ulcerative colitis in combination with biologic	15 (oral) or 25 (SC)	10 to 15 mg/m² maximum; 15 to 25 mg once weekly (oral or SC)

For all indications an additional oral therapy with folic acid (either 1 mg daily or 5 mg weekly) and 4 mg ondansetron orally before the weekly MTX application is recommended.

Methotrexate Monotherapy in Crohn's Disease

MTX monotherapy applied at a dose of 25 mg IM weekly, in conjunction with a steroid taper over 10 weeks, induces remission in patients with CD.[2] In the North American Crohn's Study Group's landmark trial, significantly more patients receiving MTX were in clinical remission at week 16 compared to placebo (39% vs 19%). In the pivotal maintenance of remission trial, the MTX dose was reduced to 15 mg IM weekly, which was superior to placebo in maintaining remission for 40 weeks in 65% of patients on MTX vs 39% on placebo.[3] However, a subset of patients relapsed on the reduced dose of 15 mg MTX and could be brought back into remission on the higher dose of 25 mg MTX/week.[3] Thus, a reduction of MTX from 25 to 15 mg weekly is associated with a risk of relapse, and nowadays it is generally recommended to keep patients who responded to MTX induction therapy with 25 mg MTX weekly on the same dose for maintenance (a reduction to 15 mg weekly can be considered in select patients). MTX monotherapy has been shown to be similarly effective in patients who are failing or intolerant to thiopurine therapy as well as in pediatric patients at a dose of 10 to 15 mg/m² (body surface area; maximal dosing 15 to 25 mg).[1] There are no controlled prospective data available describing the efficacy of MTX regarding mucosal healing in CD aside of 2 small uncontrolled case series including a total of 22 patients with CD and with a mucosal healing rate of around 35% in a time frame of 3 to 60 months after start of MTX.[1]

Methotrexate Monotherapy in Ulcerative Colitis

The use of MTX monotherapy to induce and maintain remission in patients with active UC has been debated for decades.[4] Two large placebo-controlled multicenter trials in Europe and the United States have recently reported that MTX at a dose of 25 mg SC once weekly is not more effective compared to placebo in either inducing or maintaining remission.[5,6] The results of both studies show that in contrast to CD, the use of MTX as monotherapy in patients with UC cannot be recommended.

Methotrexate in Combination With Biologics in IBD

Based on the SONIC (Study of Biologic and Immunomodulator Naive Patients in Crohn's Disease) and UC-SUCCESS (Infliximab, Azathioprine, or Infliximab + Azathioprine for Treatment of Moderate to Severe Ulcerative Colitis) trial, a combination therapy of infliximab (IFX) with a thiopurine (azathioprine or 6-mercaptopurine) is recommended for patients with active CD or UC.[7,8] In cases of thiopurine intolerance, MTX in combination with a biologic is recommended. The COMMIT (Combination of Maintenance Methotrexate-Infliximab Trial) demonstrated an effect of MTX 25 mg SC once weekly on IFX trough and significant prevention of anti-IFX antibody (aIFX-AB) levels (IFX trough and detectable aIFX-AB [%]: 6.4 mg/mL and 4% on MTX/IFX vs 3.8 mg/mL and 20% on IFX mono; $P < .01$).[9] In contrast to SONIC, the COMMIT study did not demonstrate a benefit of a combination therapy IFX/MTX vs a monotherapy with IFX only (steroid-free remission IFX/MTX vs IFX monotherapy 76% vs 77% at week 14 and 56% vs 57% at week 50, respectively). The study was remarkable in that the rate of steroid-free remission was twice that observed in other pivotal studies in patients with CD. The presumably absent additive effect of MTX in COMMIT may have been due to trial design, patient population (inclusion criteria, duration of disease, previous exposure to immunosuppression), or a short follow-up period. Interestingly, in IBD, apart from the combination of IFX and azathioprine, no additional clinical efficacy of a combination therapy with adalimumab, certolizumab, or golimumab has been reported.[10] Retrospective studies in pediatric CD and adult IBD patients showed a longer persistence of IFX therapy in combination with MTX at doses > 12.5 mg MTX/week.[11,12] There are no prospectively controlled data available comparing a combination therapy of a biologic using 2 different dosing regimen of MTX (25 mg MTX SC vs 15 mg MTX orally weekly) or showing an advantage of a combination therapy vs a biologic monotherapy using MTX in patients with UC.

Methotrexate: Adverse Events, Toxicity, and Recommended Concomitant Therapies

The most commonly observed adverse events during MTX therapy are nausea and vomiting (20% to 30%) and hepatotoxicity (around 10% to 15%). Adverse events such as anorexia, bone marrow suppression, stomatitis, MTX-induced diarrhea, or opportunistic infections occur less often. Hypersensitivity pneumonitis is rare (< 1%), but a new onset chronic cough during MTX therapy should always raise suspicion for this serious adverse event. Impaired kidney function or drugs impairing tubular secretion such as probenecid can result in an increase in circulating MTX with consecutive toxic adverse event (stomatitis, enteritis, bone marrow toxicity). Other factors associated with MTX toxicity include a decrease in serum albumin and serum folate levels. Also, MTX should not be applied in patients with preexisting liver disease or excess alcohol intake.

Folic acid or folinic acid reduce potential gastrointestinal (including the incidence of stomatitis) and liver toxicity of MTX.[1] Patients on MTX should be treated either concomitantly with 5 mg folic or folinic acid weekly or 1 mg folic acid daily, which for the patient is easier to remember. The therapeutic efficacy of MTX is neither affected by this supplementation nor does it matter if the folic acid is given on the same day as MTX or delayed by 24 hours (in case of weekly administration of folic acid). Checking serum folate levels prior to therapy is normally not necessary. To prevent nausea, patients should be treated with ondansetron (4 mg) before the weekly MTX administration and as needed 8 to 12 hours after MTX administration.

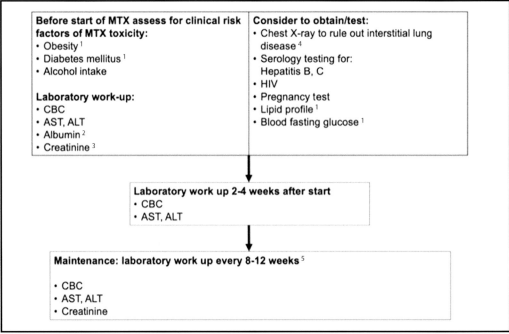

Figure 12-1. Recommended tests before starting MTX therapy. 1 = Associated with hepatotoxicity in the context of nonalcoholic fatty liver disease (NAFLD) and the risk of preexisting liver fibrosis. 2 = Low albumin is associated with thrombocytopenia, liver, and pulmonary toxicity. 3 = Creatinine clearance < 79 mL/min reduces methotrexate clearance and is associated with higher risk of toxicity. 4 = Consider mainly in patients > 50 years or Hx of pulmonary problems. 5 = Consider transient elastography yearly after 2 to 3 years of therapy. (ALT = alanine aminotransferase; AST = aspartate transaminase; CBC = complete blood count; MTX = methotrexate.)

Methotrexate: Elective Surgery, Cancer Risk, and Pregnancy

Preoperative exposure to MTX has not been associated with an increased risk of postoperative complications in the setting of abdominal surgery in patients with IBD.[13] Also, guideline recommendations for patients with rheumatoid arthritis undergoing elective orthopedic surgery recommend continuation of MTX.[14]

In contrast to thiopurines, there is no reported increased risk of solid cancers or lymphoma associated with MTX.[15] MTX is contraindicated in pregnancy and should be stopped 3 months before planned pregnancy in men and women. The recommendations for men to stop MTX 3 months before pregnancy is solely based on expert opinion, but recently abnormalities in the DNA integrity of sperm have been reported.[14,16] Thus far, several cohort studies have not shown an increased risk for newborns of fathers exposed to MTX.[17]

Methotrexate Monitoring

Before and after starting MTX or increasing the dose it is recommended to check complete blood count, liver chemistries, and creatinine (Figure 12-1). In the case of normal liver function tests and no risk factors for cirrhosis (nonalcoholic steatohepatitis, alcohol), there is no requirement for a liver biopsy following a certain duration of therapy or cumulative thresholds (eg, 3 g after approximately 3 years of 25 mg MTX weekly). If persistently abnormal liver-associated chemistries occur, MTX should be discontinued and a liver biopsy should be considered.[1] Longitudinal evaluations of liver fibrosis with transient elastography (FibroScan) may offer a noninvasive method to measure liver stiffness in patients on concurrent MTX, but standardized prospective studies of this approach are lacking.[18]

So far studies in patients with rheumatoid arthritis and IBD have not found any meaningful correlation between the clinical efficacy of MTX and serum or plasma levels of either intact MTX or its metabolites, suggesting that there is little clinical value in monitoring these levels. Recent research evaluated the role of MTX polyglutamates in erythrocytes, which appears to better correlate with effectiveness in patients with rheumatoid arthritis, but this approach can be still considered experimental.[19]

References

1. Herfarth HH, Kappelman MD, Long MD, et al. Use of methotrexate in the treatment of inflammatory bowel diseases. *Inflamm Bowel Dis*. 2016;22(1):224-233.
2. Feagan BG, Rochon J, Fedorak RN, et al. Methotrexate for the treatment of Crohn's disease. *N Engl J Med*. 1995;332(5):292-297.
3. Feagan BG, Fedorak RN, Irvine EJ, et al. A comparison of methotrexate with placebo for the maintenance of remission in Crohn's disease. *N Engl J Med*. 2000;342:1627-1632.
4. Herfarth HH, Osterman MT, Isaacs KL, et al. Efficacy of methotrexate in ulcerative colitis: failure or promise. *Inflamm Bowel Dis*. 2010;16(8):1421-1430.
5. Herfarth H, Barnes EL, Valentine JF, et al. Methotrexate is not superior to placebo in maintaining steroid-free response or remission in ulcerative colitis. *Gastroenterology*. 2018;155(4):1098-1108.e9.
6. Carbonnel F, Colombel JF, Filippi J, et al. Methotrexate is not superior to placebo for inducing steroid-free remission, but induces steroid-free clinical remission in a larger proportion of patients with ulcerative colitis. *Gastroenterology*. 2016;150(2):380-388.e4.
7. Colombel JF, Sandborn WJ, Reinisch W, et al. Infliximab, azathioprine, or combination therapy for Crohn's disease. *N Engl J Med*. 2010;362:1383-1395.
8. Panaccione R, Ghosh S, Middleton S, et al. Combination therapy with infliximab and azathioprine is superior to monotherapy with either agent in ulcerative colitis. *Gastroenterology*. 2014;146(2):392-400.e3.
9. Feagan BG, McDonald JW, Panaccione R, et al. Methotrexate in combination with infliximab is no more effective than infliximab alone in patients with Crohn's disease. *Gastroenterology*. 2014;146(3):681-688.e1.
10. Lichtenstein GR, Loftus EV, Isaacs KL, et al. ACG clinical guideline: management of Crohn's disease in adults. *Am J Gastroenterol*. 2018;113(4):481-517.
11. Grossi V, Lerer T, Griffiths A, et al. Concomitant use of immunomodulators affects the durability of infliximab therapy in children with Crohn's disease. *Clin Gastroenterol Hepatol*. 2015;13(10):1748-1756.
12. Colman RJ, Rubin DT. Optimal doses of methotrexate combined with anti-TNF therapy to maintain clinical remission in inflammatory bowel disease. *J Crohns Colitis*. 2015;9(4):312-317.
13. Afzali A, Park CJ, Zhu K, et al. Preoperative use of methotrexate and the risk of early postoperative complications in patients with inflammatory bowel disease. *Inflamm Bowel Dis*. 2016;22(8):1887-1895.
14. Visser K, Katchamart W, Loza E, et al. Multinational evidence-based recommendations for the use of methotrexate in rheumatic disorders with a focus on rheumatoid arthritis: integrating systematic literature research and expert opinion of a broad international panel of rheumatologists in the 3E Initiative. *Ann Rheum Dis*. 2009;68(7):1086-1093.
15. Beaugerie L, Itzkowitz SH. Cancers complicating inflammatory bowel disease. *N Engl J Med*. 2015;372:1441-1452.
16. Ley D, Jones J, Parrish J, et al. Methotrexate reduces DNA integrity in sperm from men with inflammatory bowel disease. *Gastroenterology*. 2018;154(8):2064-2067.e3.
17. Grosen A, Kelsen J, Hvas CL, et al. The influence of methotrexate treatment on male fertility and pregnancy outcome after paternal exposure. *Inflamm Bowel Dis*. 2017;23(4):561-569.
18. Laharie D, Seneschal J, Schaeverbeke T, et al. Assessment of liver fibrosis with transient elastography and FibroTest in patients treated with methotrexate for chronic inflammatory diseases: a case-control study. *J Hepatol*. 2010;53(6):1035-1040.
19. Fischer M, Siva S, Cook GK, et al. Methotrexate polyglutamate monitoring in patients with Crohn's disease. *Clin Pharmacol Drug Dev*. 2017;6(3):240-245.

QUESTION 13

WHAT IS THE EVOLVING ROLE OF CALCINEURIN INHIBITORS IN IBD?

Ralley Prentice, MBBS and
Britt Christensen, BSc, MBBS (Hons), MPH, PhD

Ulcerative colitis (UC) and Crohn's disease (CD) are immune-mediated conditions characterized by inappropriate intestinal T-cell activation and inflammation, with a complex and incompletely defined pathogenesis. T-cell activation, which ultimately results in mucosal damage, is dependent on multiple intracellular signaling mechanisms responsible for translating and perpetuating cytokine-mediated cellular replication and inflammatory activity. Tacrolimus and cyclosporine, via slightly different intermediaries, inhibit the action of calcineurin, which is responsible for the dephosphorylation of nuclear factor of activated T cells. These transcription factors induce production of interleukin 2, a key cytokine in promoting T-cell survival and proliferation,[1] with its inhibition consequently dampening the inflammatory response significantly.

Cyclosporine Therapy in Ulcerative Colitis

Cyclosporine has been employed in the management of inflammatory bowel disease (IBD) for many years, most extensively in patients with acute severe ulcerative colitis (ASUC) refractory to 3 to 5 days of intravenous (IV) corticosteroids, consequently requiring rescue medical therapy or colectomy. In the first trials demonstrating efficacy in ASUC, IV cyclosporine was dosed at 4 mg/kg/day. However, a 2 mg/kg/day dosing schedule has subsequently been found to be equivalent for time to response, mean endoscopic scores, and overall response rate despite higher cyclosporine levels in 4 mg/kg/day patients, with a trend to increased complications in the higher-dosed patients.[2] Therefore, cyclosporine is usually commenced via a continuous infusion at 2 mg/kg/day, with dose adjustments based on day 2 trough levels. Patient response is assessed clinically and

Rubin DT, Friedman S, Farraye FA, eds. *Curbside Consultation in IBD:*
49 Clinical Questions, Third Edition (pp 71-76).
© 2022 Taylor & Francis Group.

biochemically and usually occurs within 4 to 10 days. Patients are then transitioned to twice daily oral cyclosporine at a total daily dose double that of the IV dose. In the short term, cyclosporine has been found to avoid colectomy in 80% to 90% of patients presenting with ASUC.[3] However, despite excellent short-term outcomes with cyclosporine, prolonged use is limited by adverse events and relapse rates are high on cessation of therapy. Therefore, when transitioning to oral cyclosporine, a gradual steroid taper with commencement of an immunomodulator (azathioprine or 6-mercaptopurine) as a maintenance therapy is advisable. In patients who have already failed treatment with an immunomodulator, failure and colectomy rates with cyclosporine are increased, hence historically cyclosporine has only been utilized as an induction agent for thiopurine naive patients as a bridge to maintenance thiopurine therapy. Care must be taken with triple immunosuppression in this setting, and *Pneumocystis carinii* prophylaxis should be considered.

Infliximab, an anti–tumor necrosis factor (TNF) monoclonal antibody, is an alternative rescue therapy in ASUC.[4] The comparable efficacy for induction of remission and prevention of colectomy of cyclosporine vs infliximab in immunomodulator-naive patients has been demonstrated at both 3 and 12 months in randomized controlled trials[4,5] and confirmed in a systematic review.[6] However, there are several advantages and disadvantages to both agents. The cost of cyclosporine is lower, potentially negated in real-world circumstances by the relative complexity of its administration and monitoring, requiring initial longer average hospital stays of 11 vs 4 days for infliximab.[7] In addition, if bridging to an immunomodulator following cyclosporine therapy, the costs and risk associated with long-term anti-TNF therapy can be avoided. Infliximab is expensive but relatively straightforward to administer; however, this can be uniquely hindered by marked intestinal loss of proteins (including therapeutic monoclonal antibody) in those with severe colitis.[8] In addition, following successful treatment with infliximab, this agent is usually continued as a maintenance therapy, resulting in long-term reliance on a biologic agent.

In patients who are commenced on cyclosporine, monitoring for side effects is pertinent. In a retrospective review of 111 patients treated with IV cyclosporine followed by oral treatment, major adverse events occurred in 15.2% of patients, including nephrotoxicity in 5.4%.[9] Serious infections were noted in 6.3% and seizures in 3.6%. More minor side effects, including hypomagnesaemia, hypertension, hypertrichosis, headaches, hyperkalemia, and gingival swelling also occur.[9] Importantly, calcineurin inhibitors (CNIs) are not known to affect male or female fertility, with no teratogenic effects and minimal placental passage.[9]

Sequential Therapy With Cyclosporine and Infliximab

The use of sequential therapy with infliximab to cyclosporine or vice versa in refractory ASUC patients has also been explored, enabling short-term avoidance of colectomy in up to 60% of patients.[10] However, this strategy has been associated with a substantial risk of serious adverse events, including mortality,[10] and should be used very cautiously. Infliximab followed by cyclosporine is recommended as the preferred sequence due to the short half-life of cyclosporine and hence more limited duration of immunosuppression.[10]

Tacrolimus Therapy in Ulcerative Colitis

The role of tacrolimus in the management of UC has been less extensively investigated and defined. In IBD, tacrolimus is usually dosed at 0.1 to 0.2 mg/kg orally, targeting a trough of 10 to 15 ng/mL for induction and 5 to 10 ng/mL for maintenance.[1,11] In a single-center retrospective analysis comparing tacrolimus to anti-TNF therapy in patients with moderate to severe UC requiring hospitalization, clinical response and remission rates were equivalent, as were short-term colectomy rates, and in the small number of patients assessed, endoscopic healing rates.[11] These findings have been supported by a review of 5 nonrandomized studies, with no significant difference in rates of serious adverse events identified.[12]

Tacrolimus in Crohn's Disease

Tacrolimus is occasionally utilized in the management of luminal CD, although randomized controlled trial evidence to support this is currently limited. McSharry et al[13] reviewed 6 small-case series that included 70 patients in total and found that 44.3% (range 7% to 69%) of patients achieved complete remission with the use of oral tacrolimus. The studies were of poor quality but suggest that oral tacrolimus may be of benefit in some patients with CD. With a more robust evidence base, severe fistulizing CD has been treated with tacrolimus for more than 15 years, following pivotal randomized trials that demonstrate significant fistula improvement (more than 50% closure of fistulas draining at baseline with maintenance of closure at 4 weeks) of 43% with tacrolimus compared to only 8% in the placebo arm.[14] This is maintained as being highly significant when potential confounders of concomitant treatments and antecedent anti-TNF were considered. However, this response is not typically prolonged due to short duration of therapy as necessitated by side effect profile, with anti-TNF therapies preferentially considered standard of care in the treatment of complex fistulizing disease.

Cyclosporine in Crohn's Disease

Cyclosporine, although used less widely and currently lacking supportive randomized controlled trial evidence, has demonstrated efficacy in fistulizing CD with initial fistula closure rates of 33% to 100%.[15] Study designs vary, but most utilize an initial IV 4 mg/kg infusion for 10 days followed by 8 mg/kg/day of orally administered cyclosporine.[15]

Topical Calcineurin Inhibitors

Topical CNI therapy in ulcerating perianal CD and left-sided UC has retrospectively been shown to induce clinical improvement in disease activity, without demonstrable systemic absorption or toxicity, through various methods of application.[16,17] In the context of refractory ulcerative proctitis, a recent 4-week induction randomized controlled trial that included 85 patients, compared 2 mg daily tacrolimus suppositories to 3 mg daily beclomethasone suppositories. The 2 agents showed similar rates of clinical remission (46% and 38%, respectively, $P = .638$), endoscopic remission (30% vs 13%, $P = .92$), and adverse events.[18]

Combination Therapy With Vedolizumab: The Evolving Role of Calcineurin Inhibitors

Despite the efficacy of CNIs in the short term, as previously mentioned, long-term use in maintenance is limited by safety concerns. Recently, the role of CNI co-induction or combination therapy with vedolizumab in steroid and/or anti-TNF refractory or intolerant patients has emerged as a viable therapeutic option. Vedolizumab, an $\alpha_4\beta_7$ integrin inhibitor, prevents gut-specific T cells from honing to sites of inflammation and is effective at inducing clinical response and remission in both UC and CD. However, vedolizumab use is limited in the setting of ASUC or in those intolerant or nonresponsive to steroids due to its prolonged time to maximal response, which can take up to 3 months in UC and 6 to 12 months in CD.[19] The use of concurrent CNI in this setting is hence beneficial, with their rapid onset enabling bridging to maintenance vedolizumab. This algorithm has been shown to be effective in UC, CD, and ASUC.[20,21] In those who enter remission or have improvement post-induction with CNI, vedolizumab is commenced. CNI therapy is usually continued for 6 to 12 weeks before halving the dose for 1 week in patients who are clinically well and ceasing if response is maintained. Vedolizumab is then continued into the maintenance phase.[20,21] The success of this strategy has been demonstrated in a cohort of 20 patients (9 CD, 11 UC, 1 anti-TNF naive) receiving concomitant CNI and vedolizumab induction for management of steroid and largely anti-TNF refractory disease or ASUC.[20] Steroid-free clinical remission was achieved in 44% of CD and 55% of UC patients at week 14 and maintained in 33% of CD and 45% of UC patients at week 52. This is equivalent to rates seen in the pivotal vedolizumab trials GEMINI 1 and 2, despite inclusion of a more treatment-resistant cohort. The average duration of dual therapy with a CNI was 64 days in this study, with all patients having ceased the CNI within 12 months. Adverse events attributable to the CNI were minimal, with minor neurotoxicity in 5 patients. Importantly, patients received prophylaxis against pneumocystis jirovecii while on concomitant steroids.[20] These positive findings have been replicated in 2 studies of patients with severe steroid refractory UC who had induction therapy with a CNI and were transitioned to vedolizumab; a 12-month colectomy free survival of 67% to 68% was demonstrated in both studies, and again adverse events were minimal.[21,22]

Finally, in patients with primary nonresponse to vedolizumab, rescue therapy with CNIs has also been effectively employed in a small number of patients. In a study by Christensen et al, 1 of 2 patients with UC and 2 of 5 patients with CD achieved steroid- and CNI-free remission following rescue therapy with CNIs after failing induction therapy with vedolizumab (Figure 13-1).[20]

Conclusion

The role of CNIs in the treatment of IBD is rapidly evolving. Currently they can be utilized in the treatment of the following:

- Patients with ASUC who are immunomodulator naive as a bridge to immunomodulatory therapy
- Patients with ASUC as a bridge to vedolizumab maintenance
- Moderate to severe CD or UC patients who are refractory to or intolerant of steroids, or as steroid-sparing agents, in the context of bridging to vedolizumab
- Rescue therapy in patients with CD or UC with primary nonresponse to vedolizumab
- Patients with refractory CD fistulas
- ASUC refractory/failing anti-TNF therapy, although the infective risks inherent in this degree of immunosuppression are considerable and should be taken seriously
- Ulcerative perianal CD, distal UC, pyoderma gangrenosum, and oral CD as a topical agent

As their use expands, appropriate selection of patients for treatment with CNIs, considering the side effect profile, remains essential.

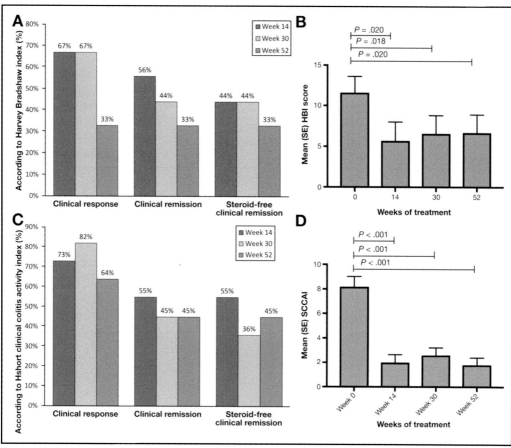

Figure 13-1. Responses to CNI induction with vedolizumab bridging. (Reproduced with permission from Christensen B, Gibson PR, Micic D, et al. Safety and efficacy of combination treatment with calcineurin inhibitors and vedolizumab in patients with refractory inflammatory bowel disease. *Clin Gastroenterol Hepatol.* 2019;17[3]:486-493.)

References

1. Matsuoka K, Saito E, Fujii T, et al. Tacrolimus for the treatment of ulcerative colitis. *Intest Res.* 2015;13(3):219-226.
2. Van Assche G, D'Haens G, Noman M, et al. Randomized, double-blind comparison of 4 mg/kg versus 2 mg/kg intravenous cyclosporine in severe ulcerative colitis. *Gastroenterology.* 2003;125(4):1025-1031.
3. Stack W, Long R, Hawkey C. Short- and long-term outcome of patients treated with cyclosporin for severe acute ulcerative colitis. *Alimentary Pharmacol Ther.* 1998;12(10):973-978.
4. Jarnerot G, Hertervig E, Friis-Liby I, et al. Infliximab as rescue therapy in severe to moderately severe ulcerative colitis: a randomized, placebo-controlled study. *Gastroenterology.* 2005;128(7):1805-1811.
5. Laharie D, Bourreille A, Branche J, et al. Ciclosporin versus infliximab in patients with severe ulcerative colitis refractory to intravenous steroids: a parallel, open-label randomized controlled trial. *Lancet.* 2012;380(9857):1909-1915.
6. Narula N, Marshall JK, Colombel J-F, et al. Systematic review and meta-analysis: infliximab or cyclosporine as rescue therapy in patients with severe ulcerative colitis refractory to steroids. *Am J Gastroenterol.* 2016;111(4):477-491.
7. Löwenberg M, Duijvis N, Ponsioen C, et al. Length of hospital stay and associated hospital costs with infliximab versus cyclosporine in severe ulcerative colitis. *Eur J of Gastroenterol Hepatol.* 2014;26(11):1240-1246.
8. Brandse JF, Brink GRvd, Wildenberg ME, et al. Loss of infliximab into feces is associated with lack of response to therapy in patients with severe ulcerative colitis. *Gastroenterology.* 2015;149(2):350-355.e352.

9. Sternthal M, Murphy S, George J, Kornbluth A, Lichtiger S, Present D. Adverse events associated with the use of cyclosporine in patients with inflammatory bowel disease. *Am J Gastroenterol.* 2008;103(4):937-943.

10. Leblanc S, Allez M, Seksik P, et al. Successive treatment with cyclosporine and infliximab in steroid-refractory ulcerative colitis. *Am J Gastroenterol.* 2011;106(4):771-777.

11. Yamamoto T, Shimoyama T, Umegae S, Matsumoto K. Tacrolimus vs anti-tumour necrosis factor agents for moderately to severely active ulcerative colitis: a retrospective observational study. *Alimentary Pharmacol Ther.* 2016;43(6):705-716.

12. Takeuchi K, Shimoyama T, Yamamoto T. Comparison of safety and efficacy of tacrolimus versus infliximab for active ulcerative colitis. *Dig Dis.* 2018;36(2):106-112.

13. McSharry K, Dalzell AM, Leiper K, El-Matary W. Systematic review: the role of tacrolimus in the management of Crohn's disease. *Alimentary Pharmacol Ther.* 2011;34(11-12):1282-1294.

14. Sandborn W, Present D, Isaacs K, et al. Tacrolimus for the treatment of fistulas in patients with Crohn's disease: a randomized, placebo-controlled trial. *Gastroenterology.* 2003;125(2):380-388.

15. Present D, Lichtiger S. The efficacy of cyclosporine in the treatment of the fistula of Crohn's disease. *Gastroenterology.* 1992;102:A680.

16. Dieren Jv, Bodegraven Av, Kuipers E, et al. Local application of tacrolimus in distal colitis: feasible and safe. *Inflamm Bowel Dis.* 2009;15(2):193-198.

17. Sandborn W, Tremaine W, Schroeder K, Steiner B, Batts K, Lawson G. Cyclosporine enemas for treatment-resistant, mildly to moderately active, left-sided ulcerative colitis. *Am J Gastroenterol.* 1993;88(5):640-645.

18. Lie MRKL, Kreijne JE, Dijkstra G, et al. No superiority of tacrolimus suppositories vs beclomethasone suppositories in a randomized trial of patients with refractory ulcerative proctitis. *Clin Gastroenterol Hepatol.* 2019;3565(19):1777-1784.

19. Vasudevan A, Gibson PR, Langenberg DRv. Time to clinical response and remission for therapeutics in inflammatory bowel diseases: what should the clinician expect, what should patients be told? *World J Gastroenterol.* 2017;23(35):6385-6402.

20. Christensen B, Gibson P, Micic D, et al. Safety and efficacy of combination treatment with calcineurin inhibitors and vedolizumab in patients with refractory inflammatory bowel disease. *Clin Gastroenterol Hepatol.* 2019;17(3):486-493.

21. Pellet G, Stefanescu C, Carbonnel F, et al. Efficacy and safety of induction therapy with calcineurin inhibitors in combination with vedolizumab in patients with refractory ulcerative colitis. *Clin Gastroenterol Hepatol.* 2019;17(3):494-501.

22. Ollech JE, Dwadasi S, Rai V, et al. Efficacy and safety of induction therapy with calcineurin inhibitors followed by vedolizumab maintenance in 71 patients with severe steroid-refractory ulcerative colitis. *Aliment Pharmacol Ther.* 2019;51(6):637-643.

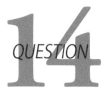

WHAT PREPARATIONS SHOULD OCCUR BEFORE INITIATING BIOLOGIC THERAPY?

Akriti P. Saxena, MD and Mark T. Osterman, MD, MSCE

The last decade marks an exciting era in the field of inflammatory bowel disease (IBD) as a wave of new biologic agents has been approved by the US Food and Drug Administration (FDA). Together with an expanding therapeutic armamentarium comes greater responsibility in the care of patients with IBD, encompassing both preventative measures and health maintenance. As newer biologics with different mechanisms of action are introduced into practice, prescribers have to be increasingly vigilant about preventing and quickly recognizing adverse events. As new treatment paradigms of top-down and treat-to-target approaches permeate clinical practice, we anticipate an uptake in the use of biologic agents early in the course of disease.

This chapter focuses on preventative measures prior to initiating biologic therapy due to the underlying immunomodulatory mechanism of these agents. The literature to support these practices originates primarily from anti–tumor necrosis factors (TNFs). The risk of opportunistic infections, hepatitis B reactivation, and tuberculosis infection appears to be lower with the newer generation of biologic agents such as vedolizumab (anti-integrin)[1] and ustekinumab (anti–interleukin [IL] 12/IL-23)[2] based on preliminary studies. However, it would be prudent to follow the same precautionary practices as applicable to anti-TNF therapy until further data become available. Baseline blood tests, including a complete blood count and comprehensive metabolic panel, are obtained prior to initiating biologic therapy and are monitored regularly while on treatment, although the appropriate frequency of these tests has not been determined.

Rubin DT, Friedman S, Farraye FA, eds. *Curbside Consultation in IBD: 49 Clinical Questions, Third Edition* (pp 77-80).
© 2022 Taylor & Francis Group.

Hepatitis B Infection

Hepatitis B vaccination is recommended for all nonimmune patients with IBD. In patients with prior exposure to the virus, hepatitis B reactivation is a potentially devastating and preventable consequence of immunosuppressive therapy. It is advisable to check the following panel of hepatitis B virus (HBV) studies in all patients with IBD, and particularly before initiating biologic therapy, as the immune response to vaccination is often lowered[3]: HBV surface antibody (HBsAb), HBV surface antigen (HBsAg), and HBV core antibody (anti-HBc).

An isolated HBsAb results from vaccination, without prior exposure to the virus. The level of antibody titer, which confers immunity, is controversial and ranges from 10 IU/l to 100 IU/l. A recent American College of Gastroenterology guideline recommends a single-booster vaccination in patients with low titers and to administer the 3-dose vaccination series if patients do not respond appropriately to the booster.[4] Ongoing surveillance of titers is controversial, and in the absence of risk factors, checking HBV studies prior to the initiation of biologic therapy is likely sufficient.

It is imperative to consider hepatitis B reactivation in patients with HBsAg or anti-HBc. According to the 2015 American Gastroenterological Association guideline on HBV reactivation, patients treated with anti-TNFs who are anti-HBc positive (and either HBsAg positive or negative) are considered at moderate risk of HBV reactivation, defined as an anticipated incidence of 1% to 10%. Antiviral prophylaxis is recommended for this group (weak recommendation, moderate quality of evidence) and should be continued for 6 months beyond immunosuppressive therapy.[5]

We recognize that patients with anti-HBc antibody but no HBsAg are at lower risk for reactivation (compared to HBsAg-positive patients), and clinical monitoring may be reasonable in this setting.

Screening for Latent Tuberculosis Infection

Another potentially devastating complication of immunosuppressive therapy is the reactivation of latent tuberculosis infection (LTBI), which often masquerades as disseminated disease. Current guidelines recommend screening for LTBI prior to initiating biologic therapy and deferring therapy at least until treatment for LTBI has commenced. The screening modality of choice, however, remains controversial.

Interferon-γ release assays (IGRAs) have emerged as the preferred screening modality for latent tuberculosis infection in recent years. These assays measure sensitization to mycobacterium tuberculosis through interferon-γ release in whole blood (QuantiFERON-TB Gold and QuantiFERON-TB Gold In-Tube [QFT-GIT]; Cellestis) or peripheral blood (T-SPOT.TB; Oxford Immunotec). While tuberculin skin testing (TST) is an acceptable alternative,[6] it has fallen out of favor for several reasons, including the need for a second office visit and subjectivity in interpreting the results. IGRAs are also thought to perform better than TST in patients who have been exposed to nontuberculous mycobacteria, have received the Bacillus Calmette–Guérin vaccine,[7] or are on immunosuppressive therapy.[8] However, an indeterminant result on the QFT-GIT test has been associated with delays in initiation of biologic therapy.[9] In addition to a thorough medical history, physical examination, and the testing indicated, a chest radiograph[10] should be obtained.

Treatment is advised in conjunction with an infectious disease specialist for any patient with evidence of latent tuberculosis infection (either with a positive IGRA or TST), or an abnormal chest radiograph, and biologic therapy is typically delayed by at least 4 weeks in this scenario. After completion of therapy for LTBI, repeat testing is not advised. For patients on long-term biologic therapy, it is reasonable to consider annual testing for latent TB, although there are little data to support this practice.

Vaccines

Preventing opportunistic infections through routine vaccination is recommended for all patients with IBD. We highlight its additional importance prior to starting biologic therapy, as several studies have demonstrated that the immune response is lowered in patients on immunosuppressive medications.[11] It is most preferable to vaccinate patients at the time of diagnosis, but if not then vaccinations should be administered at least 2 weeks prior to immunosuppressive therapy.[12] Inactivated vaccines against the following pathogens are recommended: seasonal influenza, pneumococcal pneumonia (PCV13 and PPSV23), hepatitis A and B, human papilloma virus, meningococcus, and tetanus, diphtheria and pertussis. The new inactivated 2-dose herpes zoster vaccine (Shingrix) is currently approved for patients over age 50. While awaiting further guidelines specific to the IBD population, we recommend that patients with IBD under age 50 also receive Shingrix prior to starting biologic therapy, cost permitting.

Live vaccines, on the other hand, are contraindicated in patients either on biologic therapy or who are about to initiate immunosuppressive therapy in the near future. For the patient with IBD whose vaccination history is unknown, titers for measles, mumps, and rubella (MMR) are recommended. If nonimmune, vaccination may be administered if the patient has not been on immunosuppressive therapy in the preceding 3 months and therapy is not planned in the upcoming 6 weeks. Similarly, immunity to varicella zoster should be documented, and if nonimmune the live attenuated vaccine may be given if spaced apart from biologics by 1 to 3 months.[12]

A Word on Natalizumab

Natalizumab is 1 of 2 anti-integrin molecules approved for the treatment of Crohn's disease, the other being vedolizumab. The use of natalizumab has been associated with an increased risk of progressive multifocal leukoencephalopathy due to activation of the John Cunningham virus. Concurrent with its reintroduction into practice in 2005, natalizumab now has a boxed warning from the FDA and mandates specific education, monitoring, and reporting by prescribers.[13] Its use is restricted to monotherapy for 12 weeks, after which it should be discontinued if no clinical benefit is achieved. John Cunningham virus seropositivity increases the risk of progressive multifocal leukoencephalopathy and therefore must be documented prior to and at regular intervals during therapy. Vedolizumab has become the preferred anti-integrin biologic owing to its superior safety profile, even compared with the anti-TNF agents, but natalizumab may be used in select clinical scenarios.

References

1. Ng SC, Hilmi IN, Blake A, et al. Low frequency of opportunistic infections in patients receiving vedolizumab in clinical trials and post-marketing setting. *Inflamm Bowel Dis.* 2018;24(11):2431-2441.
2. Ting S-W, Chen Y-C, Huang Y-H. Risk of hepatitis B reactivation in patients with psoriasis on ustekinumab. *Clin Drug Investig.* 2018;38(9):873-880.
3. Jiang H, Wang S, Deng M, et al. Immune response to hepatitis B vaccination among people with inflammatory bowel diseases: a systematic review and meta-analysis. *Vaccine.* 2017;35(20):2633-2641.
4. Farraye FA, Melmed GY, Lichtenstein GR, Kane SV. ACG clinical guideline: preventive care in inflammatory bowel disease. *Am J Gastroenterol.* 2017;112(2):241-258.
5. Reddy KR, Beavers KL, Hammond SP, Lim JK, Falck-Ytter YT, American Gastroenterological Association Institute. American Gastroenterological Association Institute guideline on the prevention and treatment of hepatitis B virus reactivation during immunosuppressive drug therapy. *Gastroenterology.* 2015;148(1):215-219; quiz e16-7.
6. Lewinsohn DM, Leonard MK, LoBue PA, et al. Official American Thoracic Society/Infectious Diseases Society of America/Centers for Disease Control and Prevention clinical practice guidelines: diagnosis of tuberculosis in adults and children. *Clin Infect Dis.* 2017;64(2):111-115.

7. Doan TN, Eisen DP, Rose MT, Slack A, Stearnes G, McBryde ES. Interferon-gamma release assay for the diagnosis of latent tuberculosis infection: a latent-class analysis. Gao L, ed. *PLoS One*. 2017;12(11):e0188631.

8. Schoepfer AM, Flogerzi B, Fallegger S, et al. Comparison of interferon-gamma release assay versus tuberculin skin test for tuberculosis screening in inflammatory bowel disease. *Am J Gastroenterol*. 2008;103(11):2799-2806.

9. Vajravelu RK, Osterman MT, Aberra FN, et al. Indeterminate QuantiFERON-TB Gold increases likelihood of inflammatory bowel disease treatment delay and hospitalization. *Inflamm Bowel Dis*. 2018;24(1):217-226.

10. Clark M, Colombel J-F, Feagan BC, et al. American Gastroenterological Association Consensus Development Conference on the use of biologics in the treatment of inflammatory bowel disease, June 21–23, 2006. *Gastroenterology*. 2007;133(1):312-339.

11. Nguyen DL, Nguyen ET, Bechtold ML. Effect of immunosuppressive therapies for the treatment of inflammatory bowel disease on response to routine vaccinations: a meta-analysis. *Dig Dis Sci*. 2015;60(8):2446-2453.

12. Farraye FA, Melmed GY, Lichtenstein GR, Kane SV. ACG clinical guideline: preventive care in inflammatory bowel disease. *Am J Gastroenterol*. 2017;112(2):241-258.

13. Danese S, Vuitton L, Peyrin-Biroulet L. Biologic agents for IBD: practical insights. *Nat Rev Gastroenterol Hepatol*. 2015;12(9):537-545.

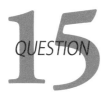

QUESTION

15

WHERE SHOULD ANTI-INTEGRIN THERAPY BE PLACED IN THE THERAPEUTIC ALGORITHM FOR CROHN'S DISEASE AND ULCERATIVE COLITIS?

Rachel W. Winter, MD, MPH and Sonia Friedman, MD

Mechanism of Action

Vedolizumab (VDZ) is an immunoglobulin G4 (IgG4) humanized anti-α4 integrin monoclonal antibody that selectively inhibits $\alpha_4\beta_7$ integrin interaction with the adhesion molecule-1 (MAdCAM-1). It selectively immunosuppresses the gut without inhibiting systemic immune responses or affecting T-cell tracking to the central nervous system. The selectivity of VDZ to the gastrointestinal tract results in targeted therapy as compared to its predecessor, natalizumab. Vedolizumab is approved for treatment of patients with moderate to severe ulcerative colitis (UC) or Crohn's disease (CD). Prior to approval of VDZ, natalizumab was the only available anti-integrin therapy approved for inflammatory bowel disease (IBD) and was positioned in the treatment algorithm for IBD after patients failed anti–tumor necrosis factor (TNF) medications. Currently, natalizumab is rarely used as VDZ, which has a more favorable safety profile, selectively targets the gastrointestinal tract and has not been associated with increased risk of progressive multifocal leukoencephalopathy (PML). Etrolizumab, a humanized monoclonal antibody that binds the β subunit of $\alpha_4\beta_7$ and $\alpha_E\beta_7$, has shown superiority to placebo in phase 2 trials, but additional trials are ongoing, and it is not yet US Food and Drug Administration–approved for therapy of CD or UC.[1]

Safety and Adverse Effects of Vedolizumab

The most serious adverse effect of natalizumab is PML, caused by the John Cunningham virus. As a result, natalizumab is currently rarely recommended for treatment of IBD. To date,

Rubin DT, Friedman S, Farraye FA, eds. *Curbside Consultation in IBD: 49 Clinical Questions, Third Edition* (pp 81-85).
© 2022 Taylor & Francis Group.

there have been no reported cases of PML associated with the use of VDZ.[2,3] The risk of PML with VDZ use was recently estimated to be no greater than 6.75 cases per 100,000 patient years (PY) of exposure, although the true risk is difficult to quantify without reported cases.[3] However, monitoring patients clinically for new neurological symptoms, including weakness, vision changes, clumsiness of limbs, and changes in personality, memory, thought processes, or orientation, is advised.

The GEMINI clinical trials showed that VDZ is effective and safe for both induction and maintenance of remission among patients with IBD.[4-7] Long-term safety studies have also been performed to demonstrate the safety of the medication beyond the trial period.[8-10] Analysis of 6 phase 2 and phase 3 clinical trials of patients with CD and UC showed a favorable safety profile for VDZ.[2] Gastrointestinal symptoms as well as infections of the gastrointestinal and upper respiratory tract were the most common side effects, but no increased risk of serious systemic or opportunistic infections were reported.[2] There were no significantly increased risks of common side effects among patients receiving VDZ compared to placebo. The reported incidence of upper respiratory infections was 28.6/100 PY and 7.4/100 PY for gastrointestinal infections among patients exposed to VDZ; among patients given placebo, rates were 34.7/100 PY for upper respiratory infections and 6.7/100 PY for gastrointestinal infections.[2] Rare complications associated with anti-TNF medications, including demyelination and exacerbation of congestive heart failure, were not observed with VDZ. Additional common side effects of VDZ include headache (11.5/100 PYs) and arthralgia (11.2/100 PYs), though rates of these side effects did not exceed those seen among patients who received placebo.[2] Similarly, 2 systematic reviews and meta-analyses report an advantageous safety profile of VDZ compared to other biologics, though head-to-head comparative studies are not available.[11,12] Due to its favorable safety profile, VDZ is now often given as a first-line therapy.

While there is less concern for systemic response or immunosuppression given the gut selectivity of the medication, infections, specifically nasal/mucosal infections and upper respiratory infections, can occur. Data from randomized controlled trials showed a numerical increase in the number of upper and lower respiratory tract infections but no statistical significance in either when compared to placebo.[13] A meta-analysis of 46 studies of real-world experience with VDZ reported that the most common adverse effects were upper respiratory infections, including nasopharyngitis (1% to 21%), arthralgia (< 1% to 20%), *Clostridioides difficile* infection (< 1% to 20%), and fatigue (1% to 19%), but there was no placebo comparison group.[14]

Positioning of Biologics

VDZ may be prescribed as a first-line biologic or after failure of a TNF antagonist in patients with CD or UC.[15] The VARSITY trial, a phase 3b, randomized, double-blind, double-dummy, active-controlled superiority trial, evaluated outcomes among patients with UC who received either VDZ or adalimumab (ADA). Results showed that at week 52, patients who were treated with VDZ were more like to be in clinical remission (31.3% VDZ vs 22.5% ADA; $P = .006$) and show endoscopic improvement (39.7% VDZ vs 27.7% ADA; $P < .001$).[15] Corticosteroid-free clinical remission was observed in 12.6% of the VDZ group and 21.8% of patients who received ADA, but the difference was not statistically significant. This paper suggests that among patients with UC, VDZ should be considered as first-line therapy and prior to treatment with ADA.

Vedolizumab and Surgery

Two meta-analyses reported no statistically significant differences in postoperative complications with VDZ use when compared to patients exposed to anti-TNF medications and to those with no preoperative biologic exposure.[16,17] No difference was seen regarding overall complications, infectious complications, surgical site infections, or need for repeat surgery. However, there are limited data regarding postoperative outcomes after exposure to VDZ, and additional studies are recommended.

Use of Vedolizumab in Pregnancy and Breastfeeding

VDZ has not been shown to be associated with increased risk of adverse birth outcomes, and current guidelines recommend that it be continued throughout pregnancy.[18] Recommendations advise that the final pregnancy infusion occur 6 to 10 weeks prior to estimated delivery date if dosed every 8 weeks and 4 to 5 weeks prior to estimated delivery date if dosed every 4 weeks.[18] Infusions can resume 24 hours after a vaginal delivery and 48 hours after cesarean delivery if there is no evidence of infection.[18] VDZ may be administered while a mother is breastfeeding as negligible levels are seen in breast milk.

Dosing of Vedolizumab

Dosing of VDZ includes 3 loading doses of 300 mg intravenously at 0, 2, and 6 weeks, followed by 300 mg intravenously every 8 weeks for maintenance. Similar to other biologics, the timing of maintenance dosing may be altered based on a patient's symptoms and metabolism of the medication. In clinical practice, VDZ is sometimes administered every 4 weeks.[8] Patients and prescribing clinicians should be aware that the time to clinical effect of VDZ may be longer than with anti-TNF agents, and patients may not see a clinical improvement until 10 to 14 weeks after initiation of the medication. One meta-analysis reported rates of clinical remission among patients with UC and CD. At weeks 6, 14, 30, and 54, clinical remission among patients with UC was achieved in 24% (95% CI, 13% to 41%), 32% (95% CI, 27% to 39%), 39% (95% CI, 30% to 48%), and 46% (95% CI, 37% to 56%), respectively; among patients with CD, clinical remission was achieved in 24% (95% CI, 20% to 27%), 30% (95% CI, 25% to 34%), 26% (95% CI, 19% to 35%), and 30% (95% CI, 20% to 42%), respectively.[14] VDZ may be used in combination with an immunomodulator or methotrexate.[19] Combination therapy reduces rated of antibody formation.[19]

In practice, VDZ trough levels often result in change in clinical management, though studies have not consistently shown a relationship between trough levels and mucosal healing.[20] Prospective studies monitoring VDZ levels demonstrate correlation of higher levels during induction with better responses to VDZ, but there are no current recommended target levels during maintenance therapy.[21] One small study suggested a level of 25 µg/mL for histological healing, though a larger study of 693 patients showed potential target VDZ concentrations to be 37.1, 18.4, and 12.7 at weeks 6, 14, and steady state, respectively.[21,22] The earliest time at which levels were associated with clinical remission at weeks 14 and 52 was at week 6.[21]

Special Considerations for Vedolizumab

While the anatomic location of disease is important to consider when choosing medical therapy for CD, VDZ is effective throughout the gastrointestinal tract and does not specifically target one region. Failure of at least one anti-TNF medication is no longer necessary prior to initiation of VDZ, and VDZ should be strongly considered over ADA among patients with UC.[15]

Given its preferable safety profile and gut selectivity, there is a strong rationale for starting VDZ as the first biologic with the following strategies:

- Patient population and type of disease: In both clinical trials and studies evaluating response in clinical practice, patients with UC treated with VDZ have been shown to have higher rates of remission than patients with CD.[8] Thus, while VDZ is effective in both CD and UC, it may be recommended more frequently as the first biologic among patients with UC as compared to CD. It could, however, be considered for first-line use in patients with either CD or UC. In addition, a prediction model for achieving corticosteroid-free remission with VDZ among patients with UC-identified 4 factors is associated with steroid-free remission, including absence of previous TNF exposure, moderate to severe baseline endoscopic activity, higher baseline albumin, and 2 years or more of disease duration.[23] Factors identified to predict decreased efficacy of VDZ included prior anti-TNF exposure and severe disease.[23]

- Fistulizing CD: Although there are few controlled studies evaluating outcomes, data support that anti-TNF medications are effective for closure of perianal fistulas. The most robust data are with infliximab in which prospective, randomized controlled trials demonstrate efficacy for induction and maintenance of fistula closure. While post hoc analysis has suggested that VDZ may be effective at fistula treatment and closure, no clinical trials are confirmatory. As a result, anti-TNF medications are often recommended before VDZ for treatment of patients with fistulizing CD.

- History of malignancy: A patient's medical history, with particular attention to history of cancer, should be considered when choosing biologic therapy for patients with IBD. VDZ should be considered as a first-line biologic for patients with a history of lymphoma or melanoma. In addition, preference may be given to initiation of VDZ among patients with a history of solid organ tumors. While treatment of IBD should be discussed with the patient's oncologist, VDZ may be a safer option for patients who are at high risk for relapse.

- Patient's age: Patients greater than 65 years of age may be at increased risk of infection and/or malignancy with anti-TNF therapy due to age alone. VDZ is gut selective and therefore less frequently associated with serious systemic infections. VDZ may be preferred among older patients, those with a history of malignancy, and those with increased susceptibility to infection.

- Comorbidities: Anti-TNF medications are contraindicated among patients with heart failure. To date, VDZ has not been shown to exacerbate congestive heart failure and is the recommended biologic among this population.

Conclusion

VDZ is a selective anti-integrin biologic therapy for treatment of moderate to severe CD and UC. VDZ should be considered for first-line biologic use among patients with IBD and in particular considered for use before ADA among patients with UC. A patient's disease phenotype, age, and comorbidities should be considered when recommending biologic therapy for CD and UC, and VDZ may be especially useful in older patients, patients with multiple comorbidities, and patients with a history of cancer. Prediction models may assist in identification of patients more likely to respond to VDZ. Etrolizumab is currently undergoing phase 3 trials, and data regarding its safety and efficacy are pending.

References

1. Zundler S, Becker E, Schulze LL, et al. Immune cell trafficking and retention in inflammatory bowel disease: mechanistic insights and therapeutic advances. *Gut*. 2019;68(9):1688-1700.
2. Colombel JF, Sands BE, Rutgeerts P, et al. The safety of vedolizumab for ulcerative colitis and Crohn's disease. *Gut*. 2017;66(5):839-851.
3. Card T, Xu J, Liang H, Bhayat F. What is the risk of progressive multifocal leukoencephalopathy in patients with ulcerative colitis or Crohn's disease treated with vedolizumab? *Inflamm Bowel Dis*. 2018;24(5):953-959.
4. Sandborn WJA, Feagan BG, Rutgeerts P, et al. Vedolizumab as induction and maintenance therapy for Crohn's disease. *N Engl J Med*. 2013;369(8):711-721.
5. Feagan BG, Rutgeerts P, Sands BE, et al. Vedolizumab as induction and maintenance therapy for ulcerative colitis. *N Engl J Med*. 2013;369(8):699-710.
6. Sands BE, Sandborn WJ, Van Assche G, et al. Vedolizumab as induction and maintenance therapy for Crohn's disease in patients naïve to or who have failed tumor necrosis factor antagonist therapy. *Inflamm Bowel Dis*. 2017;23(1):97-106.
7. Sands BE, Feagan BG, Rutgeerts P, et al. Effects of vedolizumab induction therapy for patients with Crohn's disease in whom tumor necrosis factor antagonist treatment failed. *Gastroenterology*. 2014;147(3):618-627.
8. Loftus E V, Colombel J-F, Feagan BG, et al. Long-term efficacy of vedolizumab for ulcerative colitis. *J Crohns Colitis*. 2017;11(4):400-411.
9. Chaparro M, Garre A, Ricart E, et al. Short and long-term effectiveness and safety of vedolizumab in inflammatory bowel disease: results from the ENEIDA registry. *Aliment Pharmacol Ther*. 2018;48(8):839-851.
10. Vermeire S, Loftus E V, Colombel JF, et al. Long-term efficacy of vedolizumab for Crohn's disease. *J Crohns Colitis*. 2017;11(4):412-424.
11. Singh S, Fumery M, Sandborn WJ, Murad MH. Systematic review with network meta-analysis: first- and second-line pharmacotherapy for moderate-severe ulcerative colitis. *Aliment Pharmacol Ther*. 2018;48(4):394-409.
12. Bonovas S, Lytras T, Nikolopoulos G, Peyrin-Biroulet L, Danese S. Systematic review with network meta-analysis: comparative assessment of tofacitinib and biological therapies for moderate-to-severe ulcerative colitis. *Aliment Pharmacol Ther*. 2018;47(4):454-465.
13. Feagan BG, Bhayat F, Khalid M, Blake A, Travis SPL. Respiratory tract infections in patients with inflammatory bowel disease: safety analyses from vedolizumab clinical trials. *J Crohns Colitis*. 2018;12(8):905–919.
14. Schreiber S, Dignass A, Peyrin-Biroulet L, et al. Systematic review with meta-analysis: real-world effectiveness and safety of vedolizumab in patients with inflammatory bowel disease. *J Gastroenterol*. 2018;53(9):1048-1064.
15. Sands BE, Peyrin-Biroulet L, Loftus Jr EV, et al. Vedolizumab versus adalimumab for moderate-to-severe ulcerative colitis. *N Engl J Med*. 2019;381:1215-1226.
16. Yung DE, Horesh N, Lightner AL, et al. Systematic review and meta-analysis: vedolizumab and postoperative complications in inflammatory bowel disease. *Inflamm Bowel Dis*. 2018;24(11):2327-2338.
17. Law CCY, Narula A, Lightner AL, McKenna NP, Colombel JF, Narula N. Systematic review and meta-analysis: preoperative vedolizumab treatment and postoperative complications in patients with inflammatory bowel disease. *J Crohns Colitis*. 2018;12(5):538-545.
18. Mahadevan U, Robinson C, Bernasko N, et al. Inflammatory bowel disease (IBD) in pregnancy clinical care pathway—a report from the American Gastroenterological Association IBD Parenthood Project Working Group. *Gastroenterology*. 2019;156(5):1508-1524.
19. Lichtenstein GR, Loftus EV, Isaacs KL, Regueiro MD, Gerson LB, Sands BE. ACG clinical guideline: management of Crohn's disease in adults. *Am J Gastroenterol*. 2018;113(4):481-517.
20. Al-Bawardy B, Ramos G, Willrich M, et al. Vedolizumab drug level correlation with clinical remission, biomarker normalization, and mucosal healing in inflammatory bowel disease. *Inflamm Bowel Dis*. 2019;25(3):580-586.
21. Osterman M, Rosario M, Lasch K, et al. Vedolizumab exposure levels and clinical outcomes in ulcerative colitis: determining the potential for dose optimization. *Aliment Pharmacol Ther*. 2018;49(4):408-418.
22. Pouillon L, Rousseau H, Busby-Venner H, et al. Vedolizumab trough levels and histological healing during maintenance therapy in ulcerative colitis. *J Crohns Colitis*. 2019;13(8):970-975.
23. Dulai PS, Singh S, Casteele NV, et al. Development and validation of clinical scoring tool to predict outcomes of treatment with vedolizumab in patients with ulcerative colitis. *Clin Gastroenterol Hepatol*. 2020;18(3):2952-2961.

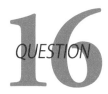

16

WHERE SHOULD ANTI–INTERLEUKIN 23 THERAPY BE PLACED IN THE THERAPEUTIC ALGORITHM FOR CROHN'S DISEASE AND ULCERATIVE COLITIS?

Joel Pekow, MD

Interleukin 23 in the Pathogenesis of IBD

Interleukin (IL) 23 is a cytokine that is produced by antigen-presenting cells, including dendritic cells and macrophages, and promotes an inflammatory signaling cascade.[1] This includes differentiation of CD4 positive T cells into T helper (Th) 17 cells, leading to release of the proinflammatory cytokines, tumor necrosis factor-α (TNF-α), IL-6, and IL-17A.[2] Likewise, IL-23 is essential for T-cell–mediated colitis in animal models.[3] Further supporting a role of IL-23 in IBD pathogenesis, several polymorphisms in the IL-23/IL-17 pathway are associated with inflammatory bowel disease (IBD).[4] In addition, IL-23 receptor transcript expression is upregulated in the tissue of patients with Crohn's disease (CD) and ulcerative colitis (UC), and IL-23 is increased in the serum of patients with UC.[5,6] Thus, there has been significant interest in developing IL-23 inhibitors for treating both CD and UC (Table 16-1).

Clinical Effectiveness of Therapies Targeting Interleukin 23 in Crohn's Disease

Ustekinumab is an immunoglobulin G1 monoclonal antibody that targets the p40 subunit common to both IL-12 and IL-23. Prior to its US Food and Drug Administration (FDA) approval for CD, randomized, placebo-controlled studies demonstrated the effectiveness of ustekinumab in the treatment of plaque psoriasis and psoriatic arthritis, leading to FDA approval of the drug

Rubin DT, Friedman S, Farraye FA, eds. *Curbside Consultation in IBD: 49 Clinical Questions, Third Edition* (pp 87-92).
© 2022 Taylor & Francis Group.

Table 16-1

Biologic Therapies Targeting IL-23 That Are Either FDA Approved or Currently in Clinical Trials for Crohn's Disease or Ulcerative Colitis

Molecule	Target	Approved Indications	Status in CD	Status in UC
Ustekinumab	P40 subunit of IL-12 and IL-23	Psoriatic arthritis, plaque psoriasis, Crohn's disease	FDA approved (2016)	FDA approved (2019)
Mirikizumab	IL-23p19 subunit	None	Phase 3	Phase 3
Risankizumab	IL-23p19 subunit	Plaque psoriasis	Phase 3	Phase 2/3
Brazikumab	IL-23p19 subunit	None	Phase 2b/3	Phase 2
Guselkumab	IL-23p19 subunit	Plaque psoriasis	Phase 2/3	Phase 2/3

for those indications.[7–9] Phase 2a and 2b trials in patients with CD did suggest a benefit.[10,11] Subsequently, 2 phase 3 trial randomized placebo-controlled trials were conducted in patients with moderate to severe CD examining induction treatment with 6 mg/kg intravenously (IV) vs 130 mg IV vs placebo. All patients in the trials were required to have objective evidence of active inflammation at baseline as defined as a C-reactive protein (CRP) > 3 mg/L, a fecal calprotectin > 250 mg/kg of body weight, or endoscopic ulcerations on ileocolonoscopy. The UNITI-1 trial included 741 patients who were primary or secondary nonresponders to anti-TNF antagonist therapy and UNITI-2 included 628 patients who failed conventional therapy. The primary end point, which was clinical response as defined by a Crohn's Disease Activity Index (CDAI) decrease > 100 or a CDAI score < 150 at week 6, was observed in 34.3%, 33.7%, and 21.5% in UNITI-1, and 51.7%, 55.5%, and 28.7% in UNITI-2 for treatment with 130 mg, 6 mg/kg, and placebo, respectively. Clinical remission at week 8 was observed for the 130 mg, 6 mg/kg, and placebo groups in 15.9%, 20.9%, and 7.3%, respectively, in UNITI-1 and 30.6%, 40.2%, and 19.6%, respectively, in UNITI-2. There were significant decreases in CRP and calprotectin during induction treatment in both ustekinumab-treated groups of patients. Responders to induction treatment from both induction trials were rerandomized to 90 mg subcutaneous dosing every 8 weeks, 90 mg every 12 weeks, or placebo for 44 weeks. Clinical response and remission were maintained in 59.4% and 53.1% of patients receiving ustekinumab every 8 weeks compared to 44.3% and 35.9% of patients treated with placebo.[12] Although endoscopic response was not an endpoint in the clinical trials, a subgroup analysis did demonstrate greater reductions in the simple endoscopic score in CD compared to baseline in patients treated with IV ustekinumab at 8 weeks compared to placebo.[13] Similarly, a separate subgroup analysis showed that histologic response occurred more frequently in patients receiving ustekinumab.[14]

Risankizumab, a humanized antibody targeting the p19 subunit of IL-23, was evaluated in a phase 2 randomized placebo control trial involving 121 patients with moderate to severe CD who had mucosal inflammation at baseline. The majority of patients in this study had been treated with and failed anti-TNF therapy. In this study, 31% of patients treated with risankizumab (pooled doses) compared to 15% who were treated with placebo (*P* = .0489) achieved clinical remission at week 12.[15] In an open-label extension study involving all patients who were not in deep remission at week 12, continued dosing with IV risankizumab increased the rates of clinical response and clinical remission at week 26.[16] Brazikumab, which similarly targets the p19 subunit of IL-23, was also evaluated in a phase 2a study in patients with moderate to severe CD who had failed TNF antagonists. In this study, patients were randomized to 700 mg IV at weeks 0 and 4 or placebo and then received open-label dosing with 210 mg subcutaneously every 4 weeks from week 12 to week 114; 49.2% of patients achieved either clinical response or remission compared to 26.7% of placebo-treated patients at week 8. When treated with open-label maintenance therapy, clinical response was seen in 53.8% and 57.7% of patients who received placebo and brazikumab, respectively, during the induction phase.[17]

Although not yet published, results of a phase 2 randomized placebo control dose ranging induction trial with mirikizumab were presented at Digestive Disease Week in 2019. This study demonstrated significantly greater endoscopic response, endoscopic remission, clinical response, and clinical remission after 12 weeks with both 600 mg and 1000 mg IV dosing given at weeks 0, 4, and 8.[18] Two other monoclonal antibodies directed against p19, guselkumab and brazikumab, are also being studied in CD, although results have not been published.

Clinical Effectiveness of Therapies Targeting Interleukin 23 in Ulcerative Colitis

A phase 3 randomized, placebo-controlled trial evaluating 8-week induction and 44-week maintenance therapy with ustekinumab in UC was published in 2018, leading to FDA approval the following year. In this study, 961 patients with moderate to severe UC were randomized to ustekinumab 130 mg IV, 6 mg/kg, or placebo for a single dose. At 8 weeks, significantly more patients treated with both ustekinumab doses (15.6% for 130 mg and 15.5% for 6 mg/kg) achieved clinical remission compared to placebo (5.3%). In addition, endoscopic healing occurred significantly more frequently in patients treated with ustekinumab at week 8, occurring in 26.3% of patients treated with 130 mg and 27% of patients treated with 6 mg/kg.[19] In this study, participants who achieved a clinical response at week 8 were randomized to placebo, 90 mg subcutaneous dosing every 8 weeks, or 90 mg subcutaneous dosing every 12 weeks. At week 44, 24%, 38.4%, and 43.8% of patients treated with placebo, 90 mg every 8 weeks, and 90 mg every 12 weeks, respectively, were in clinical remission. In addition, 51.1% of patients on ustekinumab (90 mg, 8 weeks) maintenance therapy achieved endoscopic improvement, defined as a Mayo endoscopy score of 0 or 1, compared to 28.6% of placebo-treated patients (*P* < .001).[19]

Results of a phase 2 study examining the p19 monoclonal antibody, mirikizumab, in UC were presented at Digestive Disease Week in 2018, although results have not been published. In this dose-ranging phase 2 study involving patients with moderate to severe UC, participants were treated with IV mirikizumab at weeks 0, 4, and 8. At 12 weeks, all doses were associated with a clinical response, whereas clinical remission was observed significantly more frequently only in the group receiving 200 mg. In addition, endoscopic improvement was observed significantly more frequently in patients receiving 50 mg and 200 mg of mirikizumab compared to placebo.[20] In this trial, patients who responded to mirikizumab at week 12 were then randomized to 200 mg given subcutaneously every 4 weeks or every 12 weeks; 46.8% of patients who received therapy every week for 4 weeks and 37% receiving treatment every week for 12 weeks were in clinical remission at week 52.[20] Although other selective IL-23 inhibitors are being investigated in large clinical trials, the results of these studies have not been published.

Areas of Uncertainty Regarding the Clinical Effectiveness of Interleukin 23 Blockade

There are several patient populations that have not been well studied to examine the clinical effectiveness of therapies targeting IL-23 signaling. These include the following:
- Perianal CD
- Postoperative prevention in patients with CD undergoing an ileocecectomy
- Upper gastrointestinal CD
- Severe UC

Safety of Therapies Targeting Interleukin 23

In the UNITI phase 3 trials, the rates of adverse events, serious adverse events, infections, and serious infections were similar in placebo and ustekinumab-treated patients[12]; 6.9% of individuals in the maintenance trial receiving therapy every 8 weeks, however, did report an injection site reaction. A recently published study examining long-term follow in patients in these trials receiving up to 96 weeks of treatment reported similar adverse events in ustekinumab vs placebo patients (484.39 events/100 patient years vs 447.76), serious adverse events (19.24 vs 18.82), and serious infections (4.09 vs 4.02). The number of treatment-emergent malignancies per hundred patient years of follow-up was 2.60 for placebo patients and 0.37 for ustekinumab patients.[21] Although immunogenicity is low for ustekinumab, a recent study showed that none of the patients who had anti-ustekinumab antibodies developed injection site reactions, serum sickness, or anaphylaxis.[22] Similarly, there were no major differences compared to placebo in the rate of adverse events, serious adverse events, or infections in phase 2 studies of risukizumab and brazikumab.[15] In an open-label follow-up study of risuzikumab with treatment up to 52 weeks, the most frequent reported adverse events were arthralgias (22%), headache (20%), abdominal pain (18%), nasopharyngitis (16%), nausea (16%), and pyrexia (13%).[16]

How to Position Anti–Interleukin 23 Therapies in Crohn's Disease and Ulcerative Colitis

As with other biologic agents, utilization of ustekinumab as a first-line treatment early in a patient's disease course results in higher rates of response than use in patients who previously failed biologic therapy. Unfortunately, there are no comparative effectiveness studies evaluating therapies targeting anti-IL-23 against other available treatments for either CD or UC. In addition, there is very limited understanding of clinical and biological predictors of response to therapy with any biologic agent for CD. Thus, weighing anti-IL-23 treatment against other therapeutic options should be based on several factors. These include a patient's disease phenotype, comorbidities, and cost of available options.

In patients who fail treatment with anti-TNF agents despite adequate therapeutic drug levels, treatment targeting an alternative pathway is recommended. Thus, anti-IL-23, anti-integrin therapy, or Janus kinase inhibition are attractive options in these individuals. Ustekinumab offers advantages over tofacitinib in terms of overall safety and over currently available anti-integrin therapy in its rapidity of onset and the fact that it can be given as a subcutaneous administration during maintenance dosing.

Given the effectiveness of these therapies in patients with plaque psoriasis and psoriatic arthritis and the superiority of anti-IL-23 therapy to anti-TNF agents[23-25] in plaque psoriasis, use of anti-IL-23 or IL-12/23 treatment should strongly be considered as a first-line agent in patients with both IBD and psoriasis or psoriatic arthritis. In addition, anti-IL-23 therapy should be considered first line in patients with CD with a contraindication to anti-TNF therapy, including those with multiple sclerosis. Given the favorable safety profile of ustekinumab and other IL-23 therapies in clinical trials, these therapies should also be considered in patients who at risk for infectious complications, including older patients.

There are other populations of patients where the efficacy of anti-IL-23 therapies has not been as well established. These include patients with perianal CD, treatment of CD postoperatively, patient's with inflammatory arthritis, and those hospitalized with severe UC. In these populations, there are data demonstrating the efficacy of anti-TNF inhibitors. As such, anti-TNF agents are recommended in these populations as a first-line treatment in patients without a contraindication, intolerance, or previous nonresponse until studies evaluating anti-IL-23 therapy in these populations are conducted in the future. A separate and important consideration is the understanding that joints do not express IL-23, and therefore inhibition of IL-23 is not effective for primary joint inflammation and may not be effective for the arthralgias associated with IBD or when there is inflammation of the joints associated with IBD. Further study in these types of patients is certainly needed.

Conclusion

Monoclonal antibodies targeting IL-23 are effective and safe in the treatment of CD and UC. There is a recent study in patients with plaque psoriasis demonstrating superiority of the IL-23 inhibitor, risankizumab, compared to ustekinumab.[26] Caution should be taken in extrapolating these results to CD; however, given differences in mechanisms of disease activity as a direct comparison between ustekinumab and anti-IL-23 therapy have not been performed to date in patients with IBD. As with other biologic therapies, use of ustekinumab, and likely other anti-IL-23 therapies, are more effective when used as a first-line biologic. As there are no comparative randomized controlled trials, positioning these treatments against other available therapies and considering skin and joint comorbidities in selection therapies is challenging and should be based on a patient's comorbidities, disease phenotype, and previous response as well as tolerance to other agents.

References

1. Furfaro F, Gilardi D, Allocca M, et al. IL-23 blockade for Crohn s disease: next generation of anti-cytokine therapy. *Expert Rev Clin Immunol.* 2017;13(5):457-467.
2. Aggarwal S, Ghilardi N, Xie MH, de Sauvage FJ, Gurney AL. Interleukin-23 promotes a distinct CD4 T cell activation state characterized by the production of interleukin-17. *J Biol Chem.* 2003;278(3):1910-1914.
3. Yen D, Cheung J, Scheerens H, et al. IL-23 is essential for T cell-mediated colitis and promotes inflammation via IL-17 and IL-6. *J Clin Invest.* 2006;116(5):1310-1316.
4. Kim SW, Kim ES, Moon CM, et al. Genetic polymorphisms of IL-23R and IL-17A and novel insights into their associations with inflammatory bowel disease. *Gut.* 2011;60(11):1527-1536.
5. Kobayashi T, Okamoto S, Hisamatsu T, et al. IL23 differentially regulates the Th1/Th17 balance in ulcerative colitis and Crohn's disease. *Gut.* 2008;57(12):1682-1689.
6. Mirsattari D, Seyyedmajidi M, Zojaji H, et al. The relation between the level of interleukin-23 with duration and severity of ulcerative colitis. *Gastroenterol Hepatol Bed Bench.* 2012;5(1):49-53.

7. Leonardi CL, Kimball AB, Papp KA, et al. Efficacy and safety of ustekinumab, a human interleukin-12/23 mono-clonal antibody, in patients with psoriasis: 76-week results from a randomized, double-blind, placebo-controlled trial (PHOENIX 1). *Lancet*. 2008;371(9625):1665-1674.

8. Papp KA, Langley RG, Lebwohl M, et al. Efficacy and safety of ustekinumab, a human interleukin-12/23 mono-clonal antibody, in patients with psoriasis: 52-week results from a randomized, double-blind, placebo-controlled trial (PHOENIX 2). *Lancet*. 2008;371(9625):1675-1684.

9. Gottlieb A, Menter A, Mendelsohn A, et al. Ustekinumab, a human interleukin 12/23 monoclonal antibody, for psoriatic arthritis: randomized, double-blind, placebo-controlled, crossover trial. *Lancet*. 2009;373(9664):633-640.

10. Sandborn WJ, Feagan BG, Fedorak RN, et al. A randomized trial of ustekinumab, a human interleukin-12/23 mono-clonal antibody, in patients with moderate-to-severe Crohn's disease. *Gastroenterology*. 2008;135(4):1130-1341.

11. Sandborn WJ, Gasink C, Gao LL, et al. Ustekinumab induction and maintenance therapy in refractory Crohn's disease. *N Engl J Med*. 2012;367(16):1519-1528.

12. Feagan BG, Sandborn WJ, Gasink C, et al. Ustekinumab as induction and maintenance therapy for Crohn's disease. *N Engl J Med*. 2016;375(20):1946-1960.

13. Rutgeerts P, Gasink C, Chan D, et al. Efficacy of ustekinumab for inducing endoscopic healing in patients with Crohn's disease. *Gastroenterology*. 2018;155(4):1045-1058.

14. Li K, Friedman JR, Chan D, et al. Effects of ustekinumab on histologic disease activity in patients with Crohn's disease. *Gastroenterology*. 2019;157(4):1019-1031.e7.

15. Feagan BG, Sandborn WJ, D'Haens G, et al. Induction therapy with the selective interleukin-23 inhibitor risanki-zumab in patients with moderate-to-severe Crohn's disease: a randomized, double-blind, placebo-controlled phase 2 study. *Lancet*. 2017;389(10080):1699-1709.

16. Feagan BG, Panes J, Ferrante M, et al. Risankizumab in patients with moderate to severe Crohn's disease: an open-label extension study. *Lancet Gastroenterol Hepatol*. 2018;3(10):671-680.

17. Sands BE, Chen J, Feagan BG, et al. Efficacy and safety of MEDI2070, an antibody against interleukin 23, in patients with moderate to severe Crohn's disease: a phase 2a study. *Gastroenterology*. 2017;153(1):77-86.e6.

18. Sands BE, Sandborn W, Peyrin-Biroulet L, et al. Efficacy and safety of mirikizumab (LY3074828) in a phase 2 study of patients with Crohn's disease. *Gastroenterology*. 2019;156(6):S2-216.

19. Sands BE, Sandborn WJ, Panaccione R, et al. Ustekinumab as induction and maintenance therapy for ulcerative colitis. *N Engl J Med*. 2019;381(13):1201-1214.

20. Sandborn WJ, Ferrante M, Bhandari BR, et al. Efficacy and safety of mirikizumab in a randomized phase 2 study of patients with ulcerative colitis. *Gastroenterology*. 2019;158(3):537-549.e10.

21. Sandborn WJ, Rutgeerts P, Gasink C, et al. Long-term efficacy and safety of ustekinumab for Crohn's disease through the second year of therapy. *Aliment Pharmacol Ther*. 2018;48(1):65-77.

22. Adedokun OJ, Xu Z, Gasink C, et al. Pharmacokinetics and exposure response relationships of ustekinumab in patients with Crohn's disease. *Gastroenterology*. 2018;154(6):1660-1671.

23. Griffiths CE, Strober BE, van de Kerkhof P, et al. Comparison of ustekinumab and etanercept for moderate-to-severe psoriasis. *N Engl J Med*. 2010;362(2):118-128.

24. Blauvelt A, Papp KA, Griffiths CE, et al. Efficacy and safety of guselkumab, an anti-interleukin-23 monoclonal anti-body, compared with adalimumab for the continuous treatment of patients with moderate to severe psoriasis: results from the phase III, double-blinded, placebo- and active comparator-controlled VOYAGE 1 trial. *J Am Acad Dermatol*. 2017;76(3):405-417.

25. Reich K, Papp KA, Blauvelt A, et al. Tildrakizumab versus placebo or etanercept for chronic plaque psoriasis (reSUR-FACE 1 and reSURFACE 2): results from two randomised controlled, phase 3 trials. *Lancet*. 2017;390(10091):276-288.

26. Papp KA, Blauvelt A, Bukhalo M, et al. Risankizumab versus ustekinumab for moderate-to-severe plaque psoriasis. *N Engl J Med*. 2017;376(16):1551-1560.

QUESTION 17

WHAT SHOULD CLINICIANS AND PATIENTS KNOW ABOUT BIOSIMILARS?

Ferdinando D'Amico, MD, PhD and Silvio Danese, MD, PhD

Ulcerative colitis (UC) and Crohn's disease (CD) are chronic and debilitating diseases, with a course characterized by alternating phases of remission and recurrence. The annual incidence of UC and CD in Europe ranges from 0.6 to 24.3 per 100,000 persons and from 0.3 to 12.7 per 100,000 persons, respectively.[1] The introduction of biologics has revolutionized the management and clinical course of patients with inflammatory bowel diseases (IBD). However, biologics have a very important economic impact on health care budgets, representing the main cost of the management of these patients, even overcoming hospitalization and surgery.[2]

In 2013 the patent of Remicade (infliximab) expired and Remsima and Inflectra (brand names of CT-P13) were the first infliximab biosimilars to be approved by the European Medicine Agency (EMA) for the treatment of IBD.[3,4] Subsequently 2 other molecules, such as SB2 (Flixabi) and PF-06438179/GP1111 (Zessly), have been approved by the EMA.[5,6]

Biosimilars are biological agents with a very complex production mechanism that uses living systems, including cells and tissue cultures. These molecules can vary according to the secondary, tertiary, and quaternary structure and also have different glycosylation patterns.[7] Biosimilars are drugs similar but not identical to the original product.[8] They differ from the concept of the "generic" drug, as generics are produced synthetically and are 100% reproducible.

The approval for the use of biosimilars of infliximab in IBD was pursued through the extrapolation of data from clinical studies on rheumatological diseases. A randomized, multicenter phase 1 trial (PLANETAS trial) on patients with ankylosing spondylitis and a randomized multicenter phase 3 trial (PLANETRA trial) on patients with rheumatoid arthritis showed that CT-P13 and its reference medicine (Remicade) were comparable in terms of clinical efficacy, adverse events, and immunogenicity.[9,10]

Rubin DT, Friedman S, Farraye FA, eds. *Curbside Consultation in IBD: 49 Clinical Questions, Third Edition* (pp 93-96).
© 2022 Taylor & Francis Group.

Extrapolation of data from rheumatological studies to IBD for the approval of biosimilars has raised some doubts, as patients with rheumatoid arthritis are treated with a lower dosage (3 mg/kg) of drug compared to that used in UC and CD (5 to 10 mg/kg). Furthermore, in the considered studies there was a concomitant use of immunosuppressants such as methotrexate, which may have masked efficacy data and reduced levels of anti-infliximab antibodies. Finally, another obstacle to the extrapolation mechanism is constituted by the inflammatory mechanisms underlying rheumatological diseases and chronic intestinal inflammatory diseases that cannot be overlapped, as demonstrated by the fact that some biological drugs are effective in rheumatology but not in UC and CD.[11-13]

Efficacy and Safety Data of Biosimilars in IBD

A prospective observational multicenter study evaluated efficacy and safety of CT-P13 in the setting of IBD, including patients naive to anti–tumor necrosis factor (TNF), previously treated with anti-TNF, and those switched from infliximab. The study included 547 patients (313 CD and 234 UC), of whom 311 had never been treated with anti-TNF, 139 had already been exposed to an anti-TNF, and 97 were switched from infliximab to biosimilar.

CT-P13 showed a high clinical response rate, while the occurrence of adverse events was in line with data reported with infliximab. However, analyzing by subgroups, severe adverse events occurred more frequently in patients already treated with anti-TNF or switched from infliximab compared to anti-TNF naive patients (22.3% and 12.4% vs 7.4%, respectively).[14]

A systematic review and meta-analysis assessed the efficacy and safety of CT-P13 in patients with IBD. Eleven observational studies were evaluated, including 829 patients with UC and CD. The analysis showed that the biosimilar was effective in determining the clinical response in the short (8 to 14 weeks) and medium term (24 to 30 weeks) in a high percentage of patients (79% and 75% in CD and 74% and 83% in UC, respectively), with low rates of overall adverse events (7% in CD, 8% in UC). Furthermore, patients who switched from the originator to CT-P13 had similar data on the efficacy in maintaining the clinical response.[15]

Interchangeability and Switching

Interchangeability is the possibility that the reference product can be replaced with the biosimilar product, demonstrating that both products have the same total content of drug substance and produce the same clinical results.[16]

A phase 4 multicenter Norwegian randomized study (NOR-SWITCH trial) evaluated the noninferiority of the biosimilar CT-P13 compared to the originator drug (Remicade) with regard to efficacy, safety, and immunogenicity. Four hundred eight patients with CD, UC, spondyloarthritis, rheumatoid arthritis, psoriatic arthritis, and chronic plaque psoriasis, treated with Remicade for at least 6 months, were included in the study. Patients were randomized in a 1:1 ratio to continue the infliximab originator or switch to a CT-P13 treatment. The primary endpoint was disease worsening during 52-week follow-up, considering a 30% disease worsening in each group and a noninferiority margin of 15%. Disease worsening occurred in 53 (26%) patients in the infliximab originator group and 61 (30%) patients in the CT-P13 group, confirming that CT-P13 is not inferior to the infliximab originator. Moreover, the rate of overall adverse events and the incidence of antidrug antibodies were similar between the 2 study groups (70% vs 68% and 7% vs 8% for infliximab originator and CT-P13, respectively).[17]

The efficacy and safety of infliximab biosimilar were confirmed in a 26-week open-label extension study of the NOR-SWITCH trial. In this extension study 363 patients were enrolled and divided into 2 groups: 190 patients treated with biosimilar in the main study continued treatment for further 26 weeks (maintenance group), while 173 patients treated with infliximab switched to biosimilar at week 52 (switch group). Disease worsening occurred in 32 (16.8%) patients in the maintenance group and in 20 (11.6%) patients in the switch group. No significant differences were reported in terms of adverse events or immunogenicity.[18]

Discussion

The introduction of biosimilars in the treatment of IBD, offering the prospect of a significant cost saving in health care, is a particularly hot and attractive topic. A Dutch stochastic economic model has evaluated the impact of the infliximab biosimilars on IBD-related health care costs.[19] According to this analysis, the use of biosimilars over the course of 5 years could lead to a reduction in 28% of total health care costs in The Netherlands, for a total saving of about 493 million euros.

If cost savings represent the main advantage of the use of biosimilars, the greatest doubts concern the immunogenicity, efficacy, and safety profile of these drugs, lacking long-term data. Moreover, it is essential to provide adequate and comprehensive information to patients who are faced with unclear terminologies, such as biosimilars, extrapolation, interchangeability, and switching. The decision to start a biological treatment with a biosimilar or switch from a reference drug to a biosimilar should be shared with the patient, whose preference should play a key role in the therapeutic choice.[20,21]

Furthermore, in 2018 the adalimumab (Humira) patent expired, and currently there are several biosimilars of adalimumab that have been approved and licensed by the EMA (ABP501, BI 695501, GP2017, FKB327, and SB5).[22] Clinical studies on rheumatoid arthritis and psoriasis have shown that these molecules have efficacy, safety, and immunogenicity comparable to that of the reference product and will soon be available for use. According to an European Crohn's and Colitis Organisation position statement on the use of biosimilars for IBD, biosimilarity must be verified in vitro, rather than in clinical studies, documenting the pharmacokinetic and pharmacodynamic equivalence.[20]

The next challenges for clinicians will concern the choice of a biosimilar rather than another; the possibility of performing a cross-switch, passing from one biosimilar to the other; or a reverse switch, exchanging from a biosimilar to the originator drug.

Conclusion

Biosimilars are effective and safe drugs, with an immunogenic profile comparable to that of the originator drug. The use of biosimilars will significantly reduce the health care costs, increasing the available resources and allowing the treatment of a larger number of patients. Nevertheless, further post-marketing studies have to confirm their safety profile, and randomized prospective studies are needed to clarify the role of biosimilars' interchangeability and switching with the originator drug or with other biosimilars.

References

1. Ananthakrishnan AN. Epidemiology and risk factors for IBD. *Nat Rev Gastroenterol Hepatol.* 2015 Apr;12(4):205-217.
2. van der Valk ME, Mangen MJ, Leenders M, et al. Healthcare costs of inflammatory bowel disease have shifted from hospitalization and surgery towards anti-TNFα therapy: results from the COIN study. *Gut.* 2014 Jan;63(1):72-79.
3. European Medicines Agency. *CHMP Assessment Report Remsima.* London, UK: EMA, 2013.

4. Inflectra assessment report. European Medicines Agency, 2013. http://www.ema.europa.eu/docs/en_GB/document_library/EPAR_-_Public_assessment_report/human/002778/WC500151490.pdf

5. Flixabi, European Medicines Agency, 2016. https://www.ema.europa.eu/medicines/human/EPAR/flixabi

6. Zessly. European Medicines Agency, 2018. https://www.ema.europa.eu/en/medicines/human/EPAR/zessly

7. Schiestl M, Stangler T, Torella C, Cepeljnik T, Toll H, Grau R. Acceptable changes in quality attributes of glycosylated biopharmaceuticals. *Nat Biotechnol*. 2011;29(4):310-312.

8. World Health Organization. *Expert Committee on Biological Standardization: Guidelines on Evaluation of Similar Biotherapeutic Products*. 2009. World Health Organization.

9. Park W, Hrycaj P, Jeka S, et al. A randomized, double-blind, multicenter, parallel-group, prospective study comparing the pharmacokinetics, safety, and efficacy of CT-P13 and innovator infliximab in patients with ankylosing spondylitis: the PLANETAS study. *Ann Rheum Dis*. 2013;72(10):1605-1612.

10. Yoo DH, Hrycaj P, Miranda P, et al. A randomized, double-blind, parallel-group study to demonstrate equivalence in efficacy and safety of CT-P13 compared with innovator infliximab when coadministered with methotrexate in patients with active rheumatoid arthritis: the PLANETRA study. *Ann Rheum Dis*. 2013;72(10):1613-1620.

11. Mertens M, Singh JA. Anakinra for rheumatoid arthritis: a systematic review. *J Rheumatol*. 2009;36(6):1118-1125.

12. Keating GM. Abatacept: a review of its use in the management of rheumatoid arthritis. *Drugs*. 2013;73(10):1095-1119.

13. Mok CC. Rituximab for the treatment of rheumatoid arthritis: an update. *Drug Des Devel Ther*. 2014;8:87-100.

14. Fiorino G, Manetti N, Armuzzi A, et al. The PROSIT-BIO cohort: A prospective observational study of patients with inflammatory bowel disease treated with infliximab biosimilar. *Inflamm Bowel Dis*. 2017;23(2):233-243.

15. Komaki Y, Yamada A, Komaki F, Micic D, Ido A, Sakuraba A. Systematic review with meta-analysis: the efficacy and safety of CT-P13, a biosimilar of anti-tumor necrosis factor-α agent (infliximab), in inflammatory bowel diseases. *Aliment Pharmacol Ther*. 2017;45(8):1043-1057.

16. Biosimilars: additional questions and answers regarding implementation of the Biologics Price Competition and Innovation Act of 2009: guidance for industry. FDA. http://www.federalregister.gov/documents/2015/05/13/2015-11528/biosimilars-additional-questions-and-answers-regarding-implementation-of-the-biologics-price

17. Jørgensen KK, Olsen IC, Goll GL, et al. Switching from originator infliximab to biosimilar CT-P13 compared with maintained treatment with originator infliximab (NOR-SWITCH): a 52-week, randomized, double-blind, non-inferiority trial. *Lancet*. 2017;389(10086):2304-2316.

18. Goll GL, Jørgensen KK, Sexton J, et al. Long-term efficacy and safety of biosimilar infliximab (CT-P13) after switching from originator infliximab: open-label extension of the NOR-SWITCH trial. *J Intern Med*. 2019;285(6):653-669.

19. Severs M, Oldenburg B, van Bodegraven AA, Siersema PD, Mangen MJ. Initiative of Crohn's and Colitis. The economic impact of the introduction of biosimilars in inflammatory bowel disease. *J Crohns Colitis*. 2017;11(3):289-296.

20. Danese S, Fiorino G, Raine T, et al. ECCO position statement on the use of biosimilars for inflammatory bowel disease: an update. *J Crohns Colitis*. 2017;11(1):26-34.

21. Fiorino G, Caprioli F, Daperno M, et al. Use of biosimilars in inflammatory bowel disease: a position update of the Italian Group for the Study of Inflammatory Bowel Disease (IG-IBD). *Dig Liver Dis*. 2019;51(5): P632-639.

22. Fiorino G, Gilardi D, Correale C, et al. Biosimilars of adalimumab: the upcoming challenge in IBD. *Expert Opin Biol Ther*. 2019;19(10).

WHAT ARE JANUS KINASE INHIBITORS AND WHEN SHOULD THEY BE USED IN IBD?

Roni Weisshof, MD and David T. Rubin, MD

There are limitations to the therapeutic armamentarium in inflammatory bowel disease (IBD) that include large rates of primary and secondary nonresponse rates and additional safety and tolerability issues. Although monoclonal antibody therapy has been revolutionary in IBD, there are challenges to their use. Specifically, antibodies against tumor necrosis factor-α (anti-TNF-α) have improved our ability to achieve a significant and longstanding remission and potentially influence the course of IBD. However, approximately 30% of patients are primarily nonresponsive to anti-TNF, and about one-third lose their response to the drug. Patients who fail anti-TNF are less likely response to other biologics (vedolizumab and ustekinumab) as well. The next major paradigm shift in IBD management is the multiple classes of small molecules. Small molecules, characterized by a size that enables oral delivery and absorption through the small intestinal mucosa, offer new mechanisms of action. As nonproteins, they also avoid issues of immunogenicity and of protein loss from an inflamed bowel, and therefore provide more predictable pharmacokinetic profiles. The first of these novel small molecules available in IBD are the Janus kinase inhibitors.

The Janus kinase/signal transducer and activator of transcription (JAK/STAT) is a major intracellular signaling pathway that mediates cytokine receptor activation. The JAK family includes 4 members: JAK1, JAK2, JAK3, and tyrosine kinase 2. Activation of a specific JAK by certain receptors activates 2 specific STATs and initiates the required inflammatory responses. Several inflammatory cytokines play a role in IBD pathogenesis via the JAK pathway, including interleukin (IL) 12, IL-23, IL-6, and TNF-α.[1] The first JAK inhibitor approved for treating IBD, tofacitinib, is a pan-JAK inhibitor. However, in cellular assays, it inhibits mostly the activity of JAK1 and JAK3 over JAK2, which may explain the decreased hemoglobin concentration in a minority of patients in the clinical trials.[2]

Rubin DT, Friedman S, Farraye FA, eds. *Curbside Consultation in IBD: 49 Clinical Questions, Third Edition* (pp 97-101).
© 2022 Taylor & Francis Group.

Tofacitinib was approved by the US Food and Drug Administration (FDA) on May 30, 2018, for the indication of moderately to severely active ulcerative colitis (UC).[3]

Two phase 3 induction studies, OCTAVE (Omapatrilat Cardiovascular Treatment Assessment vs Enalapril) 1 and 2, and one maintenance study, OCTAVE Sustain, were multicenter, randomized, double-blind, placebo-controlled clinical trials that evaluated tofacitinib as a treatment for adult patients with moderately to severely active UC.[4] At week 8, patients receiving tofacitinib 10 mg twice daily achieved significantly higher rates of remission, mucosal healing, and clinical response compared with placebo. Tofacitinib was the first drug to show similar efficacy in both anti-TNF-treated and anti-TNF-naive patients. However, 2 phase 2b studies failed to demonstrate clinical efficacy of tofacitinib for moderate to severe Crohn's disease.[5]

Overall, there was no difference in the rate of adverse events between treatment group and placebo in both induction and maintenance trials (including serious adverse events). However, the rates of overall infections and serious infections were higher with tofacitinib compared to placebo. Specifically, herpes zoster infection occurred in 5.1% of the patients treated with 10 mg twice daily (compared with 0.5% in the placebo group). The risk of zoster increases after the first 8 weeks and for those patients who were on the higher dose. Other infectious risks were found in large cohort studies of patients with rheumatoid arthritis, including a small increased risk for pneumonia and urinary tract infections.[6]

Dose-related increases in low-density lipoprotein (LDL) cholesterol and high-density lipoprotein (HDL) levels have been observed in tofacitinib studies performed in patients with IBD, which resolve after drug cessation. However, no increase in cardiovascular morbidity has been seen (on the basis of clinical data from more than 6000 patients, which included more than 20,000 patient years of tofacitinib exposure).[6] In fact, tofacitinib decreased carotid atherosclerosis in patients with rheumatoid arthritis, suggesting that the anti-inflammatory effects may work for atherosclerosis. Some studies also suggest that despite the increase in cholesterol level, there is no significant change in the number of small, dense LDL particles, which are considered more atherogenic than both large particles and oxidized LDL.[7] As a consequence of JAK2 inhibition, tofacitinib has the potential to cause bone marrow suppression. In the phase 3 rheumatoid arthritis clinical trials, neutrophil counts decreased modestly, but hemoglobin concentrations did not change significantly. In the OCTAVE program, there were 4 patients with UC who had thromboembolic (venous thromboembolism [VTE]) complications, all of whom were exposed to tofacitinib 10 mg during the extension phase.[8] Of note, all these patients who developed events had at least one risk factor for VTE, and none were adjudicated as being drug related.

As a small molecule, tofacitinib is likely to cross the placental barrier. Available data with drug use in pregnant women are insufficient to establish an associated risk of major birth defects, miscarriage, or adverse maternal or fetal outcomes. Based on the limited data available, exposure to tofacitinib in UC studies results in similar pregnancy result to the general population. In animal studies, teratogenic effects and fetus death were noted when pregnant rats and rabbits received tofacitinib.

Venous Thromboembolism and Label Changes

More recently, in a phase 4 safety study of tofacitinib in patients with rheumatoid arthritis over age 50 and with preexisting cardiovascular disease, an interim analysis found that patients receiving 10 mg twice daily had significantly higher rates of pulmonary embolism and mortality than those receiving 5 mg twice daily or anti-TNF therapy. Therefore, the FDA issued a boxed warning about increased risk of blood clots and death for the 10 mg twice daily dose of tofacitinib[9,10] and advised use of tofacitinib in patients who have failed anti-TNF therapy. They also encouraged screening for VTE risk and use of the lower dose when possible. The European Medicines Agency's (EMA) safety committee advised against prescribing this dose in patients who are at high risk, including patients with heart failure, cancer, inherited blood clotting disorders or a history of blood clots, as well as patients who take combined hormonal contraceptives, are receiving hormone replacement therapy, or are undergoing major surgery.[11] Severe UC was not part of the EMA contraindications. It is noteworthy that in the real-world experiences of tofacitinib in UC, there have been no reports of drug-related thromboembolic complications. This paradox is striking, given that active colitis is a risk for thrombosis, so if tofacitinib was a pro-thrombotic molecule, it would be expected to have seen multiple cases of VTE by now.

When and How to Use Tofacitinib

Tofacitinib is given for induction of remission at a dose of 10 mg twice daily for at least 8 weeks. If no response is achieved by 16 weeks of treatment, the drug should be stopped. For maintenance, the dose should be reduced to 5 mg twice daily, considering it is still effective. Otherwise, 10 mg twice daily should be continued. Patients who have a relapse after dose reduction can have their dose increased back to 10 mg twice daily. Due to the tofacitinib's distinctive character, being a small molecule over a biologic (protein-based drug), it can also be given in an intermittent manner. Starting, stopping, and restarting the drug is a valid choice if the need arises. A phase 3 withdrawal/retreatment study showed tofacitinib retreatment was effective in patients with chronic plaque psoriasis.[12]

Tofacitinib's place in the treatment algorithm for patients with moderately to severely active UC is not yet established. In our practice we have positioned it after failure of anti-TNF or vedolizumab, and the label change requires exposure to anti-TNF in the United States prior to prescribing it, but there are compelling reasons to consider it earlier for some patients, such as those with low albumin, in whom there may be exposure issues when trying to use monoclonal antibodies. Due to the unique mechanism of action and the fact that it is equally as effective in biologic-experienced as in biologic-naive patients (as oppose other therapies), it is certainly highly relevant in patients who failed multiple treatment lines. Given the rapid clinical response to the drug (significant improvements in symptoms among patients treated with tofacitinib compared with placebo was found within 3 days in the phase 3 clinical trials[13]), and the lack of the risk of immunogenicity, it might be also be used intermittently for pulse therapy, although this has not been formally studied yet.

Laboratory Monitoring

Due to the association with increases in LDL and HDL, it is recommended to assess lipid profile after starting treatment with the drug. Maximum effects are generally observed within 6 weeks. Accordingly, we recommend a baseline lipid level before starting the drug and repeat it approximately 4 to 8 weeks following initiation. Most patients with UC in our experience have not required further management of their lipids. Monitoring of complete blood count is recommended at baseline, after 4 to 8 weeks of treatment, and every 3 months thereafter in order to evaluate for the rare potential of anemia, neutropenia, or lymphopenia.

Vaccination

Patients with IBD are recommended to have vaccinations against vaccine-preventable illnesses prior to treatment with immune suppression, and with tofacitinib this includes vaccination against herpes zoster. Shingrix is a new herpes zoster vaccine that does not contain live virus. It was approved by the FDA for prevention of herpes zoster in adults age 50 and older,

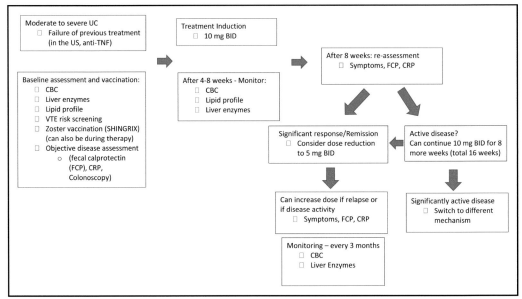

Figure 18-1. Proposed dosing and monitoring for treatment with tofacitinib in UC.

but also for "special populations" of patients who have chronic immune conditions. The vaccine contains a recombinant viral antigen (glycoprotein E) without live viral particles. It is given by 2 subcutaneous doses, 2 to 6 months apart. Data on efficacy appear promising in immunocompromised patients, despite no data specifically for patients with IBD. All patients with UC should be vaccinated prior to tofacitinib treatment. However, if needed, this vaccine can be given during treatment as well.

Screening for Venous Thromboembolism Risk

Considering the new safety data regarding VTE with tofacitinib, relevant comorbidities need to be assessed before starting tofacitinib. This should include screening for a personal and family history of clots, older age, obesity, smoking or immobilization, and prior miscarriages or other suspicions of underlying acquired or inherited clotting disorders. There are screening tools for VTE risk available online, such as the validated Caprini score, used for preoperative assessment.

Conclusion

Tofacitinib is a novel small molecule and effective for the treatment of moderately to severely active UC and has been a great addition to the armamentarium for UC. It has a unique mechanism, directing its inhibitory effect on multiple pivotal pathways in the inflammatory cascade implicated in the disease. Its efficacy has been proven in several large randomized controlled studies demonstrating rapid, significant, and sustained response in moderate to severe UC. Given the efficacy benefits of the drug, and its ease of use, one of the major factors that will eventually determine its position is the long-term safety profile. Although there have been recent label changes due to VTE events in older patients with rheumatoid arthritis, this has not been described in the UC population, so our prescribing and use has not been limited, but we do screen for risks of clots, lower the dose in maintenance when possible, and vaccinate for zoster (Figure 18-1).

References

1. Weisshof R, Golan MA, Yvellez OV, Rubin DT. The use of tofacitinib in the treatment of inflammatory bowel disease. *Immunotherapy*. 2018;10(10):837-849.
2. Meyer DM, Jesson MI, Li X, et al. Anti-inflammatory activity and neutrophil reductions mediated by the JAK1/JAK3 inhibitor, CP-690,550, in rat adjuvant-induced arthritis. *J Inflamm*. 2010;7:41.
3. FDA approves new treatment for moderately to severely active ulcerative colitis. FDA, May. 30, 2018. https://www.fda.gov/NewsEvents/Newsroom/PressAnnouncements/ucm609225.htm
4. Sandborn WJ, Su C, Sands BE, et al. Tofacitinib as induction and maintenance therapy for ulcerative colitis. *N Engl J Med*. 2017;376(18):1723-1736.
5. Panes J, Sandborn WJ, Schreiber, et al. Tofacitinib for induction and maintenance therapy of Crohn's disease: results of two phase IIb randomized placebo-controlled trials. *Gut*. 2017;66(6):1049-1059.
6. Cohen SB, Tanaka Y, Mariette X, et al. Long-term safety of tofacitinib for the treatment of rheumatoid arthritis up to 8.5 years: integrated analysis of data from the global clinical trials. *Ann Rheum Dis*. 2017;76(7):1253-1262.
7. Wolk R, Armstrong EJ, Hansen PR, et al. Effect of tofacitinib on lipid levels and lipid-related parameters in patients with moderate to severe psoriasis. *J Clin Lipidol*. 2017;11(5):1243-1256.
8. Sandborn WJ, Panes J, Sands BE, et al. Venous thromboembolic events in the tofacitinib ulcerative colitis clinical development program. *Aliment Pharmacol Ther*. 2019;50(10):1068-1076.
9. FDA approves boxed warning about increased risk of blood clots and death with higher dose of arthritis and ulcerative colitis medicine tofacitinib (Xeljanz, Xeljanz XR). FDA, 2019. https://www.fda.gov/drugs/drug-safety-and-availability/fda-approves-boxed-warning-about-increased-risk-blood-clots-and-death-higher-dose-arthritis-and
10. Increased risk of blood clots in lungs and death with higher dose of Xeljanz (tofacitinib) for rheumatoid arthritis. European Medicines Agency, March 20, 2019. https://www.ema.europa.eu/en/news/increased-risk-blood-clots-lungs-death-higher-dose-xeljanz-tofacitinib-rheumatoid-arthritis
11. Restrictions in use of Xeljanz while EMA reviews risk of blood clots in lungs. European Medicines Agency, May 17, 2019. https://www.ema.europa.eu/en/news/restrictions-use-xeljanz-while-ema-reviews-risk-blood-clots-lungs
12. Bissonnette R, Iversen L, Sofen H, et al. Tofacitinib withdrawal and retreatment in moderate-to-severe chronic plaque psoriasis: a randomized controlled trial. *Br J Dermatol*. 2015;172(5):1395-1406.
13. Hanauer S, Panaccione R, Danese S, et al. Tofacitinib induction therapy reduces symptoms within 3 days for patients with ulcerative colitis. *Clin Gastroenterol Hepatol*. 2019;17(1):139-147.

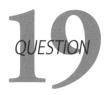

WHAT IS THE APPROACH FOR LOSS OF RESPONSE TO BIOLOGICAL THERAPY?

Konstantinos Papamichael, MD, PhD and Adam Cheifetz, MD

Secondary Loss of Response to Biological Therapy in IBD

Biological therapies are very effective for the treatment of moderate to severe inflammatory bowel disease (IBD).[1] Nevertheless, a significant proportion of patients with Crohn's disease (CD) and ulcerative colitis (UC) who had an initial clinical benefit lose response to biological therapies over time.[2] This secondary loss of response (SLR) can be defined as need for either drug optimization or discontinuation due to recurrent IBD. Most of the data regarding the incidence of SLR relate to anti–tumor necrosis factor (anti-TNF) therapies.

Based on randomized controlled trials and large observational cohort studies, SLR to anti-TNF therapy at 12 months occurs in up to 50% of patients, when defined as dose intensification, or in up to 15%, when assessed by drug discontinuation rates.[2] Defining SLR as the need for dose intensification, a systemic review of 16 infliximab studies[3] and a meta-analysis of 39 adalimumab studies[4] showed that the annual risk for SLR was 13% and 24% per patient year, respectively. Mechanisms of SLR include pharmacokinetic issues characterized by inadequate drug concentrations and often the development of anti-drug antibodies (ADA), so-called immunogenicity, or pharmacodynamic issues due to mechanistic drug failure.[3] Most SLR is due to low or undetectable drug concentrations.[5] Numerous data have shown that lower drug concentrations and ADA are associated with SLR.[6] A meta-analysis including 494 patients with CD showed that patients with antibodies to infliximab (ATI) had a risk ratio of 3.2 for SLR compared to patients without ATI.[7] Other predictors of SLR to anti-TNF therapy included male gender,[4] smoking,[4] increased body

Rubin DT, Friedman S, Farraye FA, eds. *Curbside Consultation in IBD: 49 Clinical Questions, Third Edition* (pp 103-107).
© 2022 Taylor & Francis Group.

mass index,[8] longer disease duration,[4] family history of IBD,[4] noninflammatory IBD phenotype,[9] lack of mucosal healing,[10] isolated colonic disease,[4] extraintestinal manifestations,[4] treatment with a previous anti-TNF agent,[4] increased fecal calprotectin,[11] and lack of C-reactive protein (CRP) normalization.[12]

Importantly, in order to truly diagnose SLR, physicians must first establish adherence of patients to medication and objectively document increased disease activity with biomarkers (fecal calprotectin, CRP) endoscopy, and/or imaging. Moreover, other potential reasons for abdominal pain and diarrhea, such as irritable bowel syndrome, infections, fibrostenotic strictures, bile-salt diarrhea, and small intestinal bacterial overgrowth, should be excluded.

Therapeutic Drug Monitoring and Secondary Loss of Response to Biological Therapies in IBD

Reactive therapeutic drug monitoring (TDM), defined as the assessment of biological drug concentrations and ADA in patients with clinical relapse, has rationalized the clinical management of SLR by determining the mechanism of SLR and allowing physicians to better direct care (Figure 19-1).[13-15] Additionally, it is more cost effective than empiric dose escalation.[16] Moreover, reactive TDM was also associated with higher post-adjustment clinical response and endoscopic remission and fewer hospitalizations compared to clinical decision making alone.[14]

Most of the patients with SLR to anti-TNF therapy have pharmacokinetic problems, and only in a small proportion of patients can this be attributed to pharmacodynamic issues and a mechanistic failure.[17] For patients with undetectable or low drug concentrations and no/low ADA we recommend increasing the drug dosage. Several studies have shown that a subsequent increase in drug concentrations after dose intensification for managing SLR was associated with regaining clinical response and achieving improved outcomes. In contrast, in patients who did not respond to dose intensification, drug concentrations were not elevated, and likely even more aggressive dose optimization was needed.[18,19] A post hoc analysis of a randomized clinical trial in CD regarding patients who failed infliximab and received an intensified regimen (5 mg/kg every 4 week) for 12 weeks with an increase in drug concentrations of ≥ 2.6 µg/mL was associated with regained clinical response.[19] Thus, we recommend following drug concentrations after dose optimization to ensure adequate drug concentrations are achieved.

On the other hand, those patients who have already developed high-titer ADA require a change in medication.[13] In patients who have developed high-titer ADA, we recommend switching within class prior to moving to an agent with a different mechanism of action. Additionally, the use of a concomitant immunomodulator (IMM) should be strongly considered as patients who develop ADA to one agent are more likely to develop ADA to subsequent medications.[20] In one study, ATI > 9.1 U/mL at time of LOR resulted in a likelihood ratio of 3:6 for an unsuccessful intervention implying that such high-titer ATI cannot be overcome.[21] A recent study of patients with IBD with ATI who underwent infliximab optimization to overcome immunogenicity showed that ATI titer ≥ 8.8 U/mL was associated with drug discontinuation due to SLR or serious adverse event.[22]

Patients who have adequate drug concentrations and ongoing disease activity are no longer responsive to that particular drug class and require switching to a therapy with a different mechanism of action. Yanai et al[13] showed that infliximab concentrations > 3.8 µg/mL and adalimumab concentrations > 4.5 µg/mL at time of SLR can distinguish patients who will benefit more from other therapies rather than drug optimization (dose increase, interval shortening, addition of an IMM) or switch to another anti-TNF therapy. Another prospective study showed that adalimumab trough concentrations > 4.9 µg/mL were associated with failure of 2 anti-TNF agents (adali-

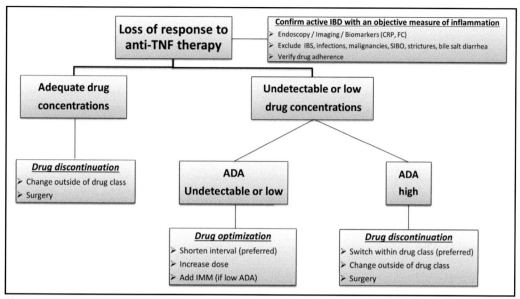

Figure 19-1. Proposed algorithm for reactive therapeutic drug monitoring of anti-TNF therapy in inflammatory bowel disease. (ADA = antidrug antibodies; CRP = C-reactive protein; FC = fecal calprotectin; IMM = immunomodulator; SIBO = small bowel bacterial overgrowth; TNF = tumor necrosis factor.)

mumab and infliximab) in 90% of cases, and in these cases switching to another drug class should be considered. However, in clinical practice we optimize patients to infliximab and adalimumab concentrations to > 10 µg/mL, as these numbers have been associated with better outcomes.[23]

Unfortunately, at the time of SLR, there is already a high percentage of patients who have developed high-titer ADA and require changing medications. Preliminary data suggest that proactive TDM, with drug titration to a target trough concentration, applied in patients with clinical response/remission, can prevent immunogenicity and SLR.[24-28] In fact, a retrospective study of proactive compared to reactive TDM of infliximab showed that proactive TDM was associated with greater drug durability, less need for IBD-related surgery or hospitalization, and lower risk of ATI or serious infusion reactions.[24] An earlier pilot observational study demonstrated that proactive TDM of infliximab compared to empiric dose escalation or reactive TDM was associated with increased drug retention.[25] Moreover, the landmark randomized controlled trial TAXIT (Trough Concentration Adapted Infliximab Treatment) showed that proactive TDM compared to clinically based dosing of infliximab was associated with a lower rate of undetectable drug concentrations and a lower risk of relapse.[26] Additionally, in patients with CD and subtherapeutic drug concentrations a one-time dose optimization improved clinical remission rates and CRP.[26] Recently, the PAILOT (Pediatric Crohn's Disease Adalimumab-Level-based Optimization Treatment) randomized controlled trial clearly demonstrated that steroid-free clinical remission at week 72 was higher in the proactive compared to the reactive TDM group (82% vs 46%; $P < .001$).[27] As such, our practice is to proactively dose to a therapeutic concentration. Moreover, proactive following reactive TDM of infliximab was associated with greater drug persistence and fewer IBD-related hospitalizations than reactive TDM alone.[28] Thus, if reactive TDM is necessary and dose optimization is feasible, we recommended following drug concentrations to confirm they are adequate.

Conclusion

SLR to biological therapies is a clinically significant problem affecting a substantial percentage of patients. Although we have several therapies in our armamentarium, we must still be aggressive with optimizing treatment strategies. Patients with IBD who fail one biological agent do not respond as well to subsequent agents, and available drugs are still limited. Though reactive TDM has been proven to be more cost effective and to better direct care than empiric dose escalation, proactive TDM may actually be able to prevent SLR to biological therapies. Nevertheless, there are still several barriers to the use of TDM in clinical practice, including the out-of-pocket cost, time lag from serum sampling to test results, and correct interpretation of the results, as clinically relevant drug thresholds may vary based on the assay used and the therapeutic outcome to target.

References

1. Miligkos M, Papamichael K, Vande Casteele N, et al. Efficacy and safety profile of anti-tumor necrosis factor-α versus anti-integrin agents for the treatment of Crohn's disease: a network meta-analysis of indirect comparisons. *Clin Ther.* 2016;38(6):1342-1358.e6.
2. Ben-Horin S, Chowers Y. Loss of response to anti-TNF treatments in Crohn's disease. *Aliment Pharmacol Ther.* 2011;33(9):987-95.
3. Gisbert JP, Panes J. Loss of response and requirement of infliximab dose intensification in Crohn's disease: a review. *Am J Gastroenterol.* 2009;104(3):760-767.
4. Billioud V, Sandborn WJ, Peyrin-Biroulet L. Loss of response and need for adalimumab dose intensification in Crohn's disease: a systematic review. *Am J Gastroenterol.* 2011;106(4):674-684.
5. Vermeire S, Dreesen E, Papamichael K, et al. How, when, and for whom should we perform therapeutic drug monitoring? *Clin Gastroenterol Hepatol.* 2020;18(6):1291-1299.
6. Fine S, Papamichael K, Cheifetz AS. Etiology and management of lack or loss of response to anti-tumor necrosis factor therapy in patients with inflammatory bowel disease. *Gastroenterol Hepatol.* 2019;15(12):656-665.
7. Nanda KS, Cheifetz AS, Moss AC. Impact of antibodies to infliximab on clinical outcomes and serum infliximab levels in patients with inflammatory bowel disease (IBD): a meta-analysis. *Am J Gastroenterol.* 2013;108(1):40-47.
8. Kurnool S, Nguyen NH, Proudfoot J, et al. High body mass index is associated with increased risk of treatment failure and surgery in biologic-treated patients with ulcerative colitis. *Aliment Pharmacol Ther.* 2018;47(11):1472-1479.
9. Sprakes MB, Ford AC, Warren L, Greer D, Hamlin J. Efficacy, tolerability, and predictors of response to infliximab therapy for Crohn's disease: a large single center experience. *J Crohns Colitis.* 2012;6(2):143-153
10. Baert F, Moortgat L, Van Assche G, et al. Mucosal healing predicts sustained clinical remission in patients with early-stage Crohn's disease. *Gastroenterology.* 2010;138(2):463-468.
11. Kallel L, Ayadi I, Matri S, et al. Fecal calprotectin is a predictive marker of relapse in Crohn's disease involving the colon: a prospective study. *Eur J Gastroenterol Hepatol.* 2010;22(3):340-345.
12. Hibi T, Sakuraba A, Watanabe M, et al. C-reactive protein is an indicator of serum infliximab level in predicting loss of response in patients with Crohn's disease. *J Gastroenterol.* 2014;49(2):254-262.
13. Yanai H, Lichtenstein L, Assa A, et al. Levels of drug and antidrug antibodies are associated with outcome of interventions after loss of response to infliximab or adalimumab. *Clin Gastroenterol Hepatol.* 2015;13(3):522-530.
14. Kelly OB, Donnell SO, Stempak JM, et al. Therapeutic drug monitoring to guide infliximab dose adjustment is associated with better endoscopic outcomes than clinical decision making alone in active inflammatory bowel disease. *Inflamm Bowel Dis.* 2017;23(7):1202-1209.
15. Guidi L, Pugliese D, Tonucci TP, et al. Therapeutic drug monitoring is more cost-effective than a clinically based approach in the management of loss of response to infliximab in inflammatory bowel disease: an observational multicenter study. *J Crohns Colitis.* 2018;12(9):1079-1088.
16. Steenholdt C, Brynskov J, Thomsen OØ, et al. Individualized therapy is more cost-effective than dose intensification in patients with Crohn's disease who lose response to anti-TNF treatment: a randomized, controlled trial. *Gut.* 2014;63(6):919-927.
17. Vande Casteele N, Herfarth H, Katz J, Falck-Ytter Y, Singh S. American Gastroenterological Association Institute technical review on the role of therapeutic drug monitoring in the management of inflammatory bowel diseases. *Gastroenterology.* 2017;153(3):835-837.
18. Hibi T, Sakuraba A, Watanabe M, et al. Retrieval of serum infliximab level by shortening the maintenance infusion interval is correlated with clinical efficacy in Crohn's disease. *Inflamm Bowel Dis.* 2012;18(8):1480-1487.

19. Steenholdt C, Bendtzen K, Brynskov J, et al. Changes in serum trough levels of infliximab during treatment intensification but not in anti-infliximab antibody detection are associated with clinical outcomes after therapeutic failure in Crohn's disease. *J Crohns Colitis.* 2015;9(3):238-245.

20. Frederiksen MT, Ainsworth MA, Brynskov J, et al. Antibodies against infliximab are associated with de novo development of antibodies to adalimumab and therapeutic failure in infliximab-to-adalimumab switchers with IBD. *Inflamm Bowel Dis.* 2014;20(10):1714-1721.

21. Vande Casteele N, Gils A, Singh S, et al. Antibody response to infliximab and its impact on pharmacokinetics can be transient. *Am J Gastroenterol.* 2013;108(6):962-971.

22. Papamichael K, Vajravelu RK, Osterman MT, et al. Long-term outcome of infliximab optimization for overcoming immunogenicity in patients with inflammatory bowel disease. *Dig Dis Sci.* 2018;63(3):761-767.

23. Papamichael K, Cheifetz AS, Melmed GY, et al. Appropriate therapeutic drug monitoring of biologic agents for patients with inflammatory bowel diseases. *Clin Gastroenterol Hepatol.* 2019;17(9):1655-1668.

24. Papamichael K, Chachu KA, Vajravelu RK, et al. Improved long-term outcomes of patients with inflammatory bowel disease receiving proactive compared with reactive monitoring of serum concentrations of infliximab. *Clin Gastroenterol Hepatol.* 2017;15(10):1580-1588.

25. Vaughn BP, Martinez-Vazquez M, Patwardhan VR, et al. Proactive therapeutic concentration monitoring of infliximab may improve outcomes for patients with inflammatory bowel disease: results from a pilot observational study. *Inflamm Bowel Dis.* 2014;20(11):1996-2003.

26. Vande Casteele N, Ferrante M, Van Assche G, et al. Trough concentrations of infliximab guide dosing for patients with inflammatory bowel disease. *Gastroenterology.* 2015;148(7):1320-1329.

27. Assa A, Matar M, Turner D, et al. Proactive monitoring of adalimumab trough concentration associated with increased clinical remission in children with Crohn's disease compared with reactive monitoring. *Gastroenterology.* 2019;157(4):985-996.

28. Papamichael K, Vajravelu RK, Vaughn BP, et al. Proactive infliximab monitoring following reactive testing is associated with better clinical outcomes than reactive testing alone in patients with inflammatory bowel disease. *J Crohns Colitis.* 2018;12(7):804-810.

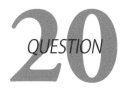

QUESTION

HOW SHOULD PROACTIVE THERAPEUTIC DRUG MONITORING BE CONSIDERED IN OUR PATIENTS?

Joseph D. Feuerstein, MD and William T. Clarke, MD, MSc

The biologic therapies have revolutionized the treatment of inflammatory bowel disease (IBD), including Crohn's disease (CD) and ulcerative colitis (UC). However, as many as 30% of patients on biologics are primary nonresponders, never achieving a true clinical benefit during induction or maintenance therapy.[1] Even in patients who have an initial response to biologics, secondary loss of response (SLR) remains a concern throughout the drug's maintenance phase. SLR to infliximab is estimated to be approximately 10% per year.[2] While these rates appear to be lower with the newer biologics, SLR remains a concern with all biologics. Biologic failure due to primary nonresponse or SLR results from low or absent serum drug concentrations.[3-5]

The concept of drug monitoring has been established in many drugs with narrow therapeutic windows (eg, tacrolimus) as well as those with significant toxicity (eg, lithium). Therapeutic drug monitoring (TDM) of biologic medications is the measurement of serum drug concentrations and antidrug antibodies to optimize biologic dosing and thereby improve IBD outcomes. However, the ideal timing of when this should be checked and how frequently it should be monitored remains unclear and is an area in need of additional research.

TDM can be used at any point in the induction or maintenance stages of biologic therapy. TDM is considered "reactive" when used in the setting of active IBD, while the term "proactive" is used when IBD is in remission and TDM is used to make sure that the drug concentration is at goal without antidrug antibodies.

Reactive TDM is widely recommended as an important tool to better understand the reason for biologic failure and guide the next steps in biologic management. Those failing biologics can be categorized as having mechanistic failure, non-immune-mediated pharmacokinetic failure, or

Rubin DT, Friedman S, Farraye FA, eds. *Curbside Consultation in IBD: 49 Clinical Questions, Third Edition* (pp 109-113).
© 2022 Taylor & Francis Group.

immune-mediated pharmacokinetic failure. Based on the TDM one can then determine the next treatment decision in a more clinically relevant manner.

While not supported by high-quality data, proactive TDM helps clinicians optimize biologic dosing and maintain adequate serum drug concentrations before patients develop non-immune-mediated pharmacokinetic failure as manifest by an IBD flare and drug failure.

Proactive drug monitoring can also help prevent formation of antidrug antibodies, which often develop in the setting of low or absent drug concentrations. Antidrug antibodies are associated with the development of immune-mediated pharmacokinetic failure. The presence of anti-infliximab antibodies was associated with a pooled risk ratio of 3.2 for loss of clinical response.[4] Patients with antidrug antibodies are also at higher risk for adverse events such as severe infusion reactions or hypersensitivity reactions.[6]

While it did not reach its primary endpoint, the TAXIT (Trough Concentration Adapted Infliximab Treatment) study showed that patients who did not receive proactive TDM had higher rates of antidrug antibodies and undetectable infliximab trough levels.[7] Importantly though, while not the primary outcome, the TAXIT study design performed TDM on all patients prior to randomization and optimized the drug concentration. In those patients who underwent an initial proactive TDM and successful drug optimization, there were higher rates of remission at the end of the study, suggesting that using proactive TDM to optimize drug concentrations may be beneficial.[6]

In a multicentered retrospective study comparing proactive TDM to reactive TDM in patients with IBD on infliximab, proactive TDM was associated with fewer IBD-related surgeries, fewer hospitalizations, longer duration on infliximab, lower risk of antibodies to infliximab, and fewer serious infusion reactions.[8] While the study was not a prospective randomized controlled trial, it fits with the intellectual rationale that knowing a drug concentration and antibodies to the drug allows clinicians to optimize their drug and prevent disease flares.

Two recent prospective studies of proactive TDM have demonstrated mixed results. In a randomized controlled trial, TAILORIX (a randomized controlled trial investigating Tailored Treatment With Infliximab for Active Luminal Crohn's Disease) demonstrated that increasing infliximab dosing based on a combination of symptoms, biomarkers, and proactive TDM was no better at maintaining corticosteroid-free remission than increasing infliximab dosing based on symptoms alone.[9] Meanwhile, the PAILOT (Pediatric Crohn's Disease Adalimumab Level-Based Optimization Treatment) trial in children with CD on adalimumab found that proactive TDM was superior to reactive TDM in maintaining corticosteroid-free remission.[10]

Societal guidelines differ in their recommendations for proactive TDM.[11,12] The recent American Gastroenterological Association (AGA) guidelines make no recommendation on proactive TDM based on limited evidence. The Australian consensus on TDM recommends proactive TDM after successful induction therapy in order to optimize biologic dosing and in patients in whom a drug break is contemplated. The Australian guidelines also state that TDM should be periodically considered in patients in clinical remission if the results are likely to impact clinical management.[8]

In our practice, we make the decision about proactive TDM on a case-by-case basis (Table 20-1). Unfortunately, financial considerations must always be made as many insurance companies will not cover routine TDM.[13] When discussing proactive TDM, we always counsel our patients about the possibility that TDM will result in an out-of-pocket expense; many patients are unable or unwilling to accept this possibility.

We consider proactive TDM in all patients following the completion of the induction phase to help guide subsequent dosing. Typically, this is checked as a week 14 level in infliximab and a week 6 level with adalimumab. Some advocate checking during induction; however, the goal trough level is less clear. Supporting the recommendation of early TDM, a study of patients starting adalimumab found that those with lower serum drug concentrations (< 8.3 μg/mL) at week 4

Table 20-1

Situations Where Therapeutic Drug Monitoring Is Most Likely to Be Beneficial

Following induction phase

More severely active IBD

Biologic used for induction without corticosteroids

Low albumin or malnutrition

High inflammatory markers (CRP, fecal calprotectin)

Previous immune-mediated pharmacokinetic failure

Extremes of body weight on non-weight-based biologics

Known low-serum drug concentrations

Low-level antidrug antibodies

Before and after discontinuing immunomodulator

of induction were more likely to develop antibodies by week 12 and more likely to have primary nonresponse or SLR.[14]

We especially encourage TDM in patients who are more likely to have low serum drug concentrations, such as those with more severe IBD, those in which corticosteroids were not used to induce remission, and those with low albumin or high inflammatory markers such as C-reactive protein or fecal calprotectin. In these patients, since the drugs are bound to albumin and excreted in the stool, it is not uncommon to inadvertently underdose these patients with biologics when routine standard dosing protocols are used.

Patients who have had immune-mediated pharmacokinetic failure to a prior biologic are likely to be at higher risk for failure of other biologics, so we recommend proactive TDM in this population at the end of the induction phase and episodically during the maintenance phase. How often it should be monitored during maintenance is unclear, but at least a yearly check seems reasonable to help prevent another drug failure.

In biologics with fixed, non-weight-based doses such as adalimumab, we encourage proactive TDM for those at the extremes of weight. Patients with obesity are likely to have higher risk of low serum drug concentrations and the most likely to benefit from proactive TDM to optimize the dosing regimen before a disease flare develops.

In patients with borderline low serum drug concentrations who opt against changing their biologic dose or interval, we recommend proactive TDM to ensure their serum drug concentrations do not continue to trend down to an unacceptably low level.

For patients on combination therapy with a biologic and an immunomodulator, we recommend TDM prior to discontinuing the immunomodulator. It is known that immunomodulators increase serum concentrations of biologics.[15] We recommend ensuring adequate biologic drug concentrations before the immunomodulator is discontinued, considering the expected drop in biologic drug concentration after immunomodulator discontinuation. In this cohort we also advocate for additional testing in the maintenance phase of the monotherapy with the biologic to make sure that the dose remains adequate even though the immunomodulator was discontinued.

Further complicating the use of TDM is the uncertainty as to what constitutes an adequate trough drug concentration.[9] Again, there are limited data, and there are no randomized controlled trials comparing different trough drug concentrations. It is also important to differentiate goal troughs in the setting of a flare and those for proactive induction and proactive maintenance time points. Patients with active inflammation and disease subtypes (eg, fistulizing CD) may require higher trough concentrations, and this should also be considered before labeling a patient as a nonresponder. Additionally, commercially available assays for trough drug concentrations have some variability, so we recommend using the same assay consistently when possible.[16]

We agree with AGA guidelines, which recommend maintenance phase trough concentrations of at least 5 µg/mL for infliximab, 7.5 µg/mL for adalimumab, and 20 µg/mL for certolizumab pegol. These concentrations are for patients in the maintenance phase of dosing and who do not have active inflammation. Patients with penetrating CD or those who are partial responders to anti–tumor necrosis factor may benefit from higher maintenance trough concentrations. At this time, there is only very early evidence to make any recommendations for goal trough drug concentrations for vedolizumab and ustekinumab, with larger studies needed.[17]

Arguments against proactive TDM include unclear target serum drug concentrations in patients in remission, the possibility for inappropriate medication changes while patients are in remission, and costs of TDM and any associated changes in treatment.

A further challenge associated with drug level and antibody testing is the lack of interassay standardization. While in theory the assays should show comparable specificity accuracy and reproducibility, in clinical practice this is not always seen. Commercial drug concentration tests appear to vary based on manufacturer and may be clinically important in certain situations of borderline drug levels. Importantly, there is no standardization for reporting of drug antibodies. While one assay may report high drug antibodies, another commercial assay may report low-level antibodies. This can make the decision surrounding the ability to overcome antibodies with higher drug doses and shorter intervals more challenging. Given these challenges, it is important to remain consistent and use the same assay, when possible.

Biologics have transformed the treatment of IBD, but their efficacy is limited by inadequate dosing. Knowledge of the drug concentration and the presence of drug antibodies is key to optimize the drug before the disease flares and one loses response to the drug. We consider proactive TDM in all patients, taking into account the situations where TDM is most likely to be beneficial or change management. Clinicians must acknowledge the overall lack of evidence and potential out-of-pocket costs associated with proactive TDM. Nevertheless, we believe proactive TDM is an important tool for improving our management of biologics by optimizing drug dosing, maintaining adequate serum drug concentrations, and reducing the formation of antidrug antibodies.

References

1. Roda G, Jharap B, Neeraj N, Colombel J-F. Loss of response to anti-TNFs: definition, epidemiology, and management. *Clin Transl Gastroenterology*. 2016;7(1):e135.
2. Gisbert JP, Panés J. Loss of response and requirement of infliximab dose intensification in Crohn's disease: a review. *Am J Gastroenterol*. 2009;104(3):760-767.
3. Seow CH, Newman A, Irwin SP, Steinhart AH, Silverberg MS, Greenberg GR. Trough serum infliximab: a predictive factor of clinical outcome for infliximab treatment in acute ulcerative colitis. *Gut*. 2010;59(1):49-54.
4. Nanda KS, Cheifetz AS, Moss AC. Impact of antibodies to infliximab on clinical outcomes and serum infliximab levels in patients with inflammatory bowel disease (IBD): a meta-analysis. *Am J Gastroenterol*. 2013;108(1):40-47; quiz 48.
5. Kennedy NA, Heap GA, Green HD, et al. Predictors of anti-TNF treatment failure in anti-TNF-naive patients with active luminal Crohn's disease: a prospective, multicenter, cohort study. *Lancet Gastroenterol Hepatol*. 2019;4(5):341-353.

6. O'Meara S, Nanda KS, Moss AC. Antibodies to infliximab and risk of infusion reactions in patients with inflammatory bowel disease: a systematic review and meta-analysis. *Inflamm Bowel Dis*. 2014;20(1):1-6.
7. Vande Casteele N, Ferrante M, Van Assche G, et al. Trough concentrations of infliximab guide dosing for patients with inflammatory bowel disease. *Gastroenterology*. 2015;148(7):1320-1329.e3.
8. Papamichael K, Chachu KA, Vajravelu RK, et al. Improved long-term outcomes of patients with inflammatory bowel disease receiving proactive compared with reactive monitoring of serum concentrations of infliximab. *Clin Gastroenterol Hepatol*. 2017;15(10):1580-1588.e3.
9. D'Haens G, Vermeire S, Lambrecht G, et al. Increasing infliximab dose based on symptoms, biomarkers, and serum drug concentrations does not increase clinical, endoscopic, and corticosteroid-free remission in patients with active luminal Crohn's disease. *Gastroenterology*. 2018;154(5):1343-1351.e1.
10. Assa A, Matar M, Turner D, et al. Proactive monitoring of adalimumab trough concentration associated with increased clinical remission in children with Crohn's disease compared with reactive monitoring. *Gastroenterology*. 2019;157(4):985-996.e2.
11. Mitrev N, Vande Casteele N, Seow CH, et al. Review article: consensus statements on therapeutic drug monitoring of anti-tumour necrosis factor therapy in inflammatory bowel diseases. *Aliment Pharmacol Ther*. 2017; 46(11-12):1037-1053.
12. Feuerstein JD, Nguyen GC, Kupfer SS, et al. American Gastroenterological Association Institute guideline on therapeutic drug monitoring in inflammatory bowel disease. *Gastroenterology*. 2017;153(3):827-834.
13. Yadav A, Vasquez P, Dolgin NH, Falchuk KR, Feuerstein JD. Variations in insurances policies regarding adherence to the AGA guideline for therapeutic drug monitoring in IBD. *J Clin Gastroenterol*. 2018;53(6):e239-e242.
14. Verstockt B, Moors G, Bian S, et al. Influence of early adalimumab serum levels on immunogenicity and long-term outcome of anti-TNF naive Crohn's disease patients: the usefulness of rapid testing. *Aliment Pharmacol Ther*. 2018;48(7):731-739.
15. Colombel JF, Adedokun OJ, Gasink C, et al. Higher levels of infliximab may alleviate the need of azathioprine comedication in the treatment of patients with Crohn's disease and Colitis Foundation disease: A Sonic post hoc analysis. *Gastroenterology*. 2017;152(5):S37-S38.
16. Bodini G, Giannini EG, Furnari M, et al. Comparison of two different techniques to assess adalimumab trough levels in patients with Crohn's disease. *J Gastrointest Liver Dis*. 2015;24(4):451-456.
17. Restellini S, Khanna R, Afif W. Therapeutic drug monitoring with ustekinumab and vedolizumab in inflammatory bowel disease. *Inflamm Bowel Dis*. 2018;24(10):2165-2172.

21
QUESTION

WHAT ARE THE RISKS OF BIOLOGIC THERAPIES AND HOW DO YOU COMMUNICATE THEM TO PATIENTS?

Susan Connor, MBBS (Hons 1), B Med Sci, PhD and
Yang (Clare) Wu, MBChB

The range of biologic therapies currently available for treating inflammatory bowel disease (IBD) include anti–tumor necrosis factor (anti-TNF) agents, infliximab, adalimumab, certolizumab, and golimumab; one anti-adhesion molecule, vedolizumab; and one interleukin (IL) 12/IL-23 antagonist, ustekinumab. The foundation of selecting the optimal treatment for a patient with IBD rests in individualized assessment of a patient's risk-to-benefit ratio.

Interpreting evidence around the safety profiles of biologic therapies is complex. Common side effects such as infusion reactions (5% in patients on combination therapy of anti-TNF agent and immunomodulator) tend to be mild.[1] Serious adverse events such as infection or malignancy are rare, but their accurate estimation is difficult. Randomized controlled trials may not always reflect the true incidence of serious complications due to short follow-up periods and inadequate power. Cohort- and population-based studies may provide better risk assessment as they involve large study populations and longer follow-up. Post-marketing studies also often provide a better reflection of how a biologic therapy is utilized in clinical practice. Overall, when conveying the incidence rates of rare side effects to patients, they should be described as best-guess estimates.

Rubin DT, Friedman S, Farraye FA, eds. *Curbside Consultation in IBD:*
49 Clinical Questions, Third Edition (pp 115-121).
© 2022 Taylor & Francis Group.

Risks of Anti–Tumor Necrosis Factor Therapy

Many studies have shown that anti-TNF therapy in patients with IBD is associated with a higher risk of serious infection. The TREAT registry is a registry that has followed 6273 patients with IBD over a median duration of 6 years.[2] Exposure to infliximab therapy compared to no exposure was associated with significantly higher risk of serious infection (HR 1.45; 95% CI, 1.12 to 1.86). In 2008, an observational study was published involving almost 200,000 patients with IBD with 900,000 person years follow-up from the French National Health Insurance database.[3] Risk of serious infection was increased with anti-TNF monotherapy (HR 1.71; 95% CI, 1.56 to 1.88) compared to thiopurine monotherapy. Combination therapy (anti-TNF and thiopurine) was associated with an increased risk of serious infection compared to both thiopurine (HR 2.11; 95% CI, 1.80 to 2.48) and anti-TNF monotherapy (HR 1.23; 95% CI, 1.05 to 1.45). Although the relative risk of serious infection in the older adult population (≥ 65 years) was similar to the younger population (18 to 64 years), the absolute risks were 2 to 3 times greater in older patients, with an incidence rate of serious infection as high as 51/1000 patient years (PY) on combination therapy.

The risk of reactivating latent tuberculosis (TB) is increased in patients treated with anti-TNFs and depends on whether the patient comes from or travels to TB-endemic countries. In France, where the annual adjusted incidence rate of TB is as low at 8.7/100,000, the RATIO registry found that patients receiving infliximab for autoimmune diseases had an annual adjusted incidence rate of 187/100,000.[4] In Korea, where TB is endemic with an annual incidence of 92/100,000 PY in the general population, the incidence of active TB in patients with IBD on anti-TNF therapy was 2484/100,000 PY.[5] Particular attention should be paid to the screening of latent TB infection and diagnosis of active TB in high-risk populations.

An association between combination therapy in patients with IBD and risk of non-Hodgkin's lymphoma has been found in numerous studies. However, whether anti-TNFs alone lead to excess risk of non-Hodgkin's lymphoma in IBD remains uncertain due to conflicting results. A meta-analysis of 26 anti-TNF studies in 2009 demonstrated an incidence rate of non-Hodgkin's lymphoma of 1.9/10,000 PY in the general population, 4/10,000 PY in patients on immunomodulator alone, and 6.1/10,000 PY in patients on combination therapy.[6] A 2014 meta-analysis of 6 studies on adalimumab exposure did not record a greater incidence rate of lymphoma in patients on adalimumab monotherapy compared to the general population.[7] A more recent observational study, following 189,289 patients over a median of 6.7 years found that compared to unexposed patients with IBD, the risk of lymphoma was higher among patients on anti-TNF monotherapy (HR 2.41; 95% CI, 1.60 to 3.64) and even higher among patients on combination therapy (HR 6.11; 95% CI, 3.46. to 10.8).[8]

There is currently no evidence that the risk of new solid malignancy is higher in patients on anti-TNF agents alone, except for skin cancer.[9] In a large nested case-control study, the incidence of melanoma was 57.1/100,000 PY in patients diagnosed with IBD compared to 44.1/100,000 PY in healthy controls.[10] On multivariate analysis, anti-TNF therapy was independently associated with melanoma (OR, 1.88; 95% CI, 1.08 to 3.29). However, it is unclear what proportion of the excess melanoma risk is due to the diagnosis of IBD itself.

The association between nonmelanoma skin cancer development and thiopurine exposure is well established and described in Question 11. Similarly, when a thiopurine is combined with adalimumab, there is a greater than expected incidence of nonmelanoma skin cancer compared to the general population with a standardized incidence ratio of 4.59 (95% CI, 2.51 to 7.70).[7] There are currently insufficient data available to draw conclusions on the risk of nonmelanoma skin cancer in patients on anti-TNF monotherapy.

Although antinuclear antibodies and double-stranded deoxyribonucleic acid antibodies are commonly seen in patients with IBD treated with anti-TNF therapy, clinical manifestations of a lupus-like illness only occur in approximately 1% of patients.[11] Other rare adverse events associated with anti-TNF therapy include congestive heart failure, psoriasiform reaction, demyelinating disease, serum sickness, and liver failure. The incidence is unknown as reports come from either single-center studies or case series.[11]

Risks of Vedolizumab

Vedolizumab, selectively targeting lymphocyte migration to the gut, has an improved safety profile compared to anti-TNF therapy.

In 2017, a meta-analysis combined data from 6 randomized controlled trials and long-term extension studies, evaluating patients who received at least one dose of vedolizumab and patients who received placebo. The incidence of infection was lower among patients receiving vedolizumab (63.5/100 PY; 95% CI, 59.6 to 67.3) compared to placebo (82.9/100 PY; 95% CI 68.3 to 97.5).[12] Half of total infections reported were minor and involved the upper respiratory tract. Higher absolute numbers of enteric infections occurred in vedolizumab-exposed patients (7.4/100 PY; 95% CI, 6.6 to 8.3) compared to placebo (6.7/100 PY; 95% CI, 3.2 to 10.1), but this did not reach statistical significance.

Cohort studies on vedolizumab exposure in the real-world setting have confirmed the relative low risk of serious infections. Of the 1087 patients with IBD treated with vedolizumab in a multicenter retrospective cohort, serious infections (requiring hospitalization) were observed at a rate of 0.79/1000 PY; 21 out of 26 cases of the serious infections were *Clostridioides difficile* colitis.[13] There is a low incidence of active TB in both patients receiving vedolizumab during clinical trials, with a reported rate of 0.1/100 PY, and in patients in the real-world setting, with 7 events reported so far.[12,14] In the event a patient is diagnosed with latent TB, specialist opinion should be sought before commencing vedolizumab.

No relationship was observed between the development of malignancy and vedolizumab exposure, including skin cancers. When the number of malignancies in the GEMINI long-term safety study and post-marketing data was standardized against the expected number of malignancies in patients with IBD from Optum's Clinformatics Data Mart database, no statistically significant difference was found.[15] The 2017 meta-analysis reported 4/2830 (0.1/100 PY) cases of colorectal cancer, and the latest post-marketing study reported 1 case of colorectal cancer in 1087 patients who retrospectively followed up for 12 months.[12,13] Further studies are needed to assess the risk of *C difficile* and colorectal cancer in vedolizumab use. A possible excess risk of gastrointestinal infection and gastrointestinal malignancy is conceivable given the gut-selective mechanism of the drug.

Table 21-1

Comparison of Biologic Drugs and Their Relative Risk of Serious Complications

Risks	Anti-TNF Therapy Monotherapy	Anti-TNF Combination Therapy	Vedolizumab	Ustekinumab
Serious infections	↑	↑	=	=
Tuberculosis	↑	↑	Low	Low
Lymphoma	Unclear	↑	Awaiting further studies	Awaiting further studies
Melanoma	↑	↑	=	=
Nonmelanoma skin cancer	Unclear	↑	=	=
Solid cancer	=	=	=	=
↑ increased risk compared to unexposed patients; = equivocal compared to unexposed patients.				

Risks of Ustekinumab

Ustekinumab, a monoclonal antibody targeting IL-12 and IL-23, is the latest biologic to become available. Registration randomized controlled trials UNITI and IM-UNITI did not reveal any significant differences in the rate of serious infections between ustekinumab and placebo arms.[16] A real-world cohort study that followed 221 patients with IBD on ustekinumab, and a median follow-up of 52 weeks, also found a low rate of serious infectious complications (3.1 per 100 PY), with all patients being on concomitant immunomodulator or corticosteroids.[17] One case of active TB occurred 10 months after a single dose of ustekinumab during IM-UNITI, and no cases of TB were reported in the real-world cohort.[16,17] In the event a patient is diagnosed with latent TB, specialist opinion should be sought before commencing ustekinumab.

There are currently no large-scale observational studies on the risk of malignancy in patients with IBD receiving ustekinumab, but studies on ustekinumab exposure in psoriasis patients have produced some reassuring results. As of 2017, the PSOLAR registry had followed 12,090 participants with psoriasis for a median of 4.17 years.[18] Treatment with ustekinumab has not been associated with any increase in the risk of solid malignancy or lymphoma. Future studies are required to determine the long-term safety profile of ustekinumab in patients with IBD.

Table 21-1 summarizes the safety profiles of different classes of biologics.

Table 21-2
Considerations When Communicating Risks to Patients
Avoid vague terms such as "common" and "rare."
Use visual aids.
Use absolute numbers rather than relative numbers.
Report percentages below 1% as fractions.
Keep to the same denominator as much as possible.
Check patient recall.
Remind the patient of potential benefits of treatment.

COMMUNICATING WITH PATIENTS

Effective communication on the risk of therapy can be challenging based on time constraints, opportunities for misunderstandings, and the lack of tools available to illustrate data. Table 21-2 outlines some practical considerations when presenting risks to patients. It is best to avoid describing adverse events as either "rare" or "common," as this can be interpreted in a wide range of ways. Instead, use numbers and pictorial displays of statistics. Over- or underexaggeration of data can occur if numbers are "framed," and this may influence patients' decisions.[11] Try to use absolute numbers rather than relative. As an example, the relative increase in risk of developing lymphoma on combination therapy compared to the unexposed is 610%. However, in absolute terms, this is an extra 5 patients per 10,000 treated over the course of 1 year. Percentages below 1% should be described as a fraction, such as using 6 in 1000 as opposed to 0.6%. If fractions are used, try to maintain the same denominator throughout the conversation.[11] Comparing risks of drugs to other real-life risks can also improve understanding; for example, the lifetime chance of dying from a motor vehicle accident is 1/102 and dying from lightning strike is 1/114,195.[19]

Visual aids have consistently been shown to be easy for patients to identify with and understand.[8] Relevant illustrations are readily found in original publications or review articles.[3,6] Figure 21-1 is an example of a Paling Palette that can be customized to show the size of each risk. During the discussion, ask the patient to recall the information you have explained. This allows you, the clinician, to check the patient's comprehension, correct misunderstandings, and improve the patient's retention of data. Lastly, whether or not the patient decides to commence a medical therapy depends on their appreciation of the trade-off between risks and benefits; do not forget to remind the patient of the potential benefit of successful treatment and encourage a preference-based decision rather than a one-sided rejection of potential side effects.

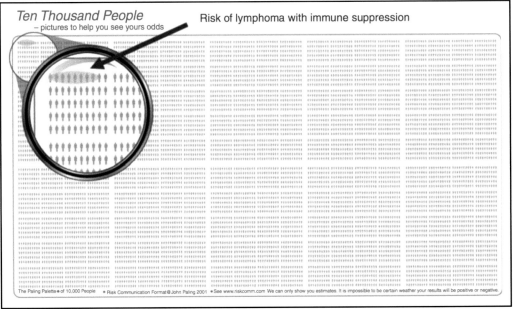

Figure 21-1. Explaining the risk of lymphoma associated with immune suppression. The number of people can be highlighted to demonstrate absolute risk. (Reproduced with permission from Siegel CA. Review article: explaining risks of inflammatory bowel disease therapy to patients. *Aliment Pharmacol Ther.* 2011;33[1]:23-32.)

References

1. Colombel JF, Sandborn WJ, Reinisch W, et al. Infliximab, azathioprine, or combination therapy for Crohn's disease. *N Engl J Med.* 2010;362(15):1383-1395.
2. Lichtenstein GR, Feagan BG, Cohen RD, et al. Infliximab for Crohn's disease: more than 13 years of real-world experience. *Inflamm Bowel Dis.* 2018;24(3):490-501.
3. Kirchgesner J, Lemaitre M, Carrat F, Zureik M, Carbonnel F, Dray-Spira R. Risk of serious and opportunistic infections associated with treatment of inflammatory bowel diseases. *Gastroenterology.* 2018;155(2):337-346.
4. Tubach F, Salmon D, Allanore PRY, Goupille P, Pallot-Prades MBB, Mariette X. Risk of tuberculosis is higher with anti-tumor necrosis factor monoclonal antibody therapy than with soluble tumor necrosis factor receptor therapy: the three-year prospective French Research Axed on Tolerance of Biotherapies registry. *Arthritis Rheum.* 2009;60(7):1884-1894.
5. Byun JM, Lee CK, Rhee SY, et al. Risks for opportunistic tuberculosis infection in a cohort of 873 patients with inflammatory bowel disease receiving a tumor necrosis factor-alpha inhibitor. *Scand J Gastroenterol.* 2015;50(3):312-320.
6. Siegel CA, Marden S, Persing SM, Larson RJ, Sands BE. Risk of lymphoma associated with combination anti-tumor necrosis factor and immunomodular therapy for the treatment of Crohn's disease: a meta-analysis. *Clin Gastroenterol Hepatol.* 2009;7(8):874-881.
7. Osterman MT, Sandborn WJ, Colombel JF, et al. Increased risk of malignancy with adalimumab combination therapy, compared with monotherapy for Crohn's disease. *Gastroenterology.* 2014;146(4):941-949.
8. Lemaitre M, Kirchgesner J, Rudnichi A, et al. Association between use of thiopurines or tumor necrosis factor antagonists alone or in combination and risk of lymphoma in patients with inflammatory bowel disease. *JAMA.* 2017;318(17):1679-1686.
9. Nyboe Andersen, N Pasternak B, Basit S, et al. Association between tumor necrosis factor-α antagonists and risk of cancer in patients with inflammatory bowel disease. *JAMA.* 2014;311(23):2406-2413.
10. Long MD, Martin CF, Pipkin CA, et al. Risk of melanoma and nonmelanoma skin cancer among patients with inflammatory bowel disease. *Gastroenterology.* 2012;143(2):390-399.
11. Siegel CA. Review article: explaining risks of inflammatory bowel disease therapy to patients. *Aliment Pharmacol Ther.* 2011;33(1):23-32.

12. Colombel JF, Sands BE, Rutgeerts P, et al. The safety of vedolizumab for ulcerative colitis and Crohn's disease. *Gut*. 2017;66(5):839-851.

13. Meserve J, Aniwan S, Koliani-Pace JL, et al. Retrospective analysis of safety of vedolizumab in patients with inflammatory bowel diseases. *Clin Gastroenterol Hepatol*. 2019;17(8):1533-1540.

14. Ng SC, Hilmi IN, Blake A, et al. Low frequency of opportunistic infections in patients receiving vedolizumab in clinical trials and post-marketing settings. *Inflamm Bowel Dis*. 2018;24(11):2431-2441. https://doi.org/10.1093/ibd/izy153

15. Card T, Ungaro R, Bhayat F, Blake A, Hantsbarger G, Travis S. Vedolizumab use is not associated with increased malignancy incidence: GEMINI LTS study results and post-marketing data. *Aliment Pharmacol Ther*. 2020;51(1):149-157.

16. Feagan BG, Sandborn WJ, Gasink C, et al. Ustekinumab as induction and maintenance therapy for Crohn's disease. *N Engl J Med*. 2016;375(20):1946-1960.

17. Biemans VBC, van der Meulen-de Jong AE, van der Woude CJ, et al. Ustekinumab for Crohn's disease: results of the ICC Registry, a nationwide prospective observational cohort study. *J Crohns Colitis*. 2020;14(1):33-45.

18. Fiorentino D, Ho V, Lebwohl MG, et al. Risk of malignancy with systemic psoriasis treatment in the Psoriasis Longitudinal Assessment Registry. *J Am Acad Dermatol*. 2017;77(5):845-854.

19. National Safety Council, National Center for Health Statistics. Mortality data for 2015. Accessed March 25, 2021. https://injuryfacts.nsc.org/all-injuries/preventable-death-overview/odds-of-dying/data-details/.

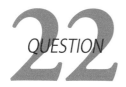

WHEN SHOULD WE CONSIDER
DEESCALATION OF THERAPY?

Seth R. Shaffer, MD, MS and David T. Rubin, MD

Introduction

Inflammatory bowel disease (IBD), including Crohn's disease (CD) and ulcerative colitis (UC), are chronic inflammatory conditions that require careful attention for individualized patient-directed management. The goal of medical management is to control inflammation and to prevent clinical symptoms and complications.[1,2] While rare, anti–tumor necrosis factor (TNF) therapies may increase the risk of infections[3] and malignancies.[4] As the benefits of medications in achieving disease remission outweigh the risks that they may carry, a gastroenterologist's goal continues to be to use the safest, most effective therapy. It is important to always assess if these medications can ever be deescalated, or withdrawn, to both reduce potential overtreatment, decrease harm to the patient, and decrease health care spending. Deescalation of therapy in IBD can be defined as either decreasing the dose of a drug or discontinuing a therapy entirely.

Patients Who Should Be Targeted for
Medication Deescalation

Recent analyses have shown no benefit of continuing 5-aminosalicylates therapy in those escalated to infliximab, vedolizumab, or tofacitinib.[5-7] American College of Gastroenterology (ACG) and American Gastroenterological Association (AGA) guidelines further recommend 5-ASA therapy can be discontinued upon escalation to anti-TNF[2,8] or tofacitinib.[8]

Rubin DT, Friedman S, Farraye FA, eds. *Curbside Consultation in IBD:*
49 Clinical Questions, Third Edition (pp 123-127).
© 2022 Taylor & Francis Group.

A patient's disease should be in deep remission, meaning the patient has achieved both clinical and objectively confirmed (often endoscopic) remission. In a meta-analysis that assessed the risk of relapse of anti-TNF discontinuation in patients with luminal CD achieving clinical remission, 40% relapsed by 12 months, while this relapse rate decreased to 26% in those achieving deep remission.[9] Patients with UC in clinical remission had a relapse rate of 50% at 12 to 24 months, while this rate decreased to 33% if endoscopic remission was a requirement. A multicenter, observational, retrospective study in Spain assessed patients with CD or UC and observed those in deep remission had relapse rates of 22% and 20%, in CD and UC patients, respectively, after 1 year of discontinuation of their therapy.[10]

A retrospective cohort study in Europe and Israel looked at adults with UC who achieved sustained clinical remission for at least 12 months on infliximab therapy and found the incidence of relapse was higher in those who discontinued infliximab therapy (HR = 3.41, 95% CI, 1.88 to 6.20) compared to those who continued therapy.[11] Rates of hospitalizations and colectomy did not differ between the groups, and of those patients who discontinued infliximab, thiopurines were protective against future relapse. Patients with CD in the STORI trial were on combination therapy (infliximab and an immunomodulator) for at least 1 year and in steroid-free remission for at least 6 months.[12] In multivariable models, Crohn's Disease Endoscopic Index of Severity (CDEIS) scores > 0 were associated with longer time to relapse (HR = 2.3, 95% CI, 1.1 to 4.9), as well as corticosteroid use between 6 to 12 months before study inclusion, hemoglobin ≤ 145 g/L, male sex, C-reactive protein (CRP) level ≥ 5 mg/L, fecal calprotectin ≥ 300 μg/g, and infliximab trough level ≥ 2 mg/L. Those in the low-risk group had a 5% (95% CI, 0.5%, 29.3%) risk of relapse over 1 year.

For patients on combination therapy (combined immunomodulator and biologic), the benefit of maintaining the immunomodulator may be mostly in the short term. Van Assche et al showed that stopping the immunomodulator after 6 months in patients with CD did not affect the 1- to 2-year remission rates compared to those who continued their immunomodulator,[13] favoring discontinuing the immunomodulator 6 to 12 months after its initiation in those with mucosal healing.

It is important that patients are in sustained (at least 1 year) clinical, endoscopic, and biochemical (CRP level < 5 mg/L; fecal calprotectin < 100 μg/g) remission before withdrawal should even be considered. For those on combination therapy, maintaining immunomodulator treatment as monotherapy, if the anti-TNF is to be withdrawn, should be discussed with the patient, as it seems to reduce the risk of relapse. Alternatively, the immunomodulator can be withdrawn after deep remission is achieved.

While there are fewer data concerning newer therapies, such as vedolizumab, ustekinumab, or tofacitinib, the same rules apply. Patients should be in deep (clinical and endoscopic) remission before this is considered an option. It is reasonable that selected patients on every 4 weeks of vedolizumab or ustekinumab be deescalated to every 8 weeks, and for patients on tofacitinib 10 mg twice daily deescalating to 5 mg twice daily is an option as well.

The Role of Therapeutic Drug Monitoring

While anti-TNF trough levels should be drawn before discontinuation, interestingly low or even undetectable infliximab levels are associated with an increased time to relapse,[12,14] perhaps indicating that those with higher trough levels in times of remission require their anti-TNF therapy and may be harmed by anti-TNF withdrawal. Another study randomized stable CD and UC patients on infliximab to receive either clinically based care or care based on infliximab trough levels.[15] Those with trough levels > 7 μg/mL were safely dose reduced to achieve infliximab trough levels of 3 to 7 μg/mL, with no difference in clinical remission rates or serum CRP levels in the short term, indicating therapeutic drug monitoring can help with safe dose reduction and withdrawal. There are no data on therapeutic drug monitoring and dose deescalating in newer biologics (vedolizumab and ustekinumab), and hence the use of therapeutic drug monitoring in aiding deescalation, or discontinuation, in these therapies is unknown.

How to Monitor These Patients

Once a patient deescalates or discontinues therapy, it is crucial to continue monitoring these patients and to try to predict relapse before clinical symptoms occur. We recommend fecal calprotectin levels be done at 3 and 9 months to monitor patients for relapse before symptom onset. Fecal calprotectin levels can be elevated up to 6 months before clinical relapse, and consistently normal levels are predictive of clinical and endoscopic remission.[16] A fecal calprotectin level ≥ 100 mcg/g was the best predictor of relapse post deescalation (AUC = 0.84; sensitivity = 0.76; specificity = 0.86, positive predictive value = 0.77, negative predictive value = 0.85).[17] If fecal calprotectin levels at 3 and 9 months are both normal, then we pursue endoscopy at 1 year to confirm their disease remains in remission. Elevated fecal calprotectin levels, despite the patient being in clinical remission, should prompt further investigations for active IBD.

Which Treatment to Resume

In patients who relapse after discontinuing anti-TNF therapy, retreatment with anti-TNF therapy is safe and effective, with clinical remission rates ranging from 78% to 90%.[10,18] Another study found that in those who had previously discontinued infliximab, 88% (38 of 43) of patients were in remission within 12 months of restarting infliximab, with no reported reactions.[12]

When restarting infliximab in those who have previously received it, premedication with hydrocortisone, and checking infliximab trough levels and antibodies after the first reinfusion, can help in predicting safety and success. The presence of antibodies against infliximab at week 6 of restarting treatment was found to be significantly different between responders and nonresponders.[19]

The University of Chicago has developed an algorithm for restarting infliximab in those who have been off of it for at least 6 months (due to intentional or unintentional discontinuation or even loss of response). Premedication with intravenous steroids, acetaminophen, and diphenhydramine with the infusion can help decrease the risk of infusion reactions. Infliximab levels should be obtained 7 to 10 days after the initial infusion, and patients with no detectable antibodies should continue with standard loading dosing regimens. Those who are found to have detectable antibodies should seek alternative therapeutic options, as infusion reactions are likely to occur if continued infliximab is administered.[20]

Initiating other biologics, such as vedolizumab or ustekinumab, for the treatment of IBD is also safe to do, as long as antibodies are absent.

Retreatment with an immunomodulator also yields good response rates in patients with relapse. In patients who had relapsed after azathioprine withdrawal followed by retreatment with azathioprine, 96% (22 of 23) patients achieved remission.[21]

In those who are on tofacitinib 5 mg twice daily and develop active disease, dose escalation back to 10 mg twice daily is safe and effective, as 49.7% of patients at 12 months may recapture clinical response.[22]

In answer to the common question from our surgical colleagues about drug holidays before or after gastrointestinal or nongastrointestinal surgery, the available data support not stopping therapy, including the recent multicenter PUCCINI (study to determine risk factors for postoperative infection in IBD) study, which demonstrated that there was no difference in postoperative infections between patients who had measurable anti-TNF and those who did not.[23] Additional studies have demonstrated similar safe outcomes for patients who had caesarean section deliveries.[24] Therefore, a careful conversation with our surgical colleagues and with patients to reassure them about the safety of continuing therapy in this setting is appropriate.

Approach to Planning Deescalation/Discontinuation

The consideration and approach to deescalation should be determined on a case-by-case basis:

1. Confirm deep remission with endoscopic evidence of mucosal healing prior to deescalation/ discontinuation. This should ideally be present for > 1 year on the current regimen at current dosage.
2. Confirm optimization of anti-TNF therapy with therapeutic drug monitoring. It is crucial to make sure this regimen is working and that the patient's trough levels are adequate.
3. Discuss risks and benefits of this approach with patients, as well as the plan if their disease becomes active after deescalation/discontinuation.
4. Deescalate the chosen therapy in dose or discontinuing altogether.
5. Monitor the patient for subclinical relapse using serial fecal calprotectin ± endoscopy.
6. If the patient requires reescalation of therapy, the prior therapy may or may not be the best agent for them at that time. Medication decisions must be made based on the current presentation.

Conclusion

Deescalation of therapy is reasonable in appropriate patients, but a careful risk assessment, shared decision making about potential relapse, and monitoring strategy of both disease and drug must occur. A rescue strategy should be discussed and identified before the deescalation. We do not support elective discontinuation of drugs prior to elective surgeries, both based on the available data as well as based on the known half-lives of these therapies. Further discussions with our surgical colleagues and our patients in these settings are very important.

References

1. Lichtenstein GR, Loftus EV, Isaacs KL, et al. ACG clinical guideline: management of Crohn's disease in adults. *Am J Gastroenterol*. 2018;113(4):481-517.
2. Rubin DT, Ananthakrishnan AN, Siegel CA, et al. ACG clinical guideline: ulcerative colitis in adults. *Am J Gastroenterol*. 2019;114(3):384-413.
3. Ford AC, Peyrin-Biroulet L. Opportunistic infections with anti-tumor necrosis factor-α therapy in inflammatory bowel disease: meta-analysis of randomized controlled trials. *Am J Gastroenterol*. 2013;108(8):1268-1276.
4. Lemaitre M, Kirchgesner J, Rudnichi A, et al. Association between use of thiopurines or tumor necrosis factor antagonists alone or in combination and risk of lymphoma in patients with inflammatory bowel disease. *JAMA*. 2017;318(17):1679-1686.
5. Singh S, Proudfoot JA, Dulai PS, et al. No benefit of concomitant 5-aminosalicylates in patients with ulcerative colitis escalated to biologic therapy: pooled analysis of individual participant data from clinical trials. *Am J Gastroenterol*. 2018;113(8):1197-1205.
6. Ma C, Kotze PG, Almutairdi A, et al. Concomitant use of aminosalicylates is not associated with improved outcomes in patients with ulcerative colitis escalated to vedolizumab. *Clin Gastroenterol Hepatol*. 2019;17(11):2374-2376.e2.
7. Hanauer S, Rubin D, Gionchetti P, et al. Tofacitinib efficacy in patients with moderate to severe ulcerative colitis: subgroup analyses of Octave Induction 1 and 2 and Octave Sustain, by 5-aminosalicylates use. *J Crohns Colitis*. 2019;13(1):S477.

8. Feuerstein JD, Isaacs KL, Schneider Y, et al. AGA clinical practice guidelines on the management of moderate to severe ulcerative colitis. *Gastroenterology*. 2020;158(5):1450-1461.

9. Gisbert JP, Marín AC, Chaparro M. The risk of relapse after anti-TNF discontinuation in inflammatory bowel disease: systematic review and meta-analysis. *Am J Gastroenterol*. 2016;111(5):632-647.

10. Casanova MJ, Chaparro M, García-Sánchez V, et al. Evolution after anti-TNF discontinuation in patients with inflammatory bowel disease: a multicenter long-term follow-up study. *Am J Gastroenterol*. 2017;112(1):120-131.

11. Fiorino G, Cortes PN, Ellul P, et al. Discontinuation of infliximab in patients with ulcerative colitis is associated with increased risk of relapse: a multinational retrospective cohort study. *Clin Gastroenterol Hepatol*. 2016;14(10): 1426-1432.e1.

12. Louis E, Mary JY, Vernier-Massouille G, et al. Maintenance of remission among patients with Crohn's disease on antimetabolite therapy after infliximab therapy is stopped. *Gastroenterology*. 2012;142(1):63-70.e5; quiz e31.

13. Van Assche G, Magdelaine-Beuzelin C, D'Haens G, et al. Withdrawal of immunosuppression in Crohn's disease treated with scheduled infliximab maintenance: a randomized trial. *Gastroenterology*. 2008;134(7):1861-1868.

14. Ben-Horin S, Chowers Y, Ungar B, et al. Undetectable anti-TNF drug levels in patients with long-term remission predict successful drug withdrawal. *Aliment Pharmacol Ther*. 2015;42(3):356-364.

15. Vande Casteele N, Ferrante M, Van Assche G, et al. Trough concentrations of infliximab guide dosing for patients with inflammatory bowel disease. *Gastroenterology*. 2015;148(7):1320-1329.e3.

16. Molander P, Färkkilä M, Ristimäki A, et al. Does fecal calprotectin predict short-term relapse after stopping TNFα-blocking agents in inflammatory bowel disease patients in deep remission? *J Crohns Colitis*. 2015;9(1):33-40.

17. Buisson A, Mak WY, Andersen MJ, et al. Fecal calprotectin is a very reliable tool to predict and monitor the risk of relapse after therapeutic de-escalation in patients with inflammatory bowel diseases. *J Crohns Colitis*. 2019;13(8):1012-1024.

18. Molander P, Färkkilä M, Kemppainen H, et al. Long-term outcome of inflammatory bowel disease patients with deep remission after discontinuation of TNFα-blocking agents. *Scand J Gastroenterol*. 2017;52(3):284-290.

19. Brandse JF, Mathôt RA, van der Kleij D, et al. Pharmacokinetic features and presence of antidrug antibodies associate with response to infliximab induction therapy in patients with moderate to severe ulcerative colitis. *Clin Gastroenterol Hepatol*. 2016;14(2):251-258.e2.

20. Sofia MA, Rubin DT. Current approaches for optimizing the benefit of biologic therapy in ulcerative colitis. *Therap Adv Gastroenterol*. 2016;9(4):548-559.

21. Treton X, Bouhnik Y, Mary JY, et al. Azathioprine withdrawal in patients with Crohn's disease maintained on prolonged remission: a high risk of relapse. *Clin Gastroenterol Hepatol*. 2009;7(1):80-85.

22. Sands BE, Armuzzi A, Marshall JK, et al. Efficacy and safety of tofacitinib dose de-escalation and dose escalation for patients with ulcerative colitis: results from OCTAVE Open. *Aliment Pharmacol Ther*. 2019;51(2):271-280.

23. Cohen BL, Fleshner P, Kane SV, et al. 415a—anti-tumor necrosis factor therapy is not associated with postoperative infection: results from prospective cohort of ulcerative colitis and Crohn's disease patients undergoing surgery to identify risk factors for postoperative infection I (Puccini). *Gastroenterology*. 2019;156(6):S-80.

24. Aboubakr A, Riggs A, Mella M, et al. Peripartum exposure to biologic therapy does not impact wound healing after caesarean section in women with inflammatory bowel disease: 635. *Am J Gastroenterol*. 2019;114:S370-S372.

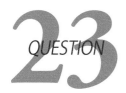

QUESTION

23

CAN YOU RESTART A BIOLOGICAL THERAPY AFTER A DRUG HOLIDAY? HOW DO YOU DO THIS?

Filip J. Baert, MD, PhD and David Drobne, MD, PhD

Biological therapy for inflammatory bowel disease (IBD) has become a mainstay of treatment due to its efficacy and safety. All 3 classes of biological therapy, namely inhibitors of tumor necrosis factor-α (TNF-α; infliximab, adalimumab, golimumab, certolizumab), anti-adhesion molecules (vedolizumab), and inhibitors of interleukin (IL) 12/IL-23 (ustekinumab) have the capacity to induce disease remission and maintain remission. Despite proven need for maintenance of remission with biological drugs there are many instances in real life when patients or physicians will stop biological drugs. In fact, every second patient interrupts treatment over 1 to 3 years of starting. After this interruption, known as a drug holiday, many patients and physicians will want to restart the same biological drug again. Here, however, is the caveat: Restarting is not the same as starting the drug for the first time. The success and safety of restarting was most profoundly studied for infliximab, although the same principles most likely apply also for other TNF inhibitors. New generation biologicals, such as vedolizumab and ustekinumab, have different immunogenicity potential.

Reason for a Drug Holiday When Restarting

When restarting the monoclonal antibody it is most important to investigate why the patient stopped the biological drug in the first place (Table 23-1). This is important because it will determine the success, and because of the safety of restarting the same drug again.

Rubin DT, Friedman S, Farraye FA, eds. *Curbside Consultation in IBD:*
49 Clinical Questions, Third Edition (pp 129-132).
© 2022 Taylor & Francis Group.

Table 23-1
Reasons for Stopping Biological Drugs

Primary nonresponse: "The patient did not have any response to the drug"
Loss of response: "The patient responded to induction, but then lost response"
Remission: "The patient was well, but stopped the drug for reasons such as pregnancy, financial constraints, etc"
Side effect: "Could be related to the drug or not"

PRIMARY NONRESPONSE

Patients who have no positive effect to induction treatment with particular class of biologic (eg, TNF inhibitor) are extremely unlikely to respond to the same drug after a drug holiday; therefore, the same drug should not be restarted. However, it should be checked if the induction dose was appropriate (for intravenous agents) and if the patient did actually apply subcutaneous injections appropriately as prescribed. Also, it should be checked if the nonresponse was objectively confirmed (eg, by performing endoscopy/magnetic resonance imaging or by lack of normalization of biomarkers, such as C-reactive protein or fecal calprotectin). Also, it is advisable to confirm that the patient had adequate concentrations of TNF inhibitors and no antidrug antibodies before declaring that the patient is a primary nonresponder.[1]

LOSS OF RESPONSE

After successful disease control by a biological drug some patients still lose response over time. Patients who discontinue TNF inhibitor due to loss of response are unlikely to have therapeutic benefit by restarting the same TNF inhibitor again (Figure 23-1A, lower curve).[2] It is similar with infusion reactions; therefore, if the reason for the drug holiday was infusion reaction the same drug should not be restarted as these will reoccur, typically during the second or third infusion in case of infliximab (the first infusion is a "booster").

REMISSION

Despite the proven need for maintenance of remission by TNF inhibitors many patients have shorter or longer drug holidays. Typical examples include patients' wish to be off the drug after prolonged remission, pregnancy, and loss of reimbursement. Fortunately, restarting these patients on TNF inhibitors is generally, but no always, successful (Figure 23-1A, upper curve).[2]

SIDE EFFECT

TNF inhibitor–induced psoriasis is one of the most common causes for stopping the TNF inhibitor. Unfortunately, psoriasiform skin lesions will reoccur after the drug holiday. This is generally a class effect, so restarting the TNF inhibitor in these cases is only exceptionally successful. Another important cause for a drug holiday is infectious complications. After treating the infection, the TNF inhibitor can usually be restarted. Here, however, it is preferred to avoid combination treatment of TNF inhibitor and azathioprine and rather use TNF monotherapy in higher doses if needed, as this seems to be equally effective but safer.[3-5]

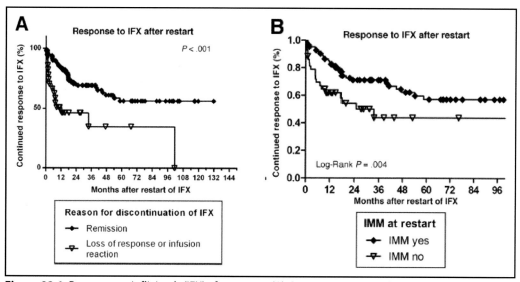

Figure 23-1. Response to infliximab (IFX) after restart. (A) Compares continued response to infliximab by reason for discontinuation. (B) Compares continued response to infliximab by concomitant use of immunomodulator (IMM) at restart. (Reproduced with permission from Baert F, Drobne D, Gils A, et al. Early trough levels and antibodies to infliximab predict safety and success of re-initiation of infliximab therapy. *Clin Gastroenterol Hepatol.* 2014;12[9]:1471-1481.e2.)

Restarting a Biological Drug

Among all biologicals, immunogenicity, the ability to induce antidrug antibody formation, is best documented for TNF inhibitors. Because of this, restarting TNF inhibitors is different than starting for the first time. By complex mechanisms, which are beyond the scope of this chapter, low concentrations of TNF inhibitors induce antidrug antibody formation.[6] A drug holiday, or even multiple drug holidays, expose the patient to the formation of antidrug antibodies; therefore, restarting can be hampered by the antidrug antibodies, which might have formed during the drug holiday. Inversely, however, high concentrations of TNF inhibitors can neutralize antidrug antibodies. Because of this, low-titer antidrug antibodies can be overcome with a high concentration of the TNF inhibitor. To be successful at restarting TNF inhibitors we thus always use induction doses (even if disease activity is low or absent; eg, in patients who start TNF inhibitor prophylactically after surgically induced remission in Crohn's disease). Another measure is to use combination treatment, as this suppresses antidrug antibodies (Figure 23-1B).[2] If combination treatment is not possible (eg, due to history of significant side effect or intolerance) or desired (eg, due to fear of infections, potential teratogenicity such as methotrexate),[7] the alternative is to use higher than normal induction doses (eg, in infliximab 10 mg/kg instead of 5 mg/kg) and proactively dose optimize (either increase dose or shorten the interval) if low concentrations of TNF inhibitor are detected after induction.[2]

Evaluating if Restart Was Successful

It is of most importance to objectively evaluate whether restarting the TNF inhibitor was successful by endoscopy and/or magnetic resonance imaging since successful treatment before a drug holiday is not a guarantee for success of restarting. Furthermore, early drug measurements can identify underdosing at restart or detect occurrence of antidrug antibodies. In the former case, dose escalation will result in long-term disease control; in the latter case, further administration of the same monoclonal antibody will be futile, and the patient should be switched to another drug.

Restarting New Generation Biologicals

Restarting new generation biologicals, such as vedolizumab and ustekinumab, is far less studied than that of TNF inhibitors. Most importantly, these drugs are far less immunogenic as it seems that they only rarely induce the formation of antidrug antibodies. For this reason, a concomitant immunomodulator is not needed during restarting nor during the induction dose regimen. However, depending on disease activity, reinduction or early dose optimization can be necessary at restart. Therapeutic drug monitoring for these drugs is not yet established, but it is very likely we will use trough-level monitoring to exclude underdosing in case of nonresponse in the near future.[8]

Conclusion

Restarting biological therapies in clinical practice is common. Patients who enjoyed disease control before a drug holiday are very likely to have good and durable response after restarting a monoclonal antibody. To suppress potential antidrug antibodies that might have developed during the drug holiday it is advised to use induction regimens and immunomodulator co-treatment during the restart of TNF inhibitors. After restart, early drug level measurements will identify patients who might have developed antidrug antibodies and also enable proactive dose escalations in case of low drug concentrations.

References

1. Papamichael K, Gils A, Rutgeerts P, et al. Role for therapeutic drug monitoring during induction therapy with TNF antagonists in IBD: evolution in the definition and management of primary nonresponse. *Inflamm Bowel Dis*. 2015;21(1):182-197.
2. Baert F, Drobne D, Gils A, et al. Early trough levels and antibodies to infliximab predict safety and success of re-initiation of infliximab therapy. *Clin Gastroenterol Hepatol*. 2014;12(9):1471-1481.e2.
3. Drobne D, Kurent T, Golob S, et al. Success and safety of high infliximab trough levels in inflammatory bowel disease. *Scand J Gastroenterol*. 2018;53(8):940-946.
4. Lega S, Phan BL, Rosenthal CJ, et al. Proactively optimized infliximab monotherapy is as effective as combination therapy in IBD. *Inflamm Bowel Dis*. 2018;25(1):134-141.
5. Greener T, Kabakchiev B, Steinhart AH, et al. Higher infliximab levels are not associated with an increase in adverse events in inflammatory bowel disease. *Inflamm Bowel Dis*. 2018;24(8):1808-1814.
6. Brandse JF, Mould D, Smeekes O, et al. A real-life population pharmacokinetic study reveals factors associated with clearance and immunogenicity of infliximab in inflammatory bowel disease. *Inflamm Bowel Dis*. 2017;23(4):650-660.
7. Strik AS, van den Brink GR, Ponsioen C, et al. Suppression of anti-drug antibodies to infliximab or adalimumab with the addition of an immunomodulator in patients with inflammatory bowel disease. *Aliment Pharmacol Ther*. 2017;45(8):1128-1134.
8. Park S, Evans E, Sandborn WJ, et al. Ustekinumab IV 6 mg/kg loading dose re-induction improves clinical and endoscopic response in Crohn's disease: a case series. *Am J Gastroenterol*. 2018;113(4):627-629.

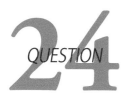

HOW CAN I GET MY PATIENTS WITH IBD THE THERAPY THEY NEED?

Shivani A. Patel, PharmD, BCPS and
Toni M. Zahorian, PharmD, BCACP

One of the major barriers to effective therapy for patients with inflammatory bowel disease (IBD) is the cost of therapy, specifically for specialty medications such as biologics and small-molecule agents. In an effort to minimize costs, patients have been known to forgo therapy, alter dosing regimens, skip doses, and/or delay filling prescriptions in order to take less medication than prescribed.[1] The financial burden associated with the cost of care adds significant stressors to our patients' health status. This can potentially influence their overall well-being by negatively impacting their adherence to therapy and chances for clinical response and remission. Therefore, care teams and providers must be knowledgeable and resourceful in order to provide safe, effective, and timely care for all patients with IBD.

There are several resources available to providers that can help minimize barriers to care. These include patient access programs, financial assistance programs, specialty pharmacies, and integrated specialty pharmacists working in collaboration with the IBD care team. The goal of this chapter is to provide a brief overview of such programs so that providers are able to successfully secure access to affordable care while maintaining a supportive environment for their patients with IBD.

The first step is securing access to therapy by obtaining insurance approval for the desired therapeutic regimen. Infusible specialty medications, such as infliximab and vedolizumab, are usually covered through a patient's medical plan. This is done via a buy-and-bill method in an outpatient setting, where the patient is billed after receiving the approved medication. For Medicare patients, infusible medications can be covered through Medicare Part B coverage. Subcutaneous injectable therapies and oral therapies are usually covered through the patient's pharmacy benefits or prescription plan. In rare cases, subcutaneous injectable therapies such as ustekinumab or cer-

Rubin DT, Friedman S, Farraye FA, eds. *Curbside Consultation in IBD:*
49 Clinical Questions, Third Edition (pp 133-139).
© 2022 Taylor & Francis Group.

tolizumab pegol can alternatively be requested and billed through the patient's medical plan if and when the doses are administered in the outpatient setting by a health care provider. This method for coverage may be investigated if a patient is not able to gain access, or approval, to the medication through the prescription plan.

As shown in Figure 24-1, obtaining approval for the desired medication regimen is the first step to securing access. Providers may be required to conduct peer-to-peer discussions with the medical reviewer affiliated with the insurance plan in order to more accurately communicate the patient's clinical status. If medically warranted therapies are inappropriately denied coverage due to variations in preferred agents or formulary alternatives, it is imperative that providers and care teams advocate for the needs of the patient and help overturn such decisions. In some cases this can be achieved by submitting a letter of medical necessity along with supporting clinical literature and rationale for the desired therapeutic regimen over other alternatives. If the medication continues to be denied inappropriately, an external review or second-level appeal with the State Department of Insurance may also be submitted. If all options of appeals are exhausted and the patient is still denied the necessary therapy, it is highly recommended to escalate the patient's case and investigate alternative avenues for coverage. These avenues include grant funding, open foundations available for patients with IBD, as well as enrollment in a manufacturer patient assistance program (PAP) for full or partial financial assistance.

In cases where the desired medication regimen is approved by the patient's insurance plan, lack of affordability due to high out-of-pocket expenses may still pose a challenge. Patients who are utilizing commercial or private insurance plans are eligible for excellent savings programs provided through the drug manufacturers. Table 24-1 lists various websites where patients can enroll into copay savings programs. These programs are meant to assist patients with their out-of-pocket expenses after the medication is primarily billed through their medical or prescription insurance coverage. Patients may receive a maximum benefit of $10,000 to $20,000 per year, depending on the medication. Funds available on copay cards are usually renewed automatically on an annual basis to provide reliable, consistent coverage throughout the duration of the therapy, barring any changes with the patient's insurance plan or medication regimen.

Unfortunately, not all patients are eligible for copay assistance programs and cards. Patients who have insurance coverage through government plans, such as Medicare, Medicaid, Medigap, Tricare, Veterans Affairs, or similar federal- or state-funded plans, are not eligible for copay savings cards. There may also be additional state restrictions for copay savings cards based on the patient's state of residence. These restrictions should be evaluated on the manufacturer website prior to enrolling patients. As a result of these limitations, ensuring affordability for specialty medications for Medicare patients is particularly challenging. Medicare patients will have a varying amount of financial responsibility based on the phase of coverage they are in at the time of the medication request. Essentially, there are 4 phases of coverage for Medicare Prescription Drug Benefit plans (Part D): deductible phase, initial coverage period, coverage gap, and catastrophic coverage. In simple terms, the out-of-pocket patient responsibility is lowest during the last phase of coverage, catastrophic coverage phase. During catastrophic coverage, patients are held responsible to pay 5% of their medication costs. While this may seem like a reasonable amount, in the context of specialty medications, this 5% can translate to a patient's responsibility ranging from $500 to $1500 per refill, depending on the medication and dose prescribed. This out-of-pocket expense is not affordable for most patients and warrants the need for active nonprofit foundations as well as reliable financial assistance programs for patients with IBD.

Table 24-2 introduces common nonprofit foundations that are intermittently open for patients with IBD. Funding provided to these foundations is relatively minimal, so coverage through such avenues may not be consistent throughout the year. Additionally, the application process is very time sensitive as the window of opportunity is short and competitive. Manufacturer-based PAPs, however, are more robust in nature and provide consistency in financial assistance for patients who

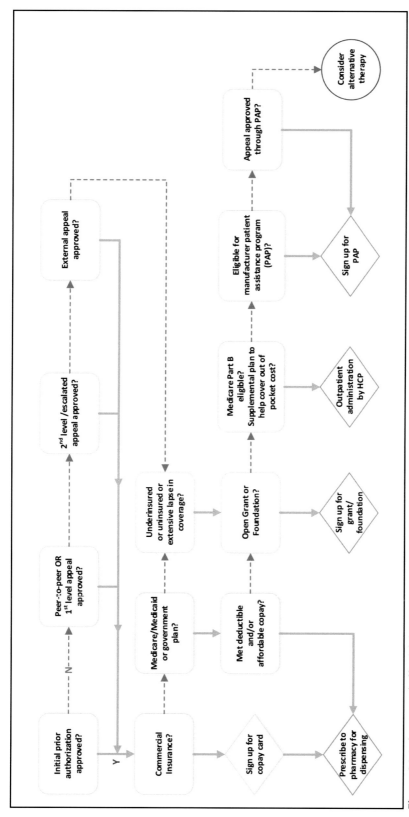

Figure 24-1. Access and affordability pathway. Start at step 1 at the top left corner. Horizontal progression, depicted by dotted lines, represents a "no" answer to the question in each square box. Vertical progression, depicted by solid lines, represents a "yes" answer to each question. Action items in the bottom row are optimal coverage plans for each unique situation.

Table 24-1
Copay Savings Card Programs

Medication	Website
Adalimumab	Humira Complete program https://www.humira.com/humira-complete/sign-up
Golimumab **Ustekinumab** **Infliximab**	Janssen CarePath https://www.myjanssencarepath.com/s/login/SelfRegister
Certolizumab pegol	Cimplicity Support program https://www.cimzia.com/signup#begin-signup
Vedolizumab	EntyvioConnect https://www.entyvio.com/financial-assistance
Infliximab-abda	Merck Copay Assistance program https://www.merckaccessprogram-renflexis.com/hcc/infusion-copay-cost-assistance/
Infliximab-dyyb	Pfizer enCompass Assistance program https://www.pfizerpro.com/product/inflectra/hcp/support/reimbursement-and-support
Tofacitinib	Copay savings card https://uc.xeljanz.com/sign-up

are eligible for coverage. Table 24-3 lists some common PAPs that can be utilized for patients who cannot afford their medications otherwise. This may include uninsured patients, underinsured patients, Medicare patients who cannot afford their copays, as well as patients who are facing a lapse in coverage due to unemployment. All PAPs have varying eligibility criteria, often involving financial eligibility through proof of income and household size. It is important for providers and care teams to be familiar with such criteria so that eligible patients can be routed to the appropriate channel for coverage in a timely manner, thus preventing further delays in therapy. In some cases, if patients are just above the eligibility criteria and denied financial assistance, it may be worthwhile to discuss the patient's unique situation with the manufacturer's assistance program and request reconsideration. If access and affordability cannot be secured by any means, it should be our responsibility as the care team to recommend the next best therapeutic alternative for the patient and follow up with the requirements for that regimen.

Given the nuances and intricacies of this process, having a dedicated care team that is specialized to undertake these responsibilities will lead to high success rates as well as higher patient satisfaction. Integrated specialty pharmacists working in collaboration with the multidisciplinary care team are well equipped to assist in this process. Pharmacists can also lead patient education initiatives, ongoing monitoring efforts, as well as side effect management for specialty medications and other complex therapeutic regimens. In the setting of increased specialty medication prescrib-

Table 24-2
Foundations Available for Patients With IBD

Foundation	Website
NeedyMeds	https://www.needymeds.org/
HealthWell	https://www.healthwellfoundation.org/patients/
Patient Advocate Foundation (CD)	http://www.patientadvocate.org/index.php
Chronic Disease Fund/Good Days (CD)	https://www.mygooddays.org/for-patients/patient-assistance/
Patient Access Network Foundation (IBD)	https://panfoundation.org/index.php/en/
National Organization for Rare Disorders (IBD)	https://rarediseases.org/
The Assistance Fund	https://tafcares.org/

ing, payer restrictions or requirements, and increased costs, it is in the interest of health systems to establish specialty pharmacies. In 2015, the University of Illinois Hospital and Health Sciences System (UI Health) described a clinical practice model in which a pharmacist was integrated into the outpatient gastroenterology clinic, working both in the clinic as well as the specialty pharmacy call center.[2] The role of the pharmacist was to improve the continuity of care by addressing gaps in the medication use process, with a goal of improving patient medication access and becoming part of the care team.

With the clinical practice model described by UI Health, pharmacists are able to ensure appropriate medication selection and monitoring, solve medication-related insurance coverage issues, provide patient medication education, screen for vaccinations, and optimize medication adherence. This delegation of tasks reduces a provider's time spent on medication-related issues and allows for more time spent engaging in direct patient care. Specialty pharmacies also often offer the additional benefits of refill reminders, direct communication with providers, same-day or next-day home delivery services, and regular adherence and/or tolerability assessments. Consequently, the demand for specialty pharmacy services and integration of pharmacists into IBD care teams has markedly increased in recent years.

Although many of us manage IBD on a regular basis and are familiar with the challenges our patients face, health care policy decisions are ultimately in the hands of federal, state, and local government officials. As a result, it is important to make the voices of patients with IBD, family members, caregivers, friends, and providers heard by advocating for particular policies impacting those with IBD and taking action to invoke change. Advocacy is a major component of the Crohn's and Colitis Foundation mission statement. In 2018, the Crohn's and Colitis Foundation public policy priorities included improved patient access to care, increased research funding, and increased membership of the Congressional Crohn's and Colitis Caucus.[3] The foundation has developed an advocacy network to help volunteers get involved via monthly action alerts, training opportunities, and legislative updates.[3]

Table 24-3
Manufacturer Patient Assistance Programs

Medication	Website/Phone
Adalimumab	Abbvie Patient Assistance Foundation https://www.abbvie.com/patients/patient-assistance.html
Golimumab **Ustekinumab** **Infliximab**	Johnson & Johnson Patient Assistance Foundation http://www.jjpaf.org/resources/jjpaf-application.pdf
Certolizumab pegol	UCB Patient Assistance Foundation 1-866-395-8366 (option 4)
Vedolizumab	EntyvioConnect PAP https://www.entyvio.com/financial-assistance
Infliximab-abda	Merck PAP https://www.merckaccessprogram-renflexis.com/hcc /merck-patient-assistance/
Infliximab-dyyb	Pfizer PAP https://www.pfizerencompassresources.com/sites/ default/files/ifa-pfizer_patient_assistance_program_ application_for-pfizer_encompass_patients.pdf
Tofacitinib	Pfizer PAP (XelSource) https://www.xeljanzhcp.com/xelsource

One example of national legislation supported by the Crohn's and Colitis Foundation that addresses barriers in the current medication approval process is bill H.R. 2077, Restoring the Patient's Voice Act of 2017.[4] This bill was introduced to the House of Representatives on April 6, 2017, and amends the Employee Retirement Income Security Act of 1974 (ERISA) to apply patient protections into step-therapy protocols.[5] Bill H.R. 2077 requires payers to implement a clear process for requesting an exception to step therapy and makes the process readily available online. It also establishes a timeline for payer responses to requests: 3 days after receipt of a non-urgent request and 24 hours after the receipt of an urgent request.[5] It is easy to see the positive impact this legislation will have on medication access, as most providers and patients have likely dealt with therapy delays as a result of denials in favor of payer-preferred medications.

References

1. Rubin DT, Feld LD, Goeppinger BS, et al. The Crohn's and Colitis Foundation of America Survey of Inflammatory Bowel Disease Patient Health Care Access. *Inflamm Bowel Dis*. 2017;23(2):224-232.
2. Bhat S, Khamo N, Abdou S, et al. The pharmacist's role in biologic management for IBD in a health system—integrated practice model. *Am J Pharm Benefits*. 2015;7(5):215-220.
3. 2018 advocacy roadmap. Crohn's and Colitis Foundation. Accessed December 6, 2019. https://www.crohnscolitisfoundation.org/sites/default/files/2020-01/2020%20Advocacy%20Roadmap.pdf
4. Co-sponsor HR 2077: Restoring the Patient's Voice Act. Crohn's and Colitis Foundation. Accessed November 15, 2018. https://www.congress.gov/bill/115th-congress/house-bill/2077
5. H.R.2077—Restoring the Patient's Voice Act of 2017. Congressional Research Service of the Library of Congress. https://www.congress.gov/bill/115th-congress/house-bill/2077, accessed November 15, 2018.

SECTION III

ALTERNATIVE TREATMENTS

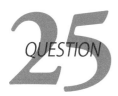

WHAT IS THE ROLE OF PROBIOTICS FOR PATIENTS WITH IBD?

Kerri Glassner, DO and Bincy P. Abraham, MD, MS

As the use of probiotics continues to increase in popularity, it is not uncommon to encounter a patient or family member inquiring about the efficacy of probiotics for inflammatory bowel disease (IBD). In recent years probiotics have gained considerable media attention and can be easily obtained from the local grocery store, pharmacy, or internet. Physicians frequently treat patients with IBD with probiotics as an adjunct to standard IBD therapy. However, despite the widespread use and popularity of probiotics, the supporting evidence is rather limited.

Probiotics are live microorganisms that when administered in sufficient amounts alter the microflora and provide a health benefit to the host. Many probiotics are derived from the normal microflora in the healthy human gut. There is evidence to suggest that probiotics have anti-inflammatory effects, restore barrier function in the gastrointestinal tract, and modulate the composition of the microbiota.[1] These mechanisms of action are relevant in IBD where the gut microbiome and its interactions with the host immune system are thought to play a significant role in disease pathogenesis.

Quality and safety are 2 important factors to consider prior to recommending the use of probiotics for patients. Despite being marketed as equivalent, different brands of probiotics vary significantly in composition and interaction with the host. In order to exert an effect in the desired location, probiotics must survive their journey through the upper gastrointestinal tract. This means coming into contact with stomach acid, bile, and digestive enzymes. In addition, probiotics must remain viable up to the time of administration. Many products being marketed have never been clinically evaluated, with claims of efficacy based on data from studies performed using different probiotic strains. The good news is that probiotics have so far been found to be safe when used in patients with IBD, a population theoretically at higher risk for infection and sepsis due to

Rubin DT, Friedman S, Farraye FA, eds. *Curbside Consultation in IBD: 49 Clinical Questions, Third Edition* (pp 143-147).
© 2022 Taylor & Francis Group.

immunosuppression and compromised mucosal barrier integrity. However, it must be noted that probiotic strains typically do not colonize the adult colon, and indefinite use is required for an ongoing effect. Long-term maintenance studies in IBD assessing efficacy and safety are needed.

There are several things that must be kept in mind when considering the use of probiotics for patients with IBD:

- All randomized controlled trials (RCTs) have included diverse species and strains, which should not be considered equivalent and cannot be compared across trials.
- IBD can be quite variable in regard to each individual's specific disease course, manifestations, and response to therapy. Two patients with IBD may respond completely differently to the same probiotic.
- It should also be noted that many studies have not controlled for confounding factors such as diet and concomitant medications, which are known to alter the microbial composition of the gut.
- The study quality of most of the RCTs is low.

We will discuss the clinical utility of probiotics in patients with Crohn's disease (CD), ulcerative colitis (UC), and pouchitis in the following sections.

Crohn's Disease: Induction of Remission

Very few studies have been performed to evaluate the efficacy of probiotics in the induction of remission in patients with CD. Two open-label studies showed improvement in Crohn's Disease Activity Index scores. However, these studies included a total of only 14 patients, and varying species were used including *Lactobacillus rhamnosus* GG in one study and a combination of *Lactobacillus* and *Bifidobacterium* in the other study.[1] A placebo-controlled trial of 11 patients who initially received concurrent antibiotic and steroid therapy for a week, and then were randomized to placebo or *Lactobacillus* GG, showed no benefit in inducing remission, with only 5 of 11 patients completing the study.[1]

Crohn's Disease: Maintenance of Remission

A study using *Lactobacillus rhamnosus* GG in children showed no benefit compared with placebo and was terminated early due to lack of efficacy and difficulty in recruitment.[2] In a large study looking at the recurrence of CD after surgery, VSL#3, a combination of *Streptococcus thermophilus*, *Bifidobacterium breve*, *Bifidobacterium longum*, *Bifidobacterium infantis*, *Lactobacillus acidophilus*, *Lactobacillus plantarum*, *Lactobacillus paracasei*, and *Lactobacillus delbrueckii subsp. bulgaricus*, showed no difference in endoscopic relapse rates 90 days after surgery compared to placebo.[3] However, there was a lower rate of recurrence and mucosal levels of inflammatory cytokines among patients who received VSL#3 for 1 year, suggesting that there might be some efficacy when continued for a longer period of time. In a randomized trial of 165 patients with CD who achieved remission on steroids or salicylates, *Saccharomyces boulardii* did not reduce recurrence rates after 52 weeks.[4] *Lactobacillus johnsonii* and *Escherichia coli Nissle 1917* also failed to show any impact on remission rates in other studies.[5,6]

Currently, the available data do not support the use of probiotics in patients with CD. Very few studies have been conducted, and of these the study sizes were quite small. The data from these trials have not shown significant efficacy for probiotic use in CD.

Ulcerative Colitis: Induction of Remission

A Cochrane review of *Saccharomyces boulardii* and VSL#3 for mild to moderate UC in 244 patients, in combination with conventional therapy, did not increase remission rates but did provide a modest benefit in terms of reducing disease activity.[7] Another study similarly found no difference in VSL#3 compared to placebo based on endoscopic scores and physician global assessment.[8] Conversely, a study of VSL#3 in addition to standard therapy with aminosalicylates or thiopurines was found to increase remission rates and mucosal healing at 12 weeks.[9] Remission was defined as reduction in the Ulcerative Colitis Disease Activity Index (UCDAI) score by more than 50%, and mucosal healing as a subscore of 0 or 1 in the sigmoidoscopy activity score of the UCDAI. This study was limited by the short duration and large dropout rate in the placebo group. An RCT of 29 children with newly diagnosed UC followed for 1 year found that VSL#3, in addition to steroids and 5-aminosalicylic acid, resulted in a remission rate of 93% compared to 36% in those treated with standard therapy plus placebo.[10]

A Japanese RCT of 20 patients with mild to moderate UC treated with a bifidobacteria-fermented milk containing *Bifidobacterium* strains and *Lactobacillus acidophilus* showed a significant reduction in endoscopic and histologic scores compared with patients who received a placebo.[11] Surprisingly, a study performed in Denmark of 100 patients with active UC randomized to ciprofloxacin or placebo for 1 week followed by *Escherichia coli Nissle* vs placebo for 7 weeks found that fewer patients on the probiotic achieved clinical remission.[12] In addition, the probiotic group had the largest number of withdrawals from the trial. This suggests that certain bacterial strains may actually be harmful for patients with IBD.

Rectal administration of probiotics for UC has also been investigated. Administration of *Escherichia coli Nissle 1917* rectally for proctitis or proctosigmoiditis did not show benefit compared to placebo.[13] However, an RCT of 40 children with mild to moderate UC confined to the rectum or sigmoid colon compared *Lactobacillus reuteri* ATCC 55730 administered as an enema with mesalamine to placebo plus mesalamine.[14] All patients in the probiotic group had a clinical response, and 31% reached remission, compared to a 53% response and 0% remission in the placebo group. Clinical response was defined as Mayo Disease Activity Index reduction of ≥ 2, and remission as a score of < 2.0. Only 31 patients completed the study due to lack of compliance with rectal enema administration, and the follow-up duration was only 8 weeks.

Ulcerative Colitis: Maintenance of Remission

Several controlled trials using *Escherichia coli Nissle 1917*, *Saccharomyces boulardii*, *Bifidobacterium breve*, and *Bifidobacterium bifidum* strains Yakult in the maintenance of remission for patients with mild to moderate UC have shown similar efficacy and safety compared to standard 5-aminosalicyclic acid regimens.[1] Three RCTs using *Escherichia coli Nissle 1917* found the probiotic to be as effective as low-dose mesalamine in maintaining remission based on histology, endoscopy, or quality of life.[1,15] Conversely, an open-label RCT comparing *Lactobacillus GG* alone and the combination of *Lactobacillus GG* and mesalamine failed to show any difference in relapse or adverse event rates between the 3 groups over a 12-month period based on UCDAI scores.[16] In children, some small studies have shown VSL#3 to be effective in maintenance of remission. The addition of VSL#3 to standard therapy decreased relapse rates (21.4% vs 73.3%) compared with placebo.[10] An open label study of 18 children with UC reported improvement in Mayo endoscopic score, inflammatory markers, and a clinical remission rate of 56% after 8 weeks of VSL#3 in addition to standard treatment.[17] Remission was defined as a simple clinical colitis activity score ≤ 3. There were several limiting factors, including lack of a placebo, small study size, short duration of follow-up, and withdrawal of 5 patients due to lack of response.

The outcomes of probiotic use in UC have been inconsistent. The current evidence suggests a trend toward the efficacy of probiotics in the induction and maintenance of remission in patients with mild to moderate UC, in particular VSL#3 in children. However, individual probiotic strains have significantly varied in efficacy. In general, the outcomes of these studies suggest that probiotics may be beneficial for mild disease, since most trials compared probiotic efficacy with low-dose mesalamine therapy.

Pouchitis

Pouchitis is a common problem after ileal pouch–anal anastomosis (IPAA) in patients with UC. Pouchitis, or inflammation within the ileal reservoir, is a process that leads to symptoms of urgency, increased frequency of bowel movements, and abdominal pain. Previous studies have shown that up to 60% of patients with IBD develop pouchitis at some time after IPAA creation. The fact that patients respond to antibiotics for treatment of pouchitis is suggestive that the microbiome may contribute to the development of pouchitis.

Several studies looking at the efficacy of *Lactobacillus*, *Bifidobacterium*, and *Clostridium butyricum* in the primary prevention of pouchitis did not show benefit.[1] Another small study evaluating the use of *Lactobacillus GG* in acute pouchitis found that although the probiotic was shown to alter pouch flora, there was no symptomatic or endoscopic improvement compared to placebo.[1] However, a study of 40 patients randomized to VSL#3 or placebo immediately after IPAA, and followed for 1 year, found that VSL#3 was effective when used as prophylactic therapy for the primary prevention of pouchitis.[18] Only 10% of patients treated with VSL#3 had an episode of acute pouchitis compared with 40% treated with placebo.

VSL#3 has been found to be superior to placebo in maintaining remission in patients who had been successfully treated with antibiotics for pouchitis. Sustained remission was observed in 85% of those treated with VSL#3 compared to 0% to 6% of placebo in 2 RCTs.[19,20] The administration of VSL#3 has been associated with a reduction in pro-inflammatory mediators, an increase in regulatory T cells in the enteric mucosa, an improved barrier function of the gut lumen, and an increase in intestinal bacterial diversity.[1]

Current evidence is suggestive that probiotics may be effective in the primary prevention of pouchitis, and maintenance of remission after successful antibiotic therapy for pouchitis, but does not support use in the induction of remission. All of the studies had limitations, including short duration, small study size, and varied probiotic dosing.

Conclusion

The strongest data to support the use of probiotics are in pouchitis, particularly with VSL#3, as there is a trend toward efficacy for the primary prevention of pouchitis after IPAA, and maintenance of remission after successful treatment for pouchitis. There are moderate and inconsistent data for use in UC with the strongest evidence in mild disease, and there is very little evidence of effectiveness in CD. The supporting data have many limitations, including the wide variety of species and strains used, confounding factors such as concomitant medications (antibiotics, proton pump inhibitors, and anti-diarrheals), diet, and small study size. There are significant concerns related to the clinical efficacy, composition, and bacterial viability of many probiotics. Due to these limitations, there are currently insufficient data to support definite recommendations on the routine use of probiotics in patients with IBD, especially in those with CD.

References

1. Abraham B, Quigley E. Probiotics in inflammatory bowel disease. *Gastroenterol Clin N Am*. 2017:46(4):769-82.
2. Bousvaros A, Guandalini S, Baldassano RN, et al. A randomized, double-blind trial of *Lactobacillus GG* versus placebo in addition to standard maintenance therapy for children with Crohn's disease. *Inflamm Bowel Dis*. 2005;11(9):833-839.
3. Fedorak RN, Feagan BG, Hotte N, et al. The probiotic VSL#3 has anti-inflammatory effects and could reduce endoscopic recurrence after surgery for Crohn's disease. *Clin Gastroenterol Hepatol*. 2015;13(5):928-935.
4. Bourreille A, Cadiot G, Le Dreau G, et al. *Saccharomyces boulardii* does not prevent relapse of Crohn's disease. *Clin Gastroenterol Hepatol*. 2013;11(8):982-987.
5. Marteau P, Lemann M, Seksik P, et al. Ineffectiveness of *Lactobacillus johnsonii* LA1 for prophylaxis of postoperative recurrences in Crohn's disease: a randomized, double blind, placebo controlled GETAID trial. *Gut*. 2006;55(6): 842-847.
6. Van Gossum A, Dewit O, Louis E, et al. Multicenter randomized-controlled clinical trial of probiotics (*Lactobacillus johnsonii*, LA1) on early endoscopic recurrence of Crohn's disease after ileo-cecal resection. *Inflamm Bowel Dis*. 2007;13(2):135-142.
7. Mallon P, McKay D, Kirk S, et al. Probiotics for induction of remission in ulcerative colitis. *Cochrane Database Syst Rev*. 2007;(4):CD005573.
8. Tursi A, Brandimarte G, Papa A, et al. Treatment of relapsing mild-to-moderate ulcerative colitis with the probiotic VSL#3 as adjunctive to a standard pharmaceutical treatment: a double-blind, randomized, placebo-controlled study. *Am J Gastroenterol*. 2010;105(10):2218-2227.
9. Sood A, Midha V, Makharia GK, et al. The probiotic preparation, VSL#3 induces remission in patients with mild-to-moderately active ulcerative colitis. *Clin Gastroenterol Hepatol*. 2009;7(11):1202-1209.
10. Miele E, Pascarella F, Giannetti E, et al. Effect of a probiotic preparation (VSL#3) on induction and maintenance of remission in children with ulcerative colitis. *Am J Gastroenterol*. 2009;104(2):437-443.
11. Kato K, Mizuno S, Umesaki Y, et al. Randomized placebo-controlled trial assessing the effect of bifidobacteria-fermented milk on active ulcerative colitis. *Aliment Pharmacol Ther*. 2004;20(10):1133-1141.
12. Petersen A, Mirsepasi H, Halkjaer S, et al. Ciprofloxacin and probiotic *Escherichia coli Nissle* add-on treatment in active ulcerative colitis: a double-blind randomized placebo controlled clinical trial. *J Crohns Colitis*. 2014;8(11):1498-1505.
13. Matthes H, Krummenerl T, Giensch M, et al. Clinical trial: probiotic treatment of acute distal ulcerative colitis with rectally administered *Escherichia coli Nissle* 1917 (EcN). *BMC Complement Altern Med*. 2010;10:13.
14. Oliva S, Di Nardo G, Ferrari F, et al. Randomized clinical trial: the effectiveness of *Lactobacillus reuteri* ATCC 55730 rectal enema in children with active distal ulcerative colitis. *Aliment Pharmacol Ther*. 2012;35(3):327-334.
15. Rembacken BJ, Snelling AM, Hawkey PM, et al. Non-pathogenic *Escherichia coli* versus mesalazine for the treatment of ulcerative colitis: a randomized trial. *Lancet*. 1999;354(9179):635-639.
16. Zocco MA, dal Verme LZ, Cremonini F, et al. Efficacy of *Lactobacillus GG* in maintaining remission of ulcerative colitis. *Aliment Pharmacol Ther*. 2006;23(11):1567-1574.
17. Huynh HQ, deBruyn J, Guan L, et al. Probiotic preparation VSL#3 induces remission in children with mild to moderate acute ulcerative colitis: a pilot study. *Inflamm Bowel Dis*. 2009;15(5):760-768.
18. Gionchetti P, Rizzello F, Helwig U, et al. Prophylaxis of pouchitis onset with probiotic therapy: a double-blind, placebo-controlled trial. *Gastroenterology*. 2003;124(5):1202-1209.
19. Gionchetti P, Rizzelo F, Venturi A, et al. Oral bacteriotherapy as maintenance treatment in patients with chronic pouchitis: a double-blind, placebo-controlled trial. *Gastroenterology*. 2000;119(2):305-309.
20. Mimura T, Rizzello F, Helwig U, et al. Once daily high dose probiotic therapy (VSL#3) for maintaining remission in recurrent or refractory pouchitis. *Gut*. 2004;53(1):108-114.

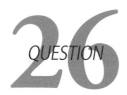

WHAT DO I TELL MY PATIENT WITH IBD WHO IS ASKING ABOUT CANNABIS AS THERAPY?

Jami Kinnucan, MD and Arun Swaminath, MD

Cannabis, colloquially referred to as marijuana, has become an increasingly frequent topic of discussion between patients with inflammatory bowel disease (IBD) and their providers in recent years. Cannabis has been classified into the category of complementary therapies, but unlike traditional complementary therapies, there are more robust data on the clinical effects in human disease states. Multiple studies have shown a high prevalence of cannabis use in IBD. In Canada, prior to national legalization in October 2018, up to 50% of patients with IBD reported current or past cannabis use to relieve abdominal pain or diarrhea and to improve appetite.[1] In the United States, data from 2013 showed 12% of patients with IBD report current use, with up to 40% with prior use.[2] One US-based study showed doubling rates of cannabis use in patients with IBD from 2012 to 2017, a period when cannabis decriminalization was widely adopted in the United States; however, the increased use appeared to wholly be for recreational use among patients with IBD.[3] A recent survey in pediatric patients (18 to 21 years old) showed 70% of pediatric IBD patients have used cannabis, and the majority (70%) of these patients did not discuss use with their provider.[4] It is important to recognize that a large fraction of patients with IBD are using or have used cannabis to treat IBD-related symptoms. As a provider, it is essential to not only ask your patient about cannabis use but to be prepared for the discussion. Following is an overview of cannabis and its potential application in patients with IBD.

Rubin DT, Friedman S, Farraye FA, eds. *Curbside Consultation in IBD: 49 Clinical Questions, Third Edition* (pp 149-155).
© 2022 Taylor & Francis Group.

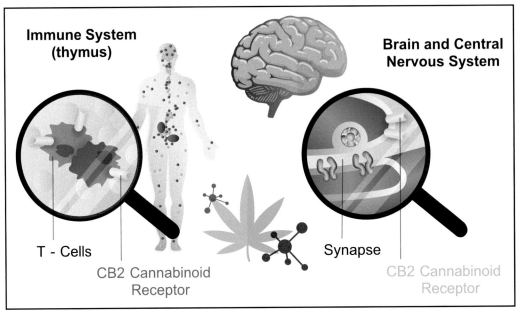

Figure 26-1. Cannabinoid receptors in the endocannabinoid system. (iStock.com.)

Cannabis Definition

Cannabis sativa (cannabis) is composed of hundreds of chemical compounds, with more than 60 phytocannabinoids (plant-based cannabinoids).[5] The most well-known cannabinoids are Δ-9-tetrhydrocannabinol (THC), thought to account for the psychoactive properties of cannabis, and cannabidiol (CBD), promoted for anti-inflammatory and immunomodulatory effects. Cannabinoids act at the endocannabinoid system (ECS), which consists of multiple receptors. CB1 receptors are highly expressed in the brain, and nervous system cells and are mainly activated by THC with weak activation by CBD. CBD may also prolong the effect of other endogenous cannabinoids. This interaction between THC and CB1 receptors in the brain is thought to contribute to the psychoactive effects of cannabis. On the other hand, CB2 receptors are absent in the brain and highly expressed in immune cells and are weakly activated by CBD. CBD is also thought to modulate the effects of THC modulation at CB1 receptor. However, CBD mainly acts through other cannabinoid receptors[6,7] (Figure 26-1). Numerous animal models of colitis have found that inflammation can be improved by modulating cannabinoid receptors.[8,9]

Cannabis Administration

Currently, cannabis comes in various formulations (% THC component) and routes of administration. The most common routes of administration are inhalation and ingestion. Inhalation can occur through cannabis wrapped in tobacco paper (cigarettes, cigars, pipes, "blunt") or vaporizer, vaping, and water pipes. Oral ingestion can occur through mixing cannabis (leaf, hashish, oil) into foods, teas, pills, or lozenges. The studies of cannabis in IBD have looked at varying doses in varying routes of administration and THC/CBD composition, making it difficult to translate into real-world use for some patients.

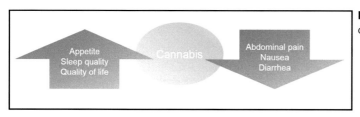

Figure 26-2. The clinical effects of cannabis in IBD.

Clinical Effects of Cannabis

The effects of cannabis have been well studied in multiple medical conditions, though prospective randomized data in IBD are limited. The most robust data for clinical use of cannabis has been done for chronic neuropathic pain and spasticity in multiple sclerosis. While it has been studied in IBD, the majority of the studies have been retrospective or observational in nature. Cannabis is currently classified as a Controlled Substance Act (CSA) schedule I drug, making it federally illegal to possess or sell. This has made cannabis difficult to study in the United States.

Human Data in Patients With IBD

Retrospective studies have identified the symptoms patients with IBD seek to mitigate with cannabis use. Patients reported improvement in pain (75% to 95%), diarrhea (29% to 85%), appetite (70% to 100%), nausea (46% to 86%), and joint pain (48%)[1,2,4,10] (Figure 26-2). While the reported effects are promising, there is a large effect size. The data lack control, and blinding and patient-reported symptom improvement is prone to significant recall bias as patients who have reported clinical benefits are more likely to be ongoing cannabis users.

CROHN'S DISEASE

To date there have been 2 prospective randomized studies assessing the effects of cannabis in Crohn's disease (CD). The first study was done by Naftali et al in Israel in 2013. They assessed the effects of cannabis in 21 patients (11 cannabis, 10 placebo) with moderate disease activity, many intolerant or primary anti–tumor necrosis factor nonresponders and all naive to cannabis use. Participants either smoked 2 cannabis (THC-containing) cigarettes per day or placebo for 8 weeks, and the primary outcome was clinical remission at 8 weeks, defined as Crohn's Disease Activity Index (CDAI) < 150. While it failed to meet the primary end point, 45% in cannabis group and 10% placebo group achieved CDAI < 150. In addition, 90% in the cannabis group and 40% in the placebo group had clinical response (CDAI Δ 100; P = .03). All patients were able to stop corticosteroid therapy, and there was a trend toward improved quality-of-life scores. However, there were no differences in hemoglobin or C-reactive protein (CRP). In addition, all patients had relapse of clinical symptoms within 2 weeks of discontinuation. The authors acknowledge limitation of true "blinding" due to psychotropic effects of THC.[11]

A follow-up study done by the same group assessed low dose-CBD in 19 medically refractory CD patients. Participants either used sublingual 10 mg CBD (no THC) or placebo for 8 weeks, and the primary outcome was clinical response (CDAI Δ 70). After 8 weeks there were no differences in CDAI scores nor laboratory parameters (blood counts, liver, or kidney function). There were no adverse events in either group, suggesting tolerability of the compound. Although it was a negative study, the low dose of CBD (10 mg compared to higher doses studied in other medical conditions), route of administration, and single cannabinoid compound might have limited the degree of clinical improvement in this small study.[12]

The following year Naftali et al presented data for use of 15% CBD: 4% THC cannabis oil in 46 patients with moderate to severe CD. They assessed cannabis oil or placebo for 8 weeks, and outcomes assessed were clinical response (CDAI), quality of life, and simple endoscopic score for CD (SES-CD). The cannabis group experienced clinical response (reduced CDAI, $P < .05$), clinical remission (65% vs 35%; $P < .05$), and improvement in quality-of-life score ($P < .05$). However, there was no change in CRP, fecal calprotectin, or SES-CD score between the groups.[13]

ULCERATIVE COLITIS

There have been 2 studies looking at the effects of cannabis in patients with ulcerative colitis (UC). The first study was the largest prospective randomized study looking at cannabis in patients with IBD to date. Irving et al assessed the efficacy and safety of once-daily oral CBD-THC 4.7% (CBD-rich extract) in 60 patients as adjuvant therapy while on stable mesalamine dosing for 10 weeks, the primary end point being clinical remission (partial Mayo score). The study had significant protocol deviation as patients were less tolerant to CBD-rich extract when compared to placebo. There were no differences in the rates of remission (28% for CBD-rich extract vs 26% for placebo). Per-protocol analysis showed improvement in partial Mayo score ($P = .038$) and a trend toward improvement in quality-of-life scores.[14] Naftali et al presented their data assessing the effects of THC cigarettes (2/day) for 8 weeks in 28 patients with UC with primary outcome assessment of clinical response (Disease Activity Index [DAI]) at the European Crohn's and Colitis Organisation annual meeting in early 2018. There was a statistically significant improvement in clinical response (DAI) over placebo; however, the placebo group also experienced clinical response. There was no change in CRP or fecal calprotectin between the 2 groups. There was endoscopic improvement (Mayo score 2 to Mayo score 1) in the cannabis group that was reported in this study. The cannabis group was more likely to experience increased memory impairment and dizziness.[15] To summarize, the theme of the human data to date appears to be improved symptom control without significant evidence of improvement in underlying inflammation. These studies are summarized in Table 26-1.

Risks of Cannabis Use in IBD

Given the low numbers of patients enrolled in IBD-specific randomized controlled trials (n = 128), the risks associated with cannabis use have mainly been reported in general population–based studies. In a large study looking at cannabis use in all patients, regular use was associated with risk for addiction to other controlled substances; abnormal brain development in youth; development of schizophrenia, anxiety, or depression; diminished life achievement; increased risk for motor vehicle accidents; chronic bronchitis; lung cancer; and cannabis hyperemesis syndrome.[16] Anecdotally, both authors have noted an uptick in the frequency of cannabis-related adverse events, specifically with cannabis hyperemesis syndrome, which may be confused with an IBD-related disease activity. The Centers for Disease Control and Prevention has recently identified that vitamin E acetate, sometimes used in THC-containing e-cigarette or vaping products, may be responsible for cases of acute lung injury.[17] Hence, we have counseled against this form of administration in our patient population.

In a few IBD studies the risks are more concerning. IBD cannabis users were more likely to stop conventional medical therapy[17] and significantly more likely to require surgery than IBD non-cannabis users.[1] The discontinuation of conventional medical therapy is known to be associated with increased risk for disease relapse, steroid requirement, and surgery.[18,19]

<u>Table 26-1</u>
Randomized Controlled Trials in Crohn's Disease and Ulcerative Colitis

Crohn's Disease

Author (Year)	Trial Design Participants	Intervention Primary Outcome	Results
Naftali (2013)	RCT x 8 weeks 21 patients*	2 THC cigs/day Clinical remission (CDAI < 150)	No difference in clinical remission Improvement CDAI (ns) No change HgB, CRP Increased QOL ($P = .05$)
Naftali (2017)	RCT x 8 weeks 19 patients*	10 mg CBD oil (SL) Clinical response (CDAI ↓ 70 pts)	No difference in clinical response
Naftali (2018 UEG)	RCT x 8 weeks 46 patients*	15% CBD; 4% THC cannabis oil Clinical response, clinical remission, QOL, SES-CD	Clinical response/remission (ss) Improved QOL (ss) No improvement CRP, FCP, SES-CD

Ulcerative Colitis

Irving (2018)	RCT x 10 weeks 60 patients**	CBD/THC 4.7% oral Clinical remission (Mayo score)	No improvement in clinical remission Intolerance in treatment group
Naftali (2018 ECCO)	RCT x 8 weeks 28 patients*	2 THC cigs/day Clinical response (Lichtiger score)	Improved clinical response (ss) Improved endoscopic score (ss) Increase memory issues, dizziness

CBD = cannabis oil; CDAI = Crohn's Disease Activity Index; Cigs = cigarettes; CRP = C-reactive protein; FCP = fecal calprotectin; HgB = hemoglobin; QOL = quality of life; SES-CD = simple endoscopic score CD; SL = sublingual; Ns = not significant; ss = statistically significant; THC = Δ-9-tetrhydrocannabinol.

*All patients continued on prior therapy with 5-aminosalicylates (5-ASA), immunomodulatory, or anti-TNF.

**All patients continued on prior 5-ASA therapy.

Legal and Personal Implications Patients Must Consider When Using Cannabis

As of December 1, 2018, there are currently 33 states and the District of Columbia that have comprehensive medicinal cannabis programs; 10 of those states and the District of Columbia have additional recreational use legalization. An additional 13 states have approved a low THC/high CBD program for medical use.[20] Despite state legislation changes, cannabis is still considered a schedule I substance through the federal CSA, which should be taken into account for potential cannabis users. Patients have to consider the legal implications (potential risk for federal prosecution) in addition to employment, school, camp, or travel regulations when planning to use cannabis to treat IBD-related symptoms. Patients should inquire about current employer cannabis policies, though it is not clear if approaching the human resources department and revealing cannabis use is not without risk. We also recommend avoiding cannabis exposure in patients with a history of schizophrenia or patients who anticipate pregnancy, as cannabis can cause paranoia and is known to negatively affect the developing brain. Currently, there are no data focusing on these issues specific to patients with IBD, and there is no vetted centralized repository of this information for patients to turn to. There is little scientific literature that can help guide providers caring for patients with IBD in suggesting dosing, formulation, and management of complications. In reality, this function is filled by the individual dispensary and the pharmacologic expertise available. The Crohn's and Colitis Foundation released a white paper and position statement reviewing the evidence of cannabis in IBD and legal and regulatory issues surrounding cannabis use in IBD.[21]

Conclusion

It is imperative that providers caring for patients with IBD be ready to discuss the potential benefits and risks of cannabis therapy, as it is not uncommon for patients with IBD to inquire about how to incorporate cannabis into their current management strategy to control symptoms. It is also not uncommon for patients to consider cannabis as a primary treatment strategy for their IBD, despite the lack of evidence to support this. It is essential for providers and patients to have an open discussion to ensure appropriate understanding of the current studies and what the data show. While cannabinoids have shown to improve inflammation in animal models, they have failed to show the same in human studies to date. In addition, all studies have looked at cannabis as adjuvant therapy to traditional IBD medical therapy, and no studies have looked at the effects of cannabis alone. It is important for providers to optimize IBD patients' medical therapy to achieve both subjective and objective remission (treat to target); if ongoing clinical symptoms are related to underlying disease activity, this should be addressed first. If patients have persistent clinical symptoms despite adequate disease control, then there might be an adjuvant role for cannabis to their current medical therapy. It is important to emphasize the importance of compliance with their standard IBD therapy. Lastly, it is important to discuss the discordance between state and federal classification of cannabis, and this could result in jeopardy at the workplace or during travel.

References

1. Lal S, Prasad N, Ryan M, et al. Cannabis use amongst patients with inflammatory bowel disease. *Eur J Gastroenterol Hepatol*. 2011;23(10):891-896.
2. Ravikoff Allegretti J, Courtwright A, Lucci M, et al. Marijuana use patterns among patients with inflammatory bowel disease. *Inflamm Bowel Dis*. 2013;19(13):2809-2814.
3. Merker AM, Riaz M, Friedman S, et al. Legalization of medicinal marijuana has minimal impact on use patterns in patients with inflammatory bowel disease. *Inflamm Bowel Dis*. 2018;24(11):2309-2314.
4. Phatak UP, Rojas-Velasquez D, Porto A, Pashankar DS. Prevalence and patterns of marijuana use in young adults with inflammatory bowel disease. *J Pediatr Gastroenterol Nutr*. 2017;64(2):261-264.
5. Turner CE, Bouwsma OJ, Billets S, Elsohly MA. Constituents of cannabis sativa L. XVIII—Electron voltage selected ion monitoring study of cannabinoids. *Biomed Mass Spectrom*. 1980;7(6):247-256.
6. Pisanti S, Bifulco M. Modern history of medical cannabis: from widespread use to prohibitionism and back. *Trends Pharmacol Sci*. 2017;38(3):195-198.
7. Lu Y, Anderson HD. Cannabinoid signaling in health and disease. *Can J Physiol Pharmacol*. 2017;95(4):311-327.
8. Jamontt JM, Molleman A, Pertwee RG, Parsons ME. The effects of Delta-tetrahydrocannabinol and cannabidiol alone and in combination on damage, inflammation and in vitro motility disturbances in rat colitis. *Br J Pharmacol*. 2010;160(3):712-723.
9. Couch DG, Maudslay H, Doleman B, Lund KN, O'Sullivan SE. The use of cannabinoids in colitis: a systematic review and meta-analysis. *Inflamm Bowel Dis*. 2018;24(4):680-697.
10. Storr M, Devlin S, Kaplan GG, Panaccione R, Andrews C. Cannabis use provides symptom relief in patients with inflammatory bowel disease but is associated with worse disease prognosis in patients with Crohn's disease. *Inflamm Bowel Dis*. 2014;20(3):472-480.
11. Naftali T, Schleider LB-L, Dotan I, Lansky EP, Benjaminov SF, Konikoff FM. Cannabis induces a clinical response in patients with Crohn's disease: a prospective placebo-controlled study. *Clin Gastroenterol Hepatol*. 2013;11(10):1276-1280.e1.
12. Naftali T, Mechulam R, Marii A, et al. Low-dose cannabidiol is safe but not effective in the treatment for Crohn's disease, a randomized controlled trial. *Dig Dis Sci*. 2017;62(6):1615-1620.
13. Naftali T, Bar-Lev Schlieder L, Konikoff F, et al. Cannabis induces clinical response but no endoscopic response in Crohn's disease patients. *Unit Euro Gastroenterol J*. 2018;6(1).
14. Irving PM, Iqbal T, Nwokolo C, et al. A randomized, double-blind, placebo-controlled, parallel-group, pilot study of cannabidiol-rich botanical extract in the symptomatic treatment of ulcerative colitis. *Inflamm Bowel Dis*. 2018;24(4):714-724.
15. Solensky R. Drug allergy: desensitization and treatment of reactions to antibiotics and aspirin. In: Lockey P, ed. *Allergens and Allergen Immunotherapy*. 3rd ed. Marcel Dekker; 2004:585-606.
16. Volkow ND, Compton WM, Weiss SW. Adverse health effects of marijuana use. *N Engl J Med*. 2014;371(9):879.
17. Outbreak of lung injury associated with the use of e-cigarette, or vaping, products. Centers for Disease Control and Prevention, November 27, 2020. https://www.cdc.gov/tobacco/basic_information/e-cigarettes/severe-lung-disease.html
18. Naftali T, Lev LB, Yablecovitch D, Half E, Konikoff, FM. Treatment of Crohn's disease with cannabis: an observational study. *Isr Med Assoc J*. 2011;13(8):455-458.
19. Gisbert JP, Marin AC, Chaparro M. Systematic review: factors associated with relapse of inflammatory bowel disease after discontinuation of anti-TNF therapy. *Aliment Pharmacol Ther*. 2015;42(4):391-405.
20. State marijuana laws—US map. Governing. http://www.governing.com/gov-data/state-marijuana-laws-map-medical-recreational.html
21. Swaminath A, Berlin EP, Cheifetz A, et al. The role of cannabis in the management of inflammatory bowel disease: a review of clinical, scientific, and regulatory information. *Inflamm Bowel Dis*. 2018;25(3):427-435.

SECTION IV

SPECIAL POPULATIONS

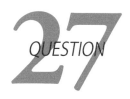

QUESTION

How Do You Treat Pouchitis and What Do You Do for Recurrent or Refractory Pouchitis?

Iris Dotan, MD and Idan Goren, MD

Despite advances in medical therapy of patients with inflammatory bowel diseases (IBD), including ulcerative colitis (UC), especially in the era of biologic therapy, the 10-year risk of colectomy is 7.5% to 10%[1,2] and over time risk is estimated to be as high as 25%.

The surgical treatment of choice for most patients with UC who require colectomy as well as for patients with familial adenomatous polyposis (FAP) is total proctocolectomy with ileal pouch–anal anastomosis (IPAA), commonly referred to as *pouch surgery*. Pouch surgery provides a major benefit compared to permanent ileostomy as it maintains the normal route of defecation and sphincter function, allowing for preserved patient's continence. Importantly, the procedure almost completely reduces the risk for UC-associated neoplasia.

The most common indications for pouch surgery in patients with UC include intractable inflammation refractory to maximal medical treatment, dysplasia, or neoplasia and complications such as hemorrhage, colonic perforation, or bowel obstruction. Rarely, extraintestinal manifestations of UC may be an indication for pouch surgery.

Surgical Technique

Pouch surgery may be done either in an open approach or laparoscopically. The colon and rectum are removed while sparing the pelvic nerves and the anal canal mucosa and sphincter mechanism. The ileal pouch is made of a segment of about 20 cm of the normal terminal ileum. Finally, the ileal reservoir (the pouch) is connected to the dentate line of the anal canal. In most cases, temporary diverting ileostomy is done to protect the anastomosis and is closed later. The

Rubin DT, Friedman S, Farraye FA, eds. *Curbside Consultation in IBD:*
49 Clinical Questions, Third Edition (pp 159-170).
© 2022 Taylor & Francis Group.

traditional 2-stage procedure includes total proctocolectomy with pouch formation and diverting ileostomy, followed by ileostomy closure as a second step. Recently, a modified 2-staged surgery, where subtotal colectomy is performed at a first stage, and completion proctectomy and formation of a pouch without protective ileostomy, thus enabling immediate pouch function, is suggested.[3]

In cases of surgery for severe disease activity, or in cases where the underlying inflammatory disease is unclear (ie, UC or Crohn's disease [CD]), subtotal colectomy and ileostomy may be done as a first stage, followed by a staged completion proctectomy and IPAA formation with protective ileostomy, and concluded by ileostomy closure as a third stage.[4] A single-staged surgery may be done in selected patients, specifically those with FAP.[5]

Normal Pouch

Pouch surgery is associated with significantly improved health-related quality of life, and most patients undergoing pouch surgery report good functional outcomes.[6]

After the first year, postoperatively, and following an adaptation of the ileal content efflux to the pouch, most patients have 5 to 8 bowel movements a day and 1 nocturnal. Full daytime continence for stool and gas is reported in 70% to 79% of patients over 10 years of follow-up, and full overnight continence in 53% to 74%.[7,8] Episodic nocturnal soiling, incontinence, and need for antidiarrheal medications to control bowel activity are relatively common.

How to Diagnose Pouchitis

The diagnosis of pouchitis is based on the combination of typical symptoms and endoscopic and histologic findings. Common symptoms are lower abdominal pain, increased frequency of bowel movements, urgency, and tenesmus. Rectal bleeding may be reported; however, this may also reflect the possibility of inflammation of the rectal cuff (cuffitis), or the rare possibility of dysplastic and neoplastic lesions. Fever, dehydration, and electrolyte imbalance are usually associated with more severe presentation of pouchitis.

Diagnosis cannot be based solely on clinical symptoms because (a) symptoms are often non-specific and may appear in conditions mimicking pouchitis, and (b) symptoms may poorly correlate with the endoscopic and histological findings. A stepwise approach to pouchitis diagnosis may include the following:

1. Stool culture, stool microscopy for parasites, and *Clostridioides difficile* toxin assay may be tested to exclude infectious process, which may resemble pouchitis clinically.

2. Endoscopic evaluation of the pouch is a key next step in diagnosis. Pouch endoscopy (pouchoscopy) should include a careful inspection of the afferent limb, pouch inlet and body, anastomosis, and the rectal cuff/anal transitional zone. Pouchoscopy with biopsies may assist in the differentiation of pouchitis and Crohn's-like disease of the pouch (CLDP) from other conditions. These may include infections and cuffitis, as mentioned. In case no significant inflammation is noticed, other differential diagnoses may be considered, including a more proximal inflammation, small intestinal bacterial overgrowth, or irritable pouch syndrome (IPS), a diagnosis of exclusion when no endoscopic and histologic evidence of inflammation are found. IPS may respond to antidiarrheal, anticholinergic, and antidepressant medications. *Cuffitis*, an inflammatory process recurring in the transitional zone remaining after IPAA and representing residual UC, may respond to topical treatment such as mesalamine suppositories or enemas. If patients with an endoscopically and histologically normal pouch experience an increase in bowel movements, antidiarrheal therapy such as loperamide may be used (loperamide 2 to 8 mg/day). If further treatment in required, specifically in patients

with a relatively new pouch, bile acid sequestrants may be used empirically. Further evaluation for noninflammatory-related causes for diarrhea, such as pancreatic insufficiency and celiac disease, may be warranted.

3. The Pouchitis Disease Activity Index (PDAI)[9] is a scoring system originally used in clinical studies to define pouchitis by incorporating clinical findings with the endoscopic and histologic features of pouchitis (Table 27-1). A PDAI score of $\geq$ 7 is used as the cut-off for the diagnosis of pouchitis. PDAI may be used to assess response to treatment as well. As in other scores of IBD, the PDAI has several disadvantages, specifically, the endoscopic distribution of findings (ie, how to quantitate diffuse disease as opposed to focal); the significance of lesions on suture lines, which may represent local ischemic changes; and the importance of short-segment pre-pouch ileitis. Furthermore, the histologic scoring included in the PDAI focuses on the acute inflammatory component (neutrophils) only, thus overlooking the potential importance of other cells, including eosinophils and the chronic component. Other scoring systems are being evaluated.[10]

How Pouchitis Can Be Classified

Idiopathic pouchitis accounts for the majority of cases and is defined when no specific etiologic factor is identified. Secondary pouchitis is defined when a causative factor, such as infection, use of nonsteroidal anti-inflammatory medications, ischemia, or CD, are identified.

A more common and more practical definition of pouchitis is according to clinical disease behavior over time. Acute pouchitis is defined as an acute flare, responding to short course (usually up to 2 weeks) of antibiotics; recurrent acute pouchitis is defined as up to 4 episodes of acute pouchitis per year; and chronic pouchitis is defined as at least 4 weeks or more of persistent symptoms or chronic antibiotic or anti-inflammatory therapy.[11] CLDP is defined as inflammation of the afferent limb, appearance of proximal small bowel strictures, which is not directly related to the surgical anastomosis, or perianal and abdominal fistulas or abscesses occurring at least a year after ileostomy take down, which are not direct complications of the IPAA surgery itself.

The mainstay treatment of idiopathic pouchitis is a 2-week course of antibiotics, specifically ciprofloxacin or metronidazole. Based on patient response to antibiotics, pouchitis may be defined as *antibiotic responsive*, *antibiotic dependent*, and *antibiotic resistant*. The latter may require a long course of anti-inflammatory medications.

Management of Acute Pouchitis

Episodes of acute pouchitis respond well to antibiotic therapy in the majority of cases. First-line therapy usually consists of a 2-week course of ciprofloxacin (500 mg twice daily), or metronidazole (500 to 1000 mg twice daily). The use of tinidazole (500 mg twice daily) may serve as an alternative in patients intolerant to metronidazole. Use of amoxicillin-clavulanic acid (875 mg twice daily) or doxycycline (100 mg twice daily) may be a reasonable alternative.

In patients who fail an initial antibiotic course, a second, longer course of 4 weeks of combination therapy with ciprofloxacin and metronidazole/tinidazole is a reasonable next step. Mesalamine and budesonide may be used alternatively (Table 27-2).

Failure to respond to antibiotics may raise a possible alternative explanation to patients' symptoms, such as CLDP, surgical complications, and vascular causes. Further evaluation with abdominal and pelvic imaging studies in addition to endoscopic evaluation may be required.

Table 27-1

Pouchitis Disease Activity Index

	Range	Score
A. Clinical		
1. Stool frequency	Usual frequency	0
	1 to 2 stools/day > usual	1
	≥ 3 stools/day > usual	2
2. Fecal urgency/abdominal cramps	None	0
	Occasional	1
	Usual	2
3. Rectal bleeding	None or rare	0
	Present daily	1
4. Fever > 37.8° C	Absent	0
	Present	1
Maximal clinical subscore: 6		
B. Endoscopic finding		
1. Edema	Absent	0
	Present	1
2. Granularity	Absent	0
	Present	1
3. Friability	Absent	0
	Present	1
4. Loss of vascular pattern	Absent	0
	Present	1
5. Mucous exudates	Absent	0
	Present	1
6. Ulcerations	Absent	0
	Present	1
Maximal endoscopic subscore: 6		

(continued)

Table 27-1 (continued)
Pouchitis Disease Activity Index

C. Histology—acute histological inflammation		
1. Polymorphonuclear infiltration	None	0
	Mild	1
	Moderate + crypt abscess	2
	Severe + crypt abscess	3
2. Ulceration per low power field (mean)	None	0
	< 25%	1
	25% to 50%	2
	> 50%	3
Maximal histological subscore: 6		
Maximal total PDAI score: 18		

Reprinted from *Mayo Clin Proc*, 69(5), Sandborn WJ, Tremaine WJ, Batts KP, Pemberton JH, Phillips SF, Pouchitis after ileal pouch-anal anastomosis: a Pouchitis Disease Activity Index, 409-415, 1994, with permission from Elsevier.

In patients responding to antibiotics, prophylaxis of pouchitis may be done using probiotics. The probiotic VSL#3 (probiotic mixture including 8 strains of lactic acid-producing bacteria: *Lactobacillus plantarum, Lactobacillus delbrueckii subsp. Bulgaricus, Lactobacillus casei, Lactobacillus acidophilus, Bifidobacterium breve, Bifidobacterium longum, Bifidobacterium infantis*, and *Streptococcus salivarius subsp. thermophilus*) was found effective for maintenance of antibiotic-induced remission of pouchitis. Of note, data based on assessment in randomized controlled trials are scarce.[12] Primary prevention of pouchitis is possible using probiotics (VSL#3) as well as tinidazole.

Management of Chronic and Antibiotic Refractory Pouchitis

Longer therapy (> 4 weeks) and a combination of ciprofloxacin and metronidazole/tinidazole/rifaximin may be effective in patients failing the first course of antibiotics (antibiotic-resistant) (Table 27-3).

In cases of antibiotic resistance or antibiotic dependence, oral budesonide (9 mg once daily) or enema (2 mg/100 mL once daily) may be used for 6 to 8 weeks, as well as oral beclomethasone (10 mg once daily).

Table 27-2

Treatment of Acute and Recurrent Acute Pouchitis

Medication	Suggested Dose	Ref	Remarks
Ciprofloxacin	1000 mg daily in divided doses for 2 weeks	20	Monotherapy. Based on a single study on 18 patients ciprofloxacin may be more effective than metronidazole for the treatment of acute pouchitis.
Metronidazole	1000 mg daily in divided doses for 2 weeks	20	Monotherapy. Based on a single study on 18 patients ciprofloxacin may be more effective than metronidazole for the treatment of acute pouchitis. Dose and duration may be limited by intolerance.
Tinidazole	1000 mg in divided doses for 2 weeks	21	
Rifaximin	400 mg 3 times daily for 4 weeks	22	No differences were found between rifaximin and placebo in rate of clinical remission, clinical improvement, or adverse events
Mesalamine	Rectal suppositories, 1000 mg 3 times per day for 8 weeks	23	
Budesonide	Enema, 2 mg/100 mL at bedtime for 6 weeks	24	Similar efficacy but better tolerability than oral metronidazole in the treatment of active pouchitis

Patients failing to improve after 6 to 8 weeks of antibiotic therapy or a course of steroids (preferably the local acting) are candidates for immunomodulators (azathioprine or 6-mercaptopurine). Biologic therapy with anti–tumor necrosis factor (TNF)-alpha (most reports are for infliximab and adalimumab) may be reserved for patients who do not respond to or are intolerant to immunomodulator treatment. Additional indications may include CLDP and inflammatory stricture of the pouch. Multiple case series were reported regarding the use of anti-TNF-αlpha agents, usually with beneficial response.[13] Recently, treatment of pouchitis with anti-integrins (vedolizumab) was reported with positive outcomes.[14]

Table 27-3

Treatment of Chronic Antibiotic Refractory Pouchitis

Medication	Suggested Dose	Ref	Remarks
Ciprofloxacin	1000 mg daily in divided doses for 2 weeks	20	In combination with metronidazole for 4 weeks
Metronidazole	1000 mg daily in divided doses for 2 weeks	20	In combination with ciprofloxacin for 4 weeks; dose and duration of therapy may be limited by intolerance
Tinidazole	1000 mg in divided doses for 2 weeks	21	
Budesonide	Enema, 2 mg/100 mL at bedtime for 6 weeks	24	Similar efficacy but better tolerability than oral metronidazole
Beclomethasone	Oral beclomethasone dipropionate 10 mg/day for 8 weeks	25	Series of 10 patients with antibiotic refractory pouchitis demonstrated 80% response rate
Infliximab/ AZA/6-MP	Infliximab 5 mg/kg for induction of remission and maintenance based on same protocol as in other IBD's. AZA/6-MP at 1 to 1.5 mg/kg daily starting dose. AZA dose may be increased to a maximal dose of 2 to 2.5 mg/kg	13	Based on systematic review the combined partial and complete response after 6 to 10 weeks of infliximab therapy is around 84% to 88%, while long-term partial and complete response rates are 45% to 58%.
Adalimumab	Adalimumab 40 mg SQ for induction of remission and maintenance based on same protocol as in other IBDs	13	Based on systematic review, the short- and long-term combined partial and complete response of 71% and 54%, respectively

(continued)

Table 27-3 (continued)
Treatment of Chronic Antibiotic Refractory Pouchitis

Medication	Suggested Dose	Ref	Remarks
Vedolizumab	14 weeks	14, 26	Of 20 patients 64% demonstrated PDAI fall of ≥ 3 points. In another study, 6 of 19 patients (32%) had symptom improvement and 14 (74%) had both endoscopic and symptomatic improvement.
Tacrolimus	Tacrolimus enema of 4 to 5 mg/100 mL daily for 8 weeks	27	9 of 10 patients improved symptomatically and one third achieved remission.
Alicaforsen	Alicaforsen enema 60 mL, 240 mg/60 mL daily for 6 weeks	28	7 of 12 patients achieved remission by week 6
FMT	Fresh or frozen samples, single FMT or repeated doses. Route via pouchoscopy, nasogastric tube, or endoscopically to the jejunum	29	5 of 23 patients achieved clinical remission. Of note, a more recent randomized, double-blinded clinical trial did not demonstrate benefit on pouchitis relapse.[30]
IVIG	At least 1 dose of IVIG (0.4 g/kg)	31	16 patients, decrease in PDAI was demonstrated after IVIG infusion
Exclusive elemental diet	4 weeks	32	Symptoms improved in some patients but was not effective for induction of remission

6-MP = 6-mercaptopurine; AZA = azathioprine; FMT = fecal microbiota transplantation; IVIG = intravenous immunoglobulins; PDAI = Pouchitis Disease Activity Index.

Noticeably, the use of most therapies mentioned is based on anecdotal reports rather than randomized placebo-controlled studies. The use of traditional IBD therapy to treat patients with chronic refractory pouchitis reflects the need to address disease burden in this selected patient population. It also reflects the notion that pouchitis may be a form of IBD, which should be treated similarly in order to prevent further tissue damage and disease burden (Figure 27-1).

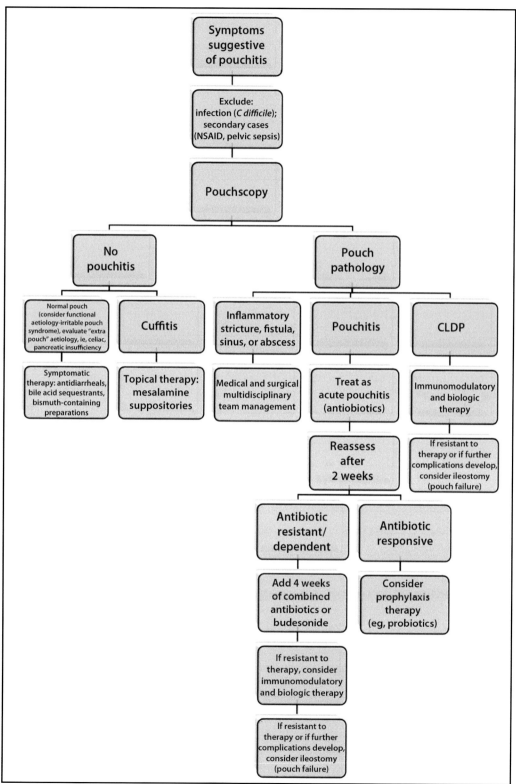

Figure 27-1. Evaluation algorithm for patients with symptoms of pouchitis. *C. difficile* = *Clostridioides difficile*; CLDP = Crohn's-like disease of the pouch; NSAID = nonsteroidal anti-inflammatory drug. (© Idan Goren, MD and Iris Dotan, MD.)

Nutrition and Diet in Pouchitis

The interaction between dietary habits and pouchitis is bidirectional. Diet modification is a commonly used strategy to manage symptoms in patients after pouch surgery. In fact, food avoidance is prevalent among patients after pouch surgery.[15] A low FODMAP diet has been shown to improve functional symptoms in patients without pouchitis. In patients with chronic pouchitis exclusive elemental nutrition has been found to improve symptoms. Diet may also play a role in the pathogenesis of pouchitis in patients with normal pouch via alterations in microbial[16] and fungal[17] composition; low fruit and vegetable consumption was shown to be associated with lower microbial diversity and with the development of pouchitis, among patients with normal pouch, thus fruit and vegetable consumption should be recommended rather than avoided.

Patients at Risk for Pouchitis

Patient stratification to those with high and low risk for idiopathic pouchitis may provide tools that enable better tailoring of therapeutic interventions. Furthermore, stratification may shed light on disease immunopathogenesis.

Patients with UC are at higher risk for pouchitis compared to patients with pouch due to FAP; this interesting observation demonstrates the importance of genetic and molecular predisposition for the development of pouchitis. This is also shown by the higher risk observed in patients with polymorphism at the NOD2/CARD15 gene; patients with refractory UC as an indication for surgery are at higher risk compared to nonrefractory indications, such as dysplasia.[18] Concurrent diagnosis of primary sclerosing cholangitis is associated with an increased risk for the development of pouchitis, as is the existence of other immune-mediated conditions.

These observations suggest that immunologic processes occurring before surgery may proceed or even progress after surgery and initiate inflammation at the previously normal pouch.

Postoperative Complications Unrelated to Pouchitis

Postoperative complications other than pouchitis may be divided into early and late, although some overlap exists, especially with regard to small bowel obstruction, which can occur at any time. Early postoperative complications are commonly related directly to the surgery. Anastomotic leaks leading to pelvic sepsis, pouch bleeding, and ileus are the most common complications. However, over time pouchitis remains the most common late complication.

Pouch Failure

Surgical complications such as pelvic sepsis, as well as inflammatory complications resistant to medical therapy, severe CLDP, and pouch dysplasia/neoplasia, may result in excision of the ileoanal pouch, formation of a permanent ileostomy, or pouch-related mortality. These outcomes are referred to as pouch failure. Of these causes, pelvic sepsis is the most common reason for pouch failure. The rate of pouch failure increases over time with 5% to 9% cumulative risk at 5 years and up to 18% over 20 years of follow-up.[19]

To summarize, total proctocolectomy and IPAA is the surgical procedure of choice for patients with intractable or complicated UC. While offering improved quality of life to most patients, and significantly decreasing the need for medications and the risk of cancer, this surgery carries several distinct short- and long-term adverse outcomes. Pouchitis is by far the most common long-term complication. The development of small intestinal inflammation in the previously normal small bowel may actually be a man-made model for the development of IBD. While pouchitis is the most antibiotic-responsive IBD, treatment with traditional IBD therapies such as mesalamine, steroids, immunomodulators, and biologics may be required in patients with chronic refractory pouchitis and CLDP. Controlled studies evaluating short- and long-term outcomes of current and newly designed interventions, including dietary ones, are much anticipated. Such studies may contribute significantly to further understanding of disease processes in patients with pouchitis, as well as in IBD.

References

1. Targownik LE, Singh H, Nugent Z, Bernstein CN. The epidemiology of colectomy in ulcerative colitis: results from a population-based cohort. *Am J Gastroenterol*. 2012;107(8):1228-1235. https://doi.org/10.1038/ajg.2012.127

2. Bohl JL, Sobba K. Indications and options for surgery in ulcerative colitis. *Surg Clin North Am*. 2015;95(6):1211–1232. doi:10.1016/j.suc.2015.07.003

3. Zittan E, Wong-Chong N, Ma GW, McLeod RS, Silverberg MS, Cohen Z. Modified two-stage ileal pouch-anal anastomosis results in lower rate of anastomotic leak compared with traditional two-stage surgery for ulcerative colitis. *J Crohns Colitis*. 2016;10(7):766-772. https://doi.org/10.1093/ecco-jcc/jjw069

4. Mège D, Figueiredo MN, Manceau G, Maggiori L, Bouhnik Y, Panis Y. Three-stage laparoscopic ileal pouch-anal anastomosis is the best approach for high-risk patients with inflammatory bowel disease: an analysis of 185 consecutive patients. *J Crohns Colitis*. 2016;10(8):898-904. https://doi.org/10.1093/ecco-jcc/jjw040

5. Joyce MR, Kiran RP, Remzi FH, Church J, Fazio VW. In a select group of patients meeting strict clinical criteria and undergoing ileal pouch-anal anastomosis, the omission of a diverting ileostomy offers cost savings to the hospital. *Dis Colon Rectum*. 2010;53(6):905-910. https://doi.org/10.1007/DCR.0b013e3181d5e0fd

6. Tulchinsky H, Dotan I, Halpern Z, Klausner JM, Rabau M. A longitudinal study of quality of life and functional outcome of patients with ulcerative colitis after proctocolectomy with ileal pouch-anal anastomosis. *Dis Colon Rectum*. 2010;53(6):866-873. https://doi.org/10.1007/DCR.0b013e3181d98d66

7. de Buck van Overstraeten A, Wolthuis AM, Vermeire S, et al. Long-term functional outcome after ileal pouch anal anastomosis in 191 patients with ulcerative colitis. *J Crohns Colitis*. 2014;8(10):1261-1266. https://doi.org/10.1016/j.crohns.2014.03.001

8. Fazio VW, Kiran RP, Remzi FH, et al. Ileal pouch anal anastomosis: analysis of outcome and quality of life in 3707 patients. *Ann Surg*. 2013;257(4):679-685. https://doi.org/10.1097/SLA.0b013e31827d99a2

9. Sandborn WJ, Tremaine WJ, Batts KP, Pemberton JH, Phillips SF. Pouchitis after ileal pouch-anal anastomosis: a Pouchitis Disease Activity Index. *Mayo Clin Proc*. 1994;69(5):409-415. https://doi.org/10.1016/s0025-6196(12)61634-6

10. Heuschen UA, Allemeyer EH, Hinz U, et al. Diagnosing pouchitis: comparative validation of two scoring systems in routine follow-up. *Dis Colon Rectum*. 2002;45(6):776-778.

11. Pardi DS, D'Haens G, Shen B, Campbell S, Gionchetti P. Clinical guidelines for the management of pouchitis. *Inflamm Bowel Dis*. 2009;15(9):1424-1431. https://doi.org/10.1002/ibd.21039

12. Nguyen N, Zhang B, Holubar SD, Pardi DS, Singh S. Treatment and prevention of pouchitis after ileal pouch-anal anastomosis for chronic ulcerative colitis. *Cochrane Database Syst Rev*. 2019;5:CD001176. https://doi.org/10.1002/14651858.CD001176.pub4

13. Herfarth HH, Long MD, Isaacs KL. Use of biologics in pouchitis a systematic review. *J Clin Gastroenterol*. 2015;49(8):647-654. https://doi.org/10.1097/MCG.0000000000000367

14. Bar F, Kuhbacher T, Dietrich NA, et al. Vedolizumab in the treatment of chronic, antibiotic-dependent or refractory pouchitis. *Aliment Pharmacol Ther*. 2018;47(5):581-587. https://doi.org/10.1111/apt.14479

15. Ianco O, Tulchinsky H, Lusthaus M, et al. Diet of patients after pouch surgery may affect pouch inflammation. *World J Gastroenterol*. 2013;19(38):6458-6464. https://doi.org/10.3748/wjg.v19.i38.6458

16. Godny L, Maharshak N, Reshef L, et al. Fruit consumption is associated with alterations in microbial composition and lower rates of pouchitis. *J Crohns Colitis*. 2019;13(10):1265-1272. https://doi.org/10.1093/ecco-jcc/jjz053

17. Goren I, Godny L, Reshef L, et al. Starch consumption may modify antiglycan antibodies and fecal fungal composition in patients with ileo-anal pouch. *Inflamm Bowel Dis*. 2019;25(4):742-749. https://doi.org/10.1093/ibd/izy370

18. Yanai H, Ben-Shachar S, Mlynarsky L, et al. The outcome of ulcerative colitis patients undergoing pouch surgery is determined by pre-surgical factors. *Aliment Pharmacol Ther*. 2017;46(5):508-515. https://doi.org/10.1111/apt.14205

19. Mark-Christensen A, Erichsen R, Brandsborg S, et al. Pouch failures following ileal pouch-anal anastomosis for ulcerative colitis. *Colorectal Dis*. 2017;20(1):44-52. https://doi.org/10.1111/codi.13802

20. Shen B, Achkar JP, Lashner BA, et al. A randomized clinical trial of ciprofloxacin and metronidazole to treat acute pouchitis. *Inflamm Bowel Dis*. 2001;7(4):301-305. https://doi.org/10.1097/00054725-200111000-00004

21. Ha CY, Bauer JJ, Lazarev M, Swaminath A, Sparrow M, Murphy SJ, et al. Early institution of tinidazole may prevent pouchitis following ileal pouch-anal anastomosis (IPAA) surgery in ulcerative colitis (UC) patients. *Gastroenterology*. 2010;138(5 Supp. doi:https://doi.org/10.1016/S0016-5085(10)60314-9

22. Isaacs KL, Sandler RS, Abreu M, et al. Rifaximin for the treatment of active pouchitis: a randomized, double-blind, placebo-controlled pilot study. *Inflamm Bowel Dis*. 2007;13(10):1250-1255. https://doi.org/10.1002/ibd.20187

23. Miglioli M, Barbara L, Di Febo G, et al. Topical administration of 5-aminosalicylic acid: a therapeutic proposal for the treatment of pouchitis. *N Engl J Med*. 1989 Jan 26;320(4):257. https://doi: 10.1056/NEJM198901263200423.

24. Sambuelli A, Boerr L, Negreira S, et al. Budesonide enema in pouchitis—a double-blind, double-dummy, controlled trial. *Aliment Pharmacol Ther*. 2002;16(1):27-34

25. Gionchetti P, Calabrese C, Calafiore A, et al. Oral beclomethasone dipropionate in chronic refractory pouchitis. *J Crohns Colitis*. 2014;8(7):649-653. https://doi:10.1016/j.crohns.2013.12.001

26. Singh A, Khan F, Lopez R, Shen B, Philpott J. Vedolizumab for chronic antibiotic-refractory pouchitis. *Gastroenterol Rep*. 2019;7(2):121-126. https://doi.org/10.1093/gastro/goz001

27. Uchino M, Ikeuchi H, Matsuoka H, et al. Topical tacrolimus therapy for antibiotic-refractory pouchitis. *Dis Colon Rectum*. 2013;56(10):1166-1173. https://doi.org/10.1097/DCR.0b013e31829ebd83

28. Miner P, Wedel M, Bane B, Bradley J. An enema formulation of alicaforsen, an antisense inhibitor of intercellular adhesion molecule-1, in the treatment of chronic, unremitting pouchitis. *Aliment Pharmacol Ther*. 2004;19(3):281-286. https://doi.org/10.1111/j.1365-2036.2004.01863.x

29. Paramsothy S, Paramsothy R, Rubin DT, et al. Fecal microbiota transplantation for inflammatory bowel disease: a systematic review and meta-analysis. *J Crohns Colitis*. 2017;11(10):1180-1199. https://doi.org/10.1093/ecco-jcc/jjx063

30. Karjalainen EK, Renkonen-Sinisalo L, Satokari R, et al. Fecal microbiota transplantation in chronic pouchitis: a randomized, parallel, double-blinded clinical trial. *Inflamm Bowel Dis*. 2021. https://doi.org/10.1093/ibd/izab001

31. Horton N, Kochhar G, Patel K, Lopez R, Shen B. Efficacy and factors associated with treatment response of intravenous immunoglobulin in inpatients with refractory inflammatory bowel diseases. *Inflamm Bowel Dis*. 2017 Jul;23(7):1080-1087. https://doi.org/10.1097/MIB.0000000000001116.

32. McLaughlin SD, Culkin A, Cole J, et al. Exclusive elemental diet impacts on the gastrointestinal microbiota and improves symptoms in patients with chronic pouchitis. *J Crohns Colitis*. 2013;7(6):460-466. https://doi.org/10.1016/j.crohns.2012.07.009

MY PATIENT WITH IBD IS COMPLAINING OF JOINT PAIN. WHAT SHOULD I DO?

Abha G. Singh, MD and Arthur Kavanaugh, MD

Joint involvement is the most common extraintestinal manifestation of inflammatory bowel disease (IBD), affecting up to 46% of patients.[1] Noninflammatory arthralgias, as well as inflammatory arthritis of the peripheral joints, can be seen; it is crucial to differentiate the two, as treatment approaches differ. Inflammatory spinal involvement (also known as *axial arthritis*) may also be seen in about one-fifth of the cases. From a rheumatologic standpoint, arthritis associated with IBD is classified within the group of conditions called *spondyloarthritis* (SpA). In addition to IBD-associated arthritis, SpA includes ankylosing spondylitis (also known as *axial SpA*), psoriatic arthritis, and reactive arthritis. Traditionally, these conditions had been called *seronegative spondyloarthropathies*, in reference to the general lack of positive test results for rheumatoid factor; however, it should be noted that positive tests for rheumatoid factor may be found in SpA patients at a greater frequency than observed in the general population (eg, > 10% as opposed to 5%). Serologic testing for anti-cyclic citrullinated peptide is also generally negative.[2] There are no specific laboratory tests for the diagnosis of IBD-associated arthritis. Inflammatory markers may be elevated and may be helpful to assess responses to treatment. However, acute phase reactant test results may reflect inflammation elsewhere (eg, concomitant gut inflammation), and a number of patients with active arthritis may have normal test results. Since IBD-associated peripheral arthritis, particularly early in the disease course, may not be associated with periarticular joint erosions, radiographs of peripheral joints may be unremarkable.

Noninflammatory arthralgias, without inflammatory swelling of the joints, have been observed in 8% to 30% of patients. Of course, with advancing age, nearly all persons will develop some signs and symptoms of osteoarthritis, also called *degenerative joint disease*, in some joints. Inflammatory arthritis of the peripheral joints, sometimes traditionally categorized as type I

Rubin DT, Friedman S, Farraye FA, eds. *Curbside Consultation in IBD:*
49 Clinical Questions, Third Edition (pp 171-175).

(pauciarticular) or type II (polyarticular) have been described in 5% to 20% patients.[3] Spinal or axial arthritis, including inflammatory back pain, frank ankylosing spondylitis, and isolated sacroiliitis, have been reported in 2% to 22% of patients. While most often arthritis develops following IBD diagnosis, in some patients articular symptoms may precede IBD.

Risk factors for joint involvement in patients with IBD include the following:

- Active bowel disease
- Family history of IBD
- History of appendectomy
- Cigarette smoking
- Presence of other extraintestinal manifestations such as erythema nodosum or pyoderma gangrenosum
- Patients with extensive colitis and Crohn's disease patients with colonic involvement

Peripheral Arthritis in IBD

TYPE 1 OR PAUCIARTICULAR/OLIGOARTICULAR

Pauciarticular peripheral arthritis is defined as arthritis affecting < 5 peripheral joints (Table 28-1). Generally this type of arthritis affects larger joints, like the knee (most common), ankle, wrist, hip, or shoulder. It often presents in an asymmetric fashion. Joint pain and swelling tends to be more acute in onset and can be migratory in nature. This type of inflammatory arthritis tends to parallel IBD disease activity, often seen early in the course of IBD. The duration of arthritis is typically from a few weeks to < 6 months.

For these patients, short courses (eg, a few weeks) of nonsteroidal anti-inflammatory drugs (NSAIDs), particularly selective cyclooxygenase-2 (COX-2) inhibitors, may be considered. Simple analgesics (eg, acetaminophen) and topical therapies (eg, topical NSAIDs, capsaicin) can be useful adjuncts, although their impact is generally limited. Local injections of corticosteroids into affected joints can be highly effective and are usually well tolerated. Short courses of oral corticosteroids at low dose (eg, < 10 mg/d of prednisone) can sometimes be helpful in rapidly gaining disease control. For patients with persistent arthritis, sulfasalazine may be an option, as it can provide benefit for both IBD as well as arthritis. Other disease-modifying antirheumatic drugs (DMARDs), such as methotrexate, are a standard rheumatologic therapy and can also provide some benefit for IBD. In particularly refractory and persistent cases, biologic agents, especially tumor necrosis factor (TNF) inhibitors, can be utilized. Treatment of underlying gastrointestinal inflammation can be effective at treating and even preventing recurrence of this type of arthritis.

TYPE 2 OR POLYARTICULAR

Polyarticular peripheral arthritis affects 5 or more, typically smaller, joints (eg, joints of the hands) often in a bilaterally symmetric manner. Metacarpophalangeal (MCP) and proximal interphalangeal (PIP) joints of hands are often involved. Knees, ankles, elbows, shoulders, wrists, and metatarsophalangeal (MTP) joints are less commonly affected. This type of arthritis tends to be independent of IBD disease activity and may persist for years with intermittent exacerbations.

Treatment of polyarticular inflammatory peripheral arthritis is often multifaceted. For many patients, NSAIDs, particularly selective COX-2 inhibitors, may be considered, with consideration of the possibility of untoward impact on the gastrointestinal tract. Simple analgesics (eg, acetaminophen) are helpful for some patients, although their impact is generally limited. Local injections of corticosteroids into affected joints can be effective if one or a few joints are more inflamed

Table 28-1

Types of Peripheral Arthritis in IBD

	Type 1 (Pauciarticular)	*Type 2 (Polyarticular)*
Prevalence	30% to 35%	20% to 25%
Pattern	• < 5 joints • Asymmetric • Mainly large joints (knee > ankle > wrist > elbow)	• 5 joints • Symmetric or asymmetric • Mainly small joints (MCPs > PIPs > wrist)
Relation to IBD	Parallels IBD disease activity	Independent of IBD disease activity
Natural history	Self-limited episodes, generally < 6 months	Persistent inflammation for months to years
Association with other EIMs	High frequency of other EIMs (erythema nodosum, uveitis)	Uveitis
EIM = extraintestinal manifestations.		

than others. Short courses of oral corticosteroids at low dose (eg, < 10 mg/d of prednisone) can sometimes be helpful in rapidly gaining disease control. For patients with persistent arthritis, sulfasalazine may be an option, as it can provide benefit for both IBD as well as arthritis. Other DMARDs such as methotrexate are more effective in this group of patients than sulfasalazine and are used as standard rheumatologic therapy; methotrexate can also provide some benefit for IBD. Thiopurines are not usually effective for the treatment of articular symptoms. In persistent cases, biologic agents, especially TNF inhibitors, can be utilized. TNF inhibitors can be effective for both peripheral arthritis and IBD. Among the 5 TNF inhibitors available worldwide, while all seem to be comparably effective for arthritis, etanercept at the doses typically used for arthritis has not been proven effective for IBD. Recent data suggest that jakinibs (eg, tofacitinib), orally available inhibitors of the Janus kinase signaling molecules, might be effective in both IBD as well as for the peripheral arthritis of SpA. Newer biologics available for the treatment of IBD, such as vedolizumab, a gut-selective anti-$\alpha_4\beta_7$ integrin, do not seem to be effective in treating peripheral arthritis of SpA; in fact, anecdotal reports of flares of arthritis among patients receiving vedolizumab have been reported. Ustekinumab, an anti–interleukin (IL) 12/IL-23 mAb, is also effective for peripheral arthritis and for IBD.[4]

Axial Arthropathies in IBD

SACROILIITIS

Isolated sacroiliitis may be observed radiographically in 25% of patients with IBD, but many of these patients may be asymptomatic or minimally symptomatic. A minority of such patients progress to ankylosing spondylitis (less than one-fifth of the time). This is most often seen on imaging (X-ray/magnetic resonance imaging [MRI]) as sclerosis, erosions, and/or ankylosis of the sacroiliac joint. MRI is more sensitive than plain X-ray and could be performed for the assessment of persistent symptoms when clinically indicated (eg, to help differentiate degenerative disease from inflammatory disease).

When symptomatic, sacroiliitis presents as inflammatory low back pain (iLBP). iLBP is classically characterized by lower back/buttock pain that occurs after rest (eg, first thing in the morning) and that improves with movement, as opposed to most cases of degenerative back pain that are aggravated by physical stress. Morning stiffness in sacroiliac area is often reported, typically lasting an hour or more. Prolonged sitting and driving are often uncomfortable with subsequent stiffness.

ANKYLOSING SPONDYLITIS/AXIAL SPONDYLOARTHRITIS

Ankylosing spondylitis is suspected, clinically based on a combination of inflammatory back pain with morning stiffness, limitation of spine flexion (Schober's test), and reduced chest expansion due to spondylitis; X-rays in established disease show sacroiliitis and proliferative changes of other areas of the spine. There appears to be a strong association between ankylosing spondylitis and IBD—approximately 5% to 10% patients with SpA develop IBD, and up to 70% of ankylosing spondylitis patients without gastrointestinal symptoms may have microscopic evidence of gut inflammation. Likewise, about 5% to 10% patients with IBD may develop SpA.[5] Presence of an elevated C-reactive protein and/or fecal calprotectin in patients with SpA has modest accuracy as a screening strategy to identify potential SpA patients with gut inflammation. Most patients with SpA are HLA-B27 positive (> 90% White ankylosing spondylitis patients); its prevalence in patients with IBD with spinal arthritis is slightly lower (50%) although still higher than that seen in the general population (8%). Radiographs of the spine and pelvis may show typical findings of ankylosing spondylitis and sacroiliitis. MRI is the gold standard for diagnosis, as it shows not only structural changes (erosions, bony proliferation) but also evidence of inflammation (eg, bone marrow edema). MRI changes may be seen before damage is evident on plain X-rays, thus leading to earlier diagnosis and treatment. However, it should be noted that MRI changes are not by themselves diagnostic of axial SpA. For example, bone marrow edema can be seen after local trauma.

Spinal or axial disease is different than peripheral arthritis in that traditional DMARDs (methotrexate, sulfasalazine, etc) are ineffective. Also, local steroid injections are more difficult and less commonly used, as are oral corticosteroids. Thus, patients often proceed from NSAIDs/COX-2 inhibitors directly to biologic DMARDs, particularly anti-TNF agents. Vedolizumab, a gut-selective anti-$\alpha_4\beta_7$ integrin, has not proven effective for axial SpA. Ustekinumab also does not appear to have efficacy for axial SpA. Jakinibs are being studied in axial SpA and may prove to have some efficacy.

Tendon Inflammation

Besides peripheral and axial arthropathies, enthesitis (inflammation at the bone insertion site of ligaments, tendons, and fascia), tenosynovitis, and dactylitis (sausage-like digits) are very commonly observed in SpA. Plantar fasciitis, causing heel pain, and Achilles tendinitis are common findings. Physical exam may not be sufficient to evaluate inflammation in the entheses. With the availability of musculoskeletal ultrasound and MRI, inflammation in these tendinous structures can be visualized and often aids with diagnosis.

Conclusion

To help facilitate early recognition of IBD-associated arthritis, certain red flags should be considered. IBD-associated arthritis, sometimes referred to as *enteropathic arthritis*, should be considered in patients with IBD with chronic low back pain (> 3 months) with morning stiffness, peripheral joint pain and swelling, enthesitis, dactylitis, or other types of tenosynovitis. Likewise, rheumatologists should be alerted to the possibility of underlying IBD in patients with spondyloarthropathies with a family history of IBD, clinical symptoms (chronic diarrhea and/or rectal bleeding, abdominal pain, weight loss, and/or persistent fever), previous perianal disease, or iron-deficiency anemia.

A high index of suspicion and early referral may decrease diagnostic delay, morbidity, and health care burden. An aggressive approach targeting better control of IBD activity with anti-TNF agents, as well as selective use of sulfasalazine, methotrexate, short-term use of COX-2 inhibitors, and physical therapy are recommended for management. While long-term use of NSAIDs may exacerbate IBD, short-term use in symptomatic patients may be reasonable.

References

1. Ott C, Schölmerich J. Extraintestinal manifestations and complications in IBD. *Nat Rev Gastroenterol Hepatol.* 2013;10(10):585-595.
2. Brakenhoff LK, van der Heijde DM, Hommes DW, et al. The joint-gut axis in inflammatory bowel diseases. *J Crohns Colitis.* 2010;4(3):257-268.
3. Colìa R, Corrado A, Cantatore FP. Rheumatologic and extraintestinal manifestations of inflammatory bowel diseases. *Ann Med.* 2016;48(8):577-558.
4. Pouillon L, Bossuyt P, Vanderstukken J. Management of patients with inflammatory bowel disease and spondyloarthritis. *Expert Rev Clin Pharmacol.* 2017;10(12):1363-1374.
5. Singh AG, Kavanaugh A. Rheumatologic complications of inflammatory bowel diseases. *Pract Gastroenterol.* 2017;41:36-39.

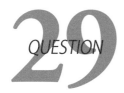

What Are the Diagnostic and Therapeutic Approaches to the Patient With IBD With Pain?

Emily Weaver, LCSW and Eva Szigethy, MD, PhD

Acute Versus Chronic Pain

While both acute and chronic pain are common in inflammatory bowel disease (IBD), they represent different phenomena and require different treatments. Acute pain, experienced in up to 80% of patients with IBD, is usually the result of a diagnosable cause that is reversible with appropriate treatment of the underlying issue.[1] Pain is considered chronic when it lasts longer than 3 months and has been reported in 30% to 50% of patients with IBD. Chronic pain, including abdominal pain, is often a progressive condition involving dysregulation of the brain-gut axis through changes in the central nervous system, autonomic nervous system, and hypothalamic pituitary adrenal axis.[2,3] Predisposing factors to chronic pain include female gender, repetitive stress, trauma history, and premorbid psychiatric diagnoses. Consequences of chronic pain include psychiatric symptoms and diagnoses, disability, and social isolation (Figure 29-1).

Types of Pain in IBD: IBD-Related Versus Generalized Pain

In visceral pain or hyperalgesia, visceral nociceptors in the gastrointestinal tract become sensitized to pain by recurrent exposure to inflammation and can remain sensitized even after intestinal inflammation subsides. Proposed mechanisms of IBD-related pain in the gut or periphery (eg, joints) include inflammatory substances such as cytokines, which can lead to sensitization

Rubin DT, Friedman S, Farraye FA, eds. *Curbside Consultation in IBD:*
49 Clinical Questions, Third Edition (pp 177-187).
© 2022 Taylor & Francis Group.

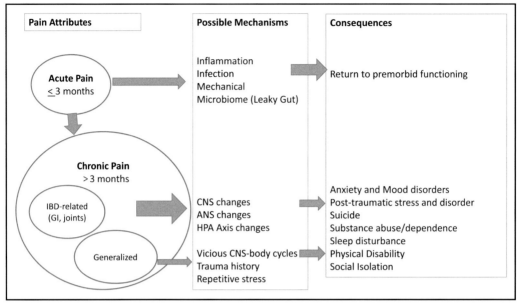

Figure 29-1. Assessing pain in IBD.

of spinal nerve endings. Changes in motility, flatus, and surgical sequelae can also contribute to additional types of gastrointestinal distress, and different etiologies are not mutually exclusive. In some patients with IBD, chronic abdominal pain is part of a central pain syndrome, whereby the brain upregulates pain signals, leading to chronic amplification of other types of pain such as headaches, back pain, and fibromyalgia.[2,4,5] This more generalized application of the nociceptive signal from the body is associated with altered brain circuitry in pathways that modulate stress and emotion regulation and requires more intensive multimodal interventions.

Diagnostic Approaches to Evaluate Chronic Pain

Due to the multifactorial nature of pain in IBD, a more thorough evaluation is necessary, especially when pain becomes chronic. This involves assessment of pain attributes such as functional impairment or disability and pain-related suffering, thus listening to the patient's "pain journey" narrative is imperative. Many patients with IBD experience pain during periods of clinical remission,[6] often referred to as *functional* pain since the etiology is not easily detected with currently available testing modalities. Functional pain in gastrointestinal disorders has recently been called *disorder of gut-brain interaction* to emphasize how important it is to consider the central nervous system in assessment and treatment. Thus, for patients with chronic functional pain, a more thorough biopsychosocial evaluation is particularly important. This evaluation needs to examine the potential impact of other physical sources of abdominal pain (celiac disease, food allergies and intolerances, colon cancer, metabolism disorders, endometriosis), other pain disorders (neuropathic, headaches, back pain, fibromyalgia, arthritis), psychiatric diagnoses (anxiety, depression, bipolar disorder, eating disorders, post-traumatic stress disorder, substance abuse/dependence), dietary and lifestyle behaviors, medication history, drug allergies and sensitivities, and evaluation of social needs, including access to basic needs and stability of social support. For patients taking opioid medication, opioid-induced hyperalgesia (narcotic bowel syndrome) must be considered.[4] Psychological factors can also influence pain perception, including low cognitive flexibility, pain catastrophizing and hypervigilance, the unconscious meaning of pain, and secondary gain, and if present should be addressed through treatment for maximum recovery. As in all patient-provider relationships, the process of evaluation and treatment is greatly enhanced by positive rapport between the clinician and the individual in pain.[7]

Self-Report Scales

While many IBD scales may include items on pain (including the Short Inflammatory Bowel Disease Questionnaire), there are multiple validated instruments dedicated to solely measuring different aspects of pain, which can be helpful for initial assessment as well as long-term measurement of the patient's functioning and improvement over time. These questionnaires measure diverse targets, from pain severity and quality to suffering and pain-related disability. The Brief Pain Inventory measures pain severity and frequency. The McGill Pain Questionnaire measures pain intensity as well as qualitative descriptions of pain. The Visceral Sensitivity Index is validated for measuring pain severity in IBS. Other common pain intensity scales include the Visual Analogue Scale and the Numeric Rating Scale (visually or audibly administered, respectively, with pediatric adaptations available), which rate pain sensation severity from 1 through 10. There are numerous scales developed for the measurement of pain as part of irritable bowel syndrome (IBS).[8] Disability scales can also be relevant when treating pain and include the Sickness Impact Profile questionnaire and the Pain Disability Index. Instruments that measure pain-related thoughts, such as the Pain Catastrophizing Scale, examine cognitive appraisals of pain (rumination, magnification, helplessness), which can also contribute to pain perception. Additionally, the National Institutes of Health's validated short self-report questionnaires, PROMIS (Patient-Reported Outcomes Measurement Information System), are available online and examine multiple areas of pain, including intensity, interference, behavior, and quality. Quality-of-life scales are also frequently utilized as an adjunct measure of functioning, such as the Short Form Health Survey 36. When opioids are utilized as part of a patient's chronic treatment plan, it is generally best practice to also utilize questionnaires that measure patient safety, such as the Current Opioid Misuse Measure and the Screener and Opioid Assessment for Patients With Pain.[2]

Psychological

Pain is frequently comorbid with mood disorders and is increasingly viewed as a consequence, cause, and correlate of emotional distress. Individuals with a history of adversity are at increased risk of developing both psychiatric problems and pain; once pain develops, individuals are also more likely to be diagnosed with psychiatric illness, including anxiety, depression, post-traumatic stress disorder, sleep disorders, and substance abuse, all of which can escalate, without adequate treatment, into suicidality with chronification of pain. Validated questionnaires measuring psychological distress include depression measures such as the Hospital Anxiety and Depression Scale (HADS), World Health Organization Well-Being Index (WBI-5), and Patient Health Questionnaire (PHQ-9); anxiety measures such as the Generalized Anxiety Disorder-7 (GAD-7); and sleep measures such as the Pittsburgh Sleep Quality Index (PSQI). The PROMIS instruments (particularly PROMIS-29 and PROMIS-43) also capture a diverse range of psychological experiences, including depression, anxiety, physical and social functioning, sleep, and pain. Validated and brief substance abuse screens include the Alcohol Use Disorders Identification Test, the Opioid Risk Tool, and the CAGE-AID questionnaire (comorbid alcohol and drug use disorders). Many of these measures are becoming increasingly available for digital administration, allowing for more ecologically valid assessments and real-time scoring and reporting capacities.

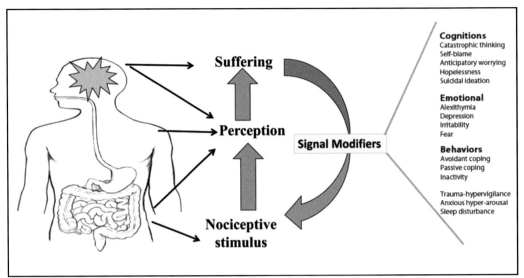

Figure 29-2. Neuropsychological modifiers of chronic abdominal pain signals. (Adapted from Srinath A, Young E, Szigethy E. Pain management in patients with inflammatory bowel disease: translational approaches from bench to bedside. *Inflamm Bowel Dis*. 2014;20[12]:2433-2449.)

The use of these types of patient-report questionnaires can be helpful to screen for pain and psychological symptoms and to track treatment response. However, patient and provider burden of such measures does not make them feasible in all settings. If time and resources are limiting factors, Figure 29-2 provides a schema that can be used to organize information obtained during the patient interview and also as a handout to explain chronic pain and its consequences to patients.

Behavioral Treatment Options

Adequate treatment of chronic pain requires a decrease in both pain intensity and pain-related disability. Behavioral treatments are considered first-line interventions for both mood disorders and chronic pain, including functional gastrointestinal disorders. The most effective nonpharmacological interventions are cognitive behavioral therapy (CBT), medical hypnosis, and mindfulness therapies such as Mindfulness Based Stress Reduction (MBSR). These therapies are time limited (between 6 and 12 sessions in general) and are increasingly being offered via virtual or online platforms as well as in-person and group sessions (Table 29-1).

CBT is a skill-focused psychotherapy that teaches individuals how to identify the impact of thoughts and feelings on behaviors and (psychologically mediated) bodily responses, which enables individuals to reframe maladaptive thought patterns (such as worrying and focusing on the negative) and behaviors (such as avoidance, excessive reassurance-seeking behaviors) that exacerbate anxiety, depression, and trauma symptoms. For those with chronic pain, CBT provides skills to identify and change the fear and avoidance cycle through thinking more adaptively about pain (decreasing pain catastrophizing and hypervigilance), increasing problem-solving and behavioral activation (instead of inactivity), and boosting acceptance, resilience, and internal locus of control. More than 18 studies compare CBT for IBS with other interventions (treatment as usual, medications, psychoeducation, or general supportive therapy), with the majority of evidence showing CBT to effectively reduce functional pain as well as improve mood.[4]

Table 29-1

Behavioral Interventions for Chronic Pain

	Cognitive Behavioral Therapy	*Hypnosis*	*Mindfulness/ Meditation*
Definition	Targets **maladaptive thoughts and behaviors to change emotions and perceptions** by teaching **coping skills** Skills such as **cognitive reframing, behavioral activation/** distraction, **exposure, relaxation**	Induction of a **trance state** = psychophysiological state where there is **relative suspension of peripheral awareness** and greater **susceptibility to suggestions** to alter relationships between **emotions, thoughts, behaviors and perceptions**	Learning **to pay attention on purpose** to present moment experience in **non-judgmental way** Attending to pain adaptively— **attention based coping and acceptance**—to buffer against secondary evaluations of physical sensations (catastrophizing)
Differentiation	Time limited, conscious; didactic problem solving	Automatic/ unconscious; social expectancy theory	Conscious and unconscious components
Dosing	8 to 20 sessions ranging from 30 to 60 minutes; individual or group; therapist guided	1 to 8 sessions ranging from 30 to 60 minutes; individual; therapist guided	8 to 12 sessions; 5 to 30 minutes; self or therapist guided
Mechanism	All 3 modalities involve **habit reversal with unlearning and new learning** with practice. Changes in thoughts, behaviors, emotions **associated with changes in underlying brain circuits**.		
Access	Requires provider training to level of fidelity and proficiency. Requires reinforcement to maintain new skill set. **Digital technology** increasing access and reach of all 3 interventions.		

With both medical hypnosis and mindfulness therapies (including MBSR and other third-wave behavioral therapies such as dialectical behavioral therapy and acceptance and commitment therapy), individuals develop skills to improve mood, increase disease self-management, and utilize active and adaptive coping when challenges arise. Hypnosis utilizes the brain's inborn ability to dissociate, and under the induced state of trance the clinician makes therapeutic suggestions that align with patient's goals to reduce susceptibility to stress, minimize pain perception and hypervigilance to bodily symptoms, and improve mood and well-being. Mindfulness therapies focus on teaching awareness and acceptance of the present moment—letting go of unnecessary thoughts and feelings and accepting reality—without judgment. This orientation to acceptance of the moment prevents individuals from catastrophizing about the future, ruminating on the past, and being hypervigilant in the here and now. Overall, evidence is strong that behavioral techniques are sufficient for the majority of individuals with concomitant IBD and anxiety, depression, or chronic pain.[5]

Increasing attention is being paid to the impact of trauma in individuals with IBD. Trauma, especially when chronic, severe, or untreated, has the power to negatively impact mood and dysregulate the brain-gut pathways through altering the autonomic nervous system, the hypothalamic-pituitary-adrenal axis, the limbic system, and the immune system, which can lead to a negative cascade of emotional and somatic distress. While trauma is common, patient-centered providers are increasingly understanding that chronic illness, including IBD diagnosis, symptoms, and associated invasive procedures such as colonoscopies and surgeries, can themselves be traumatizing events, especially when patients believe that their safety is at risk. This type of illness-related trauma, when unaddressed by the treatment team, can lead to a host of negative sequelae, including fear, isolation, nonadherence, substance abuse, hopelessness, and suicidality. However, when identified and treated through a trauma-informed, patient-centered, and, ideally, multidisciplinary treatment team, patients can overcome trauma and thrive.

Other forms of complementary alternative medicines such as exercise, yoga, and acupuncture are understudied in IBD but have some support in functional gastrointestinal disorders. A meta-analysis on acupuncture showed greater benefits from acupuncture than pharmacological therapy, but no benefits of acupuncture when it was compared to a credible "sham" acupuncture control group, possibly indicating patient preference for nonpharmacological treatment.[9] Yoga for functional gastrointestinal disorders has promising results in small studies, showing benefit above conventional treatment with decreased gastrointestinal symptom severity, improved mood, and no adverse events reported.[10]

Pharmacological Treatment Options

Multiple neuromodulators can effectively manage abdominal pain while avoiding the dangers of narcotics (Tables 29-2 and 29-3). Current guidelines indicate that tricyclic antidepressants (TCAs: amitriptyline, nortriptyline, imipramine, desipramine; side effects include drowsiness, dry mouth, arrhythmia, weight gain, and constipation) at low to moderate doses followed by serotonin noradrenergic reuptake inhibitors (SNRIs: venlafaxine, duloxetine, desvenlafaxine, milnacipran) have the most evidence of benefit for chronic abdominal pain. Selective serotonin reuptake inhibitors (SSRIs: paroxetine, fluoxetine, sertraline, citalopram, escitalopram) have less of a direct impact on pain but are helpful in managing concurrent mood disorders, which can worsen pain when untreated. SSRIs and SNRIs can include transient side effects such as nausea, diarrhea, fatigue, agitation, and headaches, while long-lasting effects can include weight gain and sexual dysfunction. Tetracyclic antidepressants (mirtazapine, trazadone; side effects include fatigue, dry mouth, weight gain, and headaches) can increase appetite, cause weight gain, and improve sleep. When first-line neuromodulators provide insufficient relief or increase in side effects at higher

Table 29-2

Antidepressants for Chronic Abdominal Pain

	Tricyclic Antidepressant	Selective Serotonin Reuptake Inhibitor	Serotonin-Norepinephrine Reuptake Inhibitor	Tetra-Cyclic (Mirtazapine)
Potential Benefits (Weeks)	Pain Depression Anxiety Insomnia	Depression Anxiety	Pain Depression	Pain Nausea/vomiting Insomnia
Adverse Effects (Days-Week)	Sedation Constipation Hypotension Dry mouth Arrhythmia/QTc Weight gain Suicidality	Agitation/restlessness Diarrhea Night sweats Headache Sexual dysfunction Suicidality Cardiovascular Bleeding SIADH	Nausea Agitation Dizziness Sleep disturbance Fatigue Liver dysfunction Suicidality	Sedation Weight gain Fatigue Dry mouth Constipation Weakness Dizziness Strange dreams
Overdose Risk	Moderate	Minimal	Minimal	Minimal

Table 29-3

Prescription of Antidepressants-Specifics

	Tricyclic Antidepressant	Selective Serotonin Reuptake Inhibitor	Serotonin-Norepinephrine Reuptake Inhibitor	Miscellaneous
Classes/dosing (mg/d)*	Amitriptyline (10-100) Imipramine (25-100) Nortriptyline (50-150) Desipramine (50-200)	Fluoxetine (20-80) Citalopram (20-40) Escitalopram (10-20) Sertaline (50-200) Paroxetine (20-50)	Venlafaxine XR (37.5-225) Duloxetine (30-120) Vortioxetine (5-20)	Mirtazapine (15-45) Bupropion SR XL (100-450)
Timing	Side effects-days Efficacy 1-3 weeks	Side effects-days Efficacy 2-4 weeks	Side effects-days Efficacy 2-4 weeks	Side effects-days Efficacy 1-2 weeks
Efficacy	Small controlled trials Analgesic effect independent of mood effect	Large randomized trials for depression and anxiety Little efficacy for direct pain reduction	Large randomized trials for depression and anxiety Small controlled studies for chronic pain	Small randomized controlled trials for depression

*For US Food and Drug Administration–approved indication which is usually depressive and anxiety disorders.
Data sources: Binion, 2014; Dekel, 2013; Drossman, 2009; Mikocka-Walus; Szigethy & Thorkelson, 2016.

doses, augmenting agents can be considered, including azapirones (buspirone—for dyspeptic features and anxiety; side effects are sedation, headache, vertigo), delta ligand agents (gabapentin, pregabalin—for neuropathic pain; side effects include fatigue, headache, vertigo, weight gain, and edema), atypical antipsychotics (quetiapine, olanzapine, sulpiride—for sleep, anxiety, nausea, fibromyalgia; side effects include sedation, dizziness, weight gain and metabolic syndrome), and atypical antidepressants (bupropion—for fatigue and depressed mood; side effects include insomnia and weight loss). Additionally, antispasmodics are commonly utilized, as well as regional or epidural analgesic injections. Effective and tolerable treatment protocols should be continued for a minimum of 6 to 12 months to prevent relapse, and all treatment should be delivered in the context of patient-centered values to maximize therapeutic rapport and effectiveness of treatment.[11]

No data support chronic opioid use in individuals with IBD, and the well-documented risks can be severe: constipation, narcotic bowel syndrome, cognitive impairment, infection, addiction, need for detoxification, and death. If opioids are utilized, they should be prescribed at the lowest dose possible and combined with behavioral and non-opioid pharmacologic therapy, following the Centers for Disease Control and Prevention's 2018 national guidelines for prescribing opioids for chronic pain.

Ideally, a referral to a multidisciplinary pain clinic can be made to optimally manage chronic pain; other best practices include thorough risk-benefit education and mutually agreed on treatment goals with signed controlled substance contract, avoiding concomitant benzodiazepine use, random toxicology screens, monitoring through state-run prescription drug monitoring programs, thorough documentation in the electronic health record, coordination with other relevant treatment providers, prescription for naloxone in the case of opioid overdose, referral to addiction medicine treatment centers if indicated, and follow-ups every 1 to 3 months to reevaluate treatment plan. Alternative treatments include partial opioid agonist agents such as methadone and suboxone. Ketamine is also an emerging treatment for chronic pain that is increasingly being utilized in outpatient clinics. With the increasing availability of medical marijuana, there is evidence that it may be a safer option for analgesia than opioids; high rates of patient-reported satisfaction but evidence of efficacy for pain in IBD is sparse, and long-term safety has not been established[12] (Table 29-4). Some studies are showing positive effects of cannabis on diarrhea, sleep, nausea, and appetite stimulation.[7]

A Multidisciplinary Approach Is Key

Due to the multifactorial complexities of IBD and pain management, patients are best treated through a holistic treatment approach such as an integrated care team. This model includes a diverse team representing the biopsychosocial spectrum of patient needs, including gastroenterologists, surgeons, pharmacists, advanced practice providers, nurses, dieticians, behavioral specialists (psychiatry, psychology, counselors, social workers, addiction specialists), researchers, case managers, and peer support specialists. While a larger team requires higher salary expenses, costs are saved and patient satisfaction is improved through high-quality preventative care, especially by reducing unplanned and preventable medical utilization through emergency room visits and hospitalizations, and increased adherence to treatment plans. The University of Pittsburgh Medical Center Total Care—IBD Program, a subspecialty IBD medical home, has found additional improvements in areas such as reduction in opioid use and depression and improved self-reported quality of life.[13,14]

Table 29-4

Opioids and Cannabis for Chronic Abdominal Pain

Opioids	Cannabis

• Avoid use
• Taper and educate about harm (physical, addiction, death)
• Non-opioid alternatives— behavioral and pharmacological
• No concomitant benzodiazepines
• Screen for misuse (questionnaires, prescription drug monitoring programs, urine toxicology)
• Brief behavioral intervention
• Refer for addiction
	• Treatment agreement
	• Track symptom targets (pain, nausea, appetite, diarrhea)
	• Screen for misuse (gateway drug)
	• Educate about side effects
	  ◦ Neurocognitive deficits
	  ◦ Future substance abuse
	  ◦ Diminished driving performance
	  ◦ Motivation
	  ◦ Paranoia
	  ◦ Depression
	  ◦ Brain development
	• Refer for addiction

Data sources: Hoffenberg, 2017; Phatak, 2017; Swaminath, 2019; Szigethy & Emerick, 2018; Szigethy et al, 2018; Wren, 2018.

Conclusion

Managing chronic pain is an essential component of IBD treatment, and many effective and safe treatments exist. Patient-centered multidisciplinary care with an emphasis on patient education and engagement is key as patients are assessed and treatment plans are created. Stepped-care approaches involving behavioral and complementary techniques and nonopioid pharmacology is best tolerated and most effective for the long-term safety and well-being of the patient with IBD with pain.

References

1. Colombel JF, Shin A, Gibson PR. AGA clinical practice update on functional gastrointestinal symptoms in patients with inflammatory bowel disease: expert review. *Clin Gastroenterol Hepatol.* 2019;17(3):380-390.
2. Szigethy E. Pain management in patients with inflammatory bowel disease. *Gastroenterol & Hepatol.* 2018;14(1):53-56.
3. Schirbel A, Reichert A, Roll S, et al. Impact of pain on health-related quality of life in patients with inflammatory bowel disease. *World J Gastroenterol.* 2010;16(25):3168-3177.
4. Srinath A, Young E, Szigethy E. Pain management in patients with inflammatory bowel disease: translational approaches from bench to bedside. *Inflamm Bowel Dis.* 2014;20(12):2433-2449.
5. Regueiro M, Greer JB, Szigethy E. Etiology and treatment of pain and psychosocial issues in patients with inflammatory bowel diseases. *Gastroenterology.* 2017;152(2):430-439.
6. Docherty MJ, Jones RC, Wallace MS. Managing pain in inflammatory bowel disease. *Gastroenterol & Hepatol.* 2011;7(9):592-601.
7. Szigethy E, Knisely M, Drossman D. Opioid misuse in gastroenterology and non-opioid management of abdominal pain. *Nat Rev Gastroenterol Hepatol.* 2018;15(3):168-180.

8. Mujagic Z, Keszthelyi D, Aziz Q, et al. Systematic review: instruments to assess abdominal pain in irritable bowel syndrome. *Aliment Pharmacol Ther*. 2015;42(9):1064-1081.

9. Manheimer E, Wieland LS, Cheng K, et al. Acupuncture of irritable bowel syndrome: systematic review and meta-analysis. *Amer J Gastroenterol*. 2010;107(6):835-847.

10. Schumann D, Anheyer D, Lauche R, Dobos G, Langhorst J, Cramer H. Effect of yoga in the therapy of irritable bowel syndrome: a systematic review. *Clin Gastroenterol Hepatol*. 2016;14(12):1720-1731.

11. Drossman DA, Tack J, Ford AC, Szigethy E, Tornblom H, Van Oudenhove L. Neuromodulators for functional gastrointestinal disorders (disorders of gut-brain interaction): a Rome Foundation working team report. *Gastroenterology*. 2018;154(4):1140-1171.

12. Swaminath A, Berlin EP, Cheifetz A, et al. The role of cannabis in the management of inflammatory bowel disease: a review of clinical, scientific, and regulatory information. *Inflammatory Bowel Dis*. 2019;25:427-435.

13. Regueiro MD, McAnallen SE, Greer JB, Perkins SE, Ramalingam S, Szigethy E. The inflammatory bowel disease specialty medical home: a new model of patient-centered care. *Inflamm Bowel Dis*. 2016;22(8):1971-1980.

14. Szigethy E, Goldblum Y, Weaver E, et al. Reduction of opioid use and depression within an IBD medical home care model. *Gastroenterology*. 2019;156:S-609-S-610.

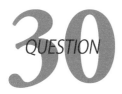

QUESTION

MY PATIENT ON TUMOR NECROSIS FACTOR ALPHA THERAPY HAS A RASH. WHAT SHOULD I DO?

Oluwakemi Onajin, MD and Diana Bolotin, MD, PhD

Cutaneous adverse effects ranging from injection site reactions to psoriasiform eruptions are commonly reported in patients on tumor necrosis factor-α (TNF-α) inhibitors. The aim of this chapter is to provide the reader with the necessary tools to diagnose and treat cutaneous adverse effects of TNF-α inhibitors. Table 30-1 lists the differential diagnosis and management of these cutaneous reactions.

Injection Site Reactions

Injection site reactions to TNF-α inhibitors are usually minor and are characterized by localized tenderness, redness, pruritus, bruising, and swelling at the site of injection. Proposed mechanisms for injection site reactions include hypersensitivity reaction and local trauma.[1] These reactions occur in 10% to 20% of patients in the first month of treatment and can last for up to 5 days.[2,3] Injection site reactions are generally self-limited and decrease in frequency with continuation of therapy. Some patients may develop a recall reaction at the site of previous injections when subsequent injections are administered at a different site.[2] Treatment includes supportive therapy with cool compresses, topical corticosteroids, and pain control. Injection site reactions can be prevented by rotating the injection sites. Discontinuation of the TNF-α inhibitor is rarely indicated.

Rubin DT, Friedman S, Farraye FA, eds. *Curbside Consultation in IBD:*
49 Clinical Questions, Third Edition (pp 189-200).
© 2022 Taylor & Francis Group.

Table 30-1

Differential Diagnosis and Management of Adverse Cutaneous Reactions to TNF-Alpha Inhibitors

Cutaneous Adverse Reaction	Clinical Presentation	Management
Injection site reaction	Localized tenderness, pruritus, erythema, swelling, bruising	Ice, pain control, and topical corticosteroids Rotate injection sites
Infusion reaction	Acute: Flushing, nausea, palpitations, fever, hives, dyspnea, wheezing, chest pain, dizziness, hypotension or hypertension Delayed: Facial edema, urticarial rash, myalgia, arthralgia, fever, and fatigue	Mild-moderate: Monitor vitals, reduce rate of infusion, IV hydration, IV diphenhydramine, acetaminophen, +/- IV corticosteroids Severe: Discontinue infliximab infusion, maintain airway, IV corticosteroids, epinephrine (if anaphylaxis)
Psoriasiform eruption	Erythematous plaques with silvery scale on scalp, trunk, and extremities Palmoplantar psoriasis: Vesicles, pustules, and brown macules with erythema and scale on the palmar hands and plantar feet	Referral to dermatology for diagnosis and management Mild-moderate: Topical therapy (emollients, corticosteroids, vitamin D analogs, retinoids, and tar), ultraviolet phototherapy (UVB and PUVA), systemic therapy (methotrexate, acitretin) Severe: Discontinue anti-TNF therapy, consider systemic agents (cyclosporine, methotrexate, IL-12/23 antagonists)

(continued)

Table 30-1 (continued)

Differential Diagnosis and Management of Adverse Cutaneous Reactions to TNF-Alpha Inhibitors

Cutaneous Adverse Reaction	*Clinical Presentation*	*Management*
Eczematous eruption	Pruritic, scaly, erythematous papules and plaques	Mild-moderate: Topical steroids and topical calcineurin inhibitors Severe: Discontinue anti-TNF therapy, referral to dermatology for diagnosis and management, systemic therapy (cyclosporine)
Vasculitis	Non-blanching, violaceous, palpable purpura on the lower extremities +/- fever, arthralgia, neuropathy and abdominal pain	Rule out systemic involvement, referral to dermatology for biopsy and management, discontinue anti-TNF therapy
Lupus and lupus-like eruption	DILE: Malar rash, discoid lesions, hair loss, photosensitivity, arthralgia, myalgia, pleuritis, pericarditis, fever, weight loss SCLE: Annular or psoriasiform scaly plaques on sun-exposed areas of the trunk and upper extremities	Referral to dermatology for biopsy and management, discontinue anti-TNF therapy, strict sun protection, topical steroids, systemic immunosuppressive therapy

(continued)

Table 30-1 (continued)

Differential Diagnosis and Management of Adverse Cutaneous Reactions to TNF-Alpha Inhibitors

Cutaneous Adverse Reaction	Clinical Presentation	Management
Granulomatous eruption	Sarcoidosis: Red-brown or violaceous macules, papules, and plaques GA and IGD: Smooth, indurated papules or annular patches and plaques	Referral to dermatology for biopsy and management, rule out infectious granulomatous dermatoses, topical steroids
Lichenoid eruption	EM: Fixed, targetoid erythematous macules and papules +/- mucosal lesions, fevers and arthralgia Lichen planus-like: Pruritic, violaceous, flat papules on the trunk and extremities	Referral to dermatology for biopsy and management Severe: Discontinue anti-TNF therapy
Infection	Bacterial: Cellulitis, erysipelas, and abscesses Mycobacterial: Tuberculosis, atypical mycobacteria Viral: Herpes zoster, herpes simplex, CMV, hepatitis B and C	Discontinue anti-TNF therapy until infection is treated, appropriate antimicrobial therapy per pathogen

(continued)

Table 30-1 (continued)

Differential Diagnosis and Management of Adverse Cutaneous Reactions to TNF-Alpha Inhibitors

Cutaneous Adverse Reaction	Clinical Presentation	Management
	Fungal: Dermatophyte, candida, deep fungal infections	
Cutaneous malignancy	Referral to dermatology for complete excision and follow-up skin surveillance	Ultraviolet protection, regular skin cancer screening exams, prompt therapy of precancerous lesions, biopsy and treatment of cutaneous malignancy

Infusion Reactions

Infusion reactions to infliximab are classified as acute and delayed reactions. Depending on the accompanying signs and symptoms, acute and delayed reactions can be further characterized as mild, moderate, or severe. Most infusion reactions to infliximab are acute.[3] Acute reactions occur during or within 24 hours of therapy and can present with pruritus, urticaria (hives), flushing, dyspnea, nausea, headache, chest pain, palpitations, and hypotension.[2,3] Alternatively, delayed reactions occur between 1 and 14 days of therapy and present with "serum sickness-like" symptoms, including facial edema, urticarial rash, myalgia, arthralgia, fever, and fatigue.[2] Infusion reactions can be managed by decreasing the rate of infusion, hydration, acetaminophen, and antihistamines (diphenhydramine or second-generation antihistamines). Severe acute reactions presenting with airway compromise may require treatment with systemic corticosteroids and discontinuation of infliximab infusion. Subsequent infusions reactions can be prevented by premedication with antihistamines and acetaminophen and systemic corticosteroids in patients with a history of severe infusion reactions. Concomitant administration of other immunosuppressive therapies (methotrexate and azathioprine) may also reduce the risk of infusion reactions.[3]

Psoriasiform Eruptions

New onset or worsening of psoriasis can occur as a paradoxical adverse effect of TNF-α inhibitors at any time during therapy. Psoriasiform eruptions in the setting of anti-TNF therapy include plaque psoriasis, guttate psoriasis, palmoplantar psoriasis, and nail and scalp psoriasis[2] (Figure 30-1). The most common subtype caused by TNF-α inhibitors is palmoplantar pustular psoriasis;[2,4] however, the other subtypes of psoriasis may also occur. Palmoplantar pustular psoriasis is characterized by vesicles, pustules, and brown macules with erythema and scale on the palmar hands and plantar feet. The most likely mechanism is the unopposed increased production

Figure 30-1. Erythematous scaly plaques of the palms in palmoplantar psoriasis.

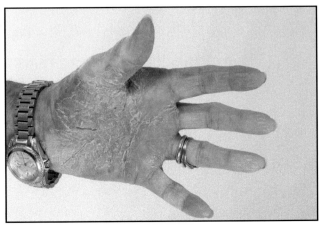

of interferon α during TNF blockade.[1,5] A genetic predisposition is also likely since only a few patients on anti-TNF therapy develop a psoriasiform rash.[1,3] A patient on TNF-α inhibitors who presents with new or worsening psoriasiform eruption should be referred to dermatology for diagnostic confirmation and management. Treatment options include topical therapy (corticosteroids, vitamin D analogs, retinoids, and tar), phototherapy (ultraviolet B, and psoralen and ultraviolet A), and systemic agents.[2] Mild to moderate cases may respond well to topical treatment and phototherapy, allowing for continuation of anti-TNF therapy, but severe cases may require cessation of treatment and alternative therapy. Switching to a different TNF-α inhibitor may lead to recurrence or persistence of psoriasiform eruptions.[3]

Eczematous Eruptions

New onset eczematous eruptions, including dyshidrotic eczema, atopic dermatitis, nummular eczema, and contact dermatitis, have been reported in patients on TNF inhibitors.[2,3] They are characterized by pruritic and scaly, ill-defined erythematous papules and plaques. Most cases can be managed with application of topical steroids and topical calcineurin inhibitors. Discontinuation of TNF inhibitor therapy is rarely indicated. In severe cases, dermatology should be consulted for diagnosis and management.

Vasculitis

Cutaneous vasculitis can be induced by TNF-α inhibitors. This reaction typically presents with nonblanching, violaceous, palpable purpura on the lower extremities and can be accompanied by systemic symptoms of fever, arthralgia, neuropathy, and abdominal pain (Figure 30-2). The proposed mechanism of TNF-α inhibitor–induced vasculitis is an immune complex–mediated inflammatory response to antibodies developed against the drug.[4] Patients on TNF-α inhibitors who present with palpable purpura should be referred to dermatology for a diagnostic skin biopsy and evaluation for systemic involvement. In confirmed cases of TNF-α inhibitor–induced vasculitis, resolution requires cessation of the offending medication.[3] Other treatment options include systemic steroids and immunosuppressive therapy.

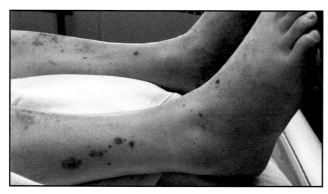

Figure 30-2. Purpuric papules of the distal lower extremities in vasculitis.

Lupus and Lupus-Like Eruption

TNF-α inhibitors can rarely cause drug-induced lupus erythematosus (DILE) and subacute cutaneous lupus erythematosus (SCLE).[3] DILE secondary to TNF-α inhibitors presents as a lupus-like syndrome and is characterized by arthralgia, myalgia, pleuritis, pericarditis, fever, and weight loss. Patients with DILE can test positive for antinuclear and anti-double stranded DNA in addition to anti-histone antibodies.[2,5] However, it is important to note that patients on anti-TNF therapy commonly test positive for these antibodies without developing symptoms of lupus erythematosus.[2,3] Unlike classic DILE, TNF-α related DILE can present with a wide range of skin findings, including malar rash, discoid lesions, hair loss, and photosensitivity.[5] In most cases, the symptoms will resolve with cessation of anti-TNF therapy. Drug-induced SCLE most commonly presents with a skin rash alone, without systemic symptoms. The skin findings are characterized by annular to psoriasiform scaly plaques on sun-exposed areas of the trunk and upper extremities (Figure 30-3). Patients will often test positive for anti-Ro/SS-A and anti-La/SSB antibodies.[6] Withdrawal of anti-TNF therapy often leads to improvement of symptoms within a few weeks. Additionally, patients with DILE may require treatment with topical or systemic steroids, antimalarials, or systemic immunosuppressive agents. Patients on TNF-α inhibitors who present with a photosensitive skin rash and lupus-like symptoms should be referred to a dermatologist for a skin biopsy and assessment for systemic involvement.

Granulomatous Eruptions

Cutaneous granulomatous reactions to TNF-α inhibitors have been described, including sarcoidosis, granuloma annulare, and interstitial granulomatous dermatitis.[2,5] Although TNF-α inhibitors can be used to treat sarcoidosis, cutaneous sarcoidosis can occur as a paradoxical reaction. Sarcoidosis is characterized by red-brown or violaceous macules, papules, and plaques (Figure 30-4). Granuloma annulare and interstitial granulomatous dermatitis present as smooth, indurated papules or annular patches and plaques on the trunk and extremities. A skin biopsy is required to diagnose granulomatous reactions and to exclude infectious granulomatous disease of the skin such as mycobacterial and atypical mycobacterial infections. Granulomatous eruptions can be treated with topical steroid. Discontinuation of anti-TNF therapy is rarely indicated, except in the case of severe and extensive eruptions.

Figure 30-3. Erythematous annular plaques on the back in SCLE.

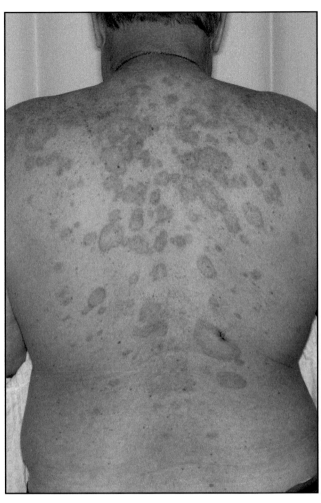

Figure 30-4. Red-brown to skin-colored papules in cutaneous sarcoidosis.

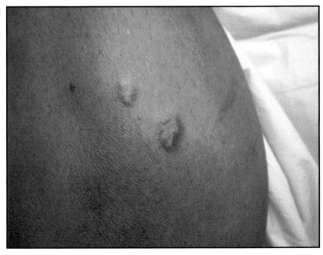

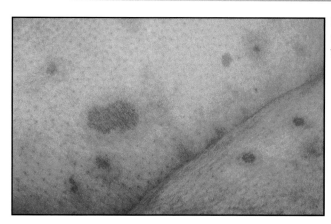

Figure 30-5. Targetoid erythematous macules and papules with dusky centers in erythema multiforme.

Lichenoid Eruptions

Lichenoid eruptions, including erythema multiforme and lichen planus-like reaction, can occur with anti-TNF therapy.[2] A few cases of Stevens-Johnson syndrome and toxic epidermal necrolysis have been reported in patients on anti-TNF therapy; however, most of the patients were on concomitant medications in addition to TNF-α inhibitors that have been implicated in Stevens-Johnson syndrome and toxic epidermal necrolysis.[1,4] Due to similar clinical features, erythema multiforme, Stevens-Johnson syndrome, and toxic epidermal necrolysis were formally considered in the same disease spectrum. However, there is now strong evidence suggesting that erythema multiforme is distinct from Stevens-Johnson syndrome and toxic epidermal necrolysis.[7] Erythema multiforme is characterized by the acute onset of fixed, targetoid erythematous macules and papules that may be accompanied by mucosal lesions, fevers, and arthralgia (Figure 30-5).

Lichen planus-like reactions present with pruritic, violaceous, flat papules on the trunk and extremities (Figure 30-6). A referral to dermatology for a skin biopsy is often required for accurate diagnosis and management. If the eruption is extensive, accompanied by mucosal involvement and/or systemic symptoms, it would be prudent to discontinue anti-TNF therapy.

Infection

TNF-α is a key factor in inflammatory and immune responses; therefore, it is established that anti-TNF therapy may increase susceptibility to systemic as well as cutaneous infections.[1,2,4,8] The skin is the second most common site of infection after the respiratory tract. Risk factors associated with infection include higher dosing, concomitant immunosuppressive therapy, age, malnutrition, and comorbidities such as pulmonary disease, rheumatoid arthritis, alcoholism, and diabetes.[1] These skin infections are typically mild, but severe skin infections requiring hospitalization can rarely occur. Prior to initiating anti-TNF therapy, patients should be screened for tuberculosis, hepatitis B, and hepatitis C. A thorough history and physical exam should be performed to screen for signs of active infections.

TNF-α inhibitor therapy has been associated with cutaneous bacterial, viral, and fungal infections. Cutaneous bacterial infections associated with anti-TNF therapy include cellulitis, erysipelas, and abscesses. Reactivation of herpetic viral infections, including herpes zoster and herpes simplex, can occur during anti-TNF therapy. There are also reported cases of cytomegalovirus infections presenting as cutaneous ulcers in the setting of anti-TNF therapy. Opportunistic fungal and mycobacterial infections may present with erythematous papules, nodules, plaques, or ulcers

Figure 30-6. Violaceous, flat papules on the legs in lichen planus-like eruption.

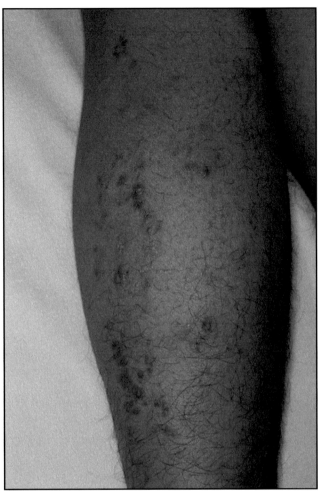

accompanied by systemic symptoms. A skin biopsy and tissue culture are necessary to make the diagnosis. Ultimately these patients should be referred to dermatology and infectious diseases for diagnostic confirmation and management.

Cutaneous Malignancy

Anti-TNF therapy can theoretically increase one's risk of cutaneous malignancy due to its effects on immune surveillance. However, studies evaluating risk of cutaneous malignancies are often confounded by the fact that many patients on anti-TNF therapy had previous or concurrent use of either azathioprine or ultraviolet phototherapy, both of which are risk factors for skin cancer development.[5] Nonetheless, several large cohort studies and a recent meta-analysis have shown an increased relative risk of nonmelanoma skin cancer (NMSC) in patients with IBD treated with anti-TNF agents.[1,5] NMSC types of skin malignancies are primarily made up of basal and squamous cell skin cancers (Figures 30-7 and 30-8). The crux of management of NMSC in patients on anti-TNF therapy is consistent routine surveillance with skin exams performed at least on an annual basis, appropriate treatment of precancerous skin lesions, and early biopsy and treatment of NMSC lesions. Patients should be counseled about self-exams and photoprotection. Risk of

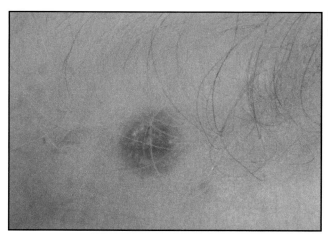

Figure 30-7. Nodular basal cell carcinoma.

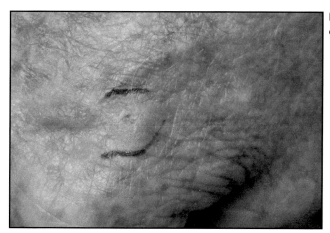

Figure 30-8. Cutaneous squamous cell carcinoma in situ.

cutaneous lymphoma or melanoma in patients on anti-TNF therapy has been debated in the literature but at this time is still uncertain. Cessation of TNF-α therapy is generally not needed for patients with a diagnosis of NMSC. Continuation of TNF-α therapy in patients with melanoma or lymphoma should be weighed against the risks of the specific features of the malignancy; often an alternative therapy for IBD is indicated in this setting.

References

1. Mocci G, Marzo M, Papa A, Armuzzi A, Guidi L. Dermatological adverse reactions during anti-TNF treatments: focus on inflammatory bowel disease. *J Crohns Colitis*. 2013;7(10):769-779. https://doi.org/10.1016/j.crohns.2013.01.009
2. Moustou A-E, Matekovits A, Dessinioti C, Antoniou C, Sfikakis PP, Stratigos AJ. Cutaneous side effects of anti-tumor necrosis factor biologic therapy: a clinical review. *J Am Acad Dermatol*. 2009;61(3):486-504. https://doi.org/10.1016/j.jaad.2008.10.060
3. Feuerstein JD, Cheifetz AS. Miscellaneous adverse events with biologic agents (excludes infection and malignancy). *Gastroenterol Clin North Am*. 2014;43(3):543-563.
4. Kerbleski JF, Gottlieb AB. Dermatological complications and safety of anti-TNF treatments. *Gut*. 2009;58(8):1033-1039. https://doi.org/10.1136/gut.2008.163683

5. Moran GW, Lim AWK, Bailey JL, et al. Review article: dermatological complications of immunosuppressive and anti-TNF therapy in inflammatory bowel disease. *Aliment Pharmacol Ther.* 2013;38(9):1002-1024. https://doi.org/10.1111/apt.12491

6. Grönhagen CM, Fored CM, Linder M, Granath F, Nyberg F. Subacute cutaneous lupus erythematosus and its association with drugs: a population-based matched case-control study of 234 patients in Sweden. *Br J Dermatol.* 2012;167(2):296-305. https://doi.org/10.1111/j.1365-2133.2012.10969.x

7. Assier H, Bastuji-Garin S, Revuz J, Roujeau JC. Erythema multiforme with mucous membrane involvement and Stevens-Johnson syndrome are clinically different disorders with distinct causes. *Arch Dermatol.* 1995;131(5):539-543.

8. Lindhaus C, Tittelbach J, Elsner P. Cutaneous side effects of TNF-alpha inhibitors. *J Dtsch Dermatol Ges.* 2017;15(3):281-288. https://doi.org/10.1111/ddg.13200

31

WHAT IS THE APPROACH TO PRIMARY SCLEROSING CHOLANGITIS IN IBD?

Bilal Hameed, MD and Norah Terrault, MD, MPH

Primary sclerosing cholangitis (PSC) is a chronic, progressive cholestatic liver disease causing inflammation and fibrosis leading to intra/extrahepatic biliary strictures. Liver disease progression to fibrosis and cirrhosis is inevitable in the majority of patients with PSC. PSC is a rare disease with a prevalence ranging from 4 to 16 per 100,000 person years, is more common in men than women (2–3:1) and typically diagnosed between 30 and 40 years of age.[1,2] Globally, PSC is more common in North America and Europe, with data suggesting the incidence and prevalence are increasing over time.[3] The median survival in patients with PSC from diagnosis until liver transplant or death is estimated to be 21.3 years in population-based cohorts.[4]

Diagnosis (Table 31-1)

For patients with chronic elevation of alkaline phosphatase, the differential diagnosis includes PSC. The diagnosis is established by magnetic resonance cholangiopancreatography (MRCP) or endoscopic retrograde cholangiopancreatography (ERCP) showing characteristic bile duct changes with strictures and beading and excluding causes of secondary cholangitis. In patients with clinical suspicion but normal cholangiogram, a liver biopsy may be considered to assess for small duct PSC. The differential diagnosis includes other conditions associated with biliary strictures (Table 31-2). Serum aminotransferase levels can be mildly elevated but if elevated more than 2 to 3 times upper limits of normal, then one needs to consider overlap syndromes (PSC with autoimmune hepatitis) or other liver diseases, and in this setting a liver biopsy is typically required. There is no role for serum antibody testing for the diagnosis of PSC.[5] P-ANCA can be positive in 26%

Rubin DT, Friedman S, Farraye FA, eds. *Curbside Consultation in IBD: 49 Clinical Questions, Third Edition* (pp 201-209).
© 2022 Taylor & Francis Group.

Table 31-1
Primary Sclerosing Cholangitis Initial Diagnosis and Routine Follow-Up

Diagnosis and Baseline
MRCP preferred (ERCP is indicated for evaluation of dominant stricture or treatment of stones)
Liver biopsy only indicated if cholangiogram normal or concern for overlap with AIH
Serum IgG4 to exclude IgG4 disease
AMA to exclude PBC
Fat-soluble vitamins
Colonoscopy if no history of IBD
Follow-Up and Surveillance
Liver enzymes 3 to 6 months; if cirrhosis include albumin, INR, total bilirubin, creatinine
Fat-soluble vitamins yearly and bone density every 2 to 3 years
Colonoscopy yearly for colon cancer surveillance if IBD
Ultrasound for gallbladder polyps annually
MRCP and CA 19-9 yearly for CAA surveillance
ERCP for dominant strictures if pruritus, cholangitis, or cholangiocarcinoma

to 94% of patients with PSC but is not disease specific nor reflects prognosis. To exclude primary biliary cholangitis (PBC), checking for antimitochondrial antibodies is recommended.

Cholangiography with MRCP is the modality of choice for the diagnosis of PSC and preferred over ERCP.[6] MRCP has a sensitivity of 86% and specificity of 94% for the diagnosis of PSC.[7] ERCP is reserved for therapeutic interventions and evaluation of dominant strictures, where there is concern for cholangiocarcinoma. Classic findings on cholangiogram include a beaded appearance reflecting multifocal stricturing of the extrahepatic or intrahepatic bile ducts or both.

Primary Sclerosing Cholangitis Subtypes

As highlighted, there are a few subtypes of PSC (Table 31-3). Most common (90%) is the classic subtype, which affects both large and small bile ducts. Small duct PSC affects only small bile ducts, resulting in a normal cholangiogram, and is seen in 5% patients. Small duct subtype has a better prognosis and lower risk of developing cholangiocarcinoma. PSC with features of autoimmune hepatitis (ie, PSC-AIH overlap) is seen more commonly in children but can be seen in up to 5% of adults.[8] Serum IgG4 is elevated in 10% patients with PSC and associated with worse outcomes than those without IgG4. Serum IgG4 level should be checked in every patient with

Table 31-2

Differential Diagnosis of PSC

Mimickers of Primary Sclerosing Cholangitis	Clinical or Laboratory Clues
Cholangiocarcinoma	Weight loss, dominant stricture, elevated CA19-9
Choledocholithiasis	Imaging evidence of stones
HIV cholangiopathy	HIV status
IgG4 cholangiopathy	IgG4 level > 1.2 ULN
Ischemic/traumatic biliary injury	History of surgery, trauma, intraarterial hepatic therapies
Recurrent biliary cholangitis	Asian origin
Choledochal cysts and biliary atresia	Imaging evidence of cystic disease
Biliary infestation (liver fluke and ascaris)	Positive stool cultures, history of time in endemic regions
Ampullary or pancreatic cancer	Imaging evidence of pancreatic duct abnormalities

suspected PSC.[9] Importantly, elevated IgG4 in PSC should not be confused with IgG4-related disease, a systemic condition with high-serum IgG4 that may include biliary stricturing but has other organ involvement. The overlapping associations of PSC with other immune conditions are shown in Figure 31-1.

IBD and Primary Sclerosing Cholangitis

Although only 8% of patients with inflammatory bowel disease (IBD) are affected by PSC, the majority (70% to 80%) of the patients with PSC have underlying IBD, mostly ulcerative colitis (UC). IBD can develop after the diagnosis of PSC. Because of this close association of PSC with IBD, all patients newly diagnosed with PSC should undergo a colonoscopy, and patients with PSC without IBD should undergo colonoscopy every 5 years to evaluate for onset of IBD. IBD activity does not correlate with liver manifestations of PSC. There is predilection for right-sided colitis, rectal sparing, and "backwash ileitis."[10] PSC patients with IBD are at higher risk of developing colonic malignancy and thus warrant annual colonoscopy.

Symptoms and Complications (Table 31-4)

About half of the patients with PSC are asymptomatic, with normal physical exam on presentation, and diagnosis is made on elevated liver enzymes in patients with IBD.[11] Common symptoms includes fatigue, pruritus, and occasional right upper quadrant pain, with symptoms more

Table 31-3

Subtypes of Primary Sclerosing Cholangitis

Subtype	Cholangiogram	Diagnosis	Other Features
Classic (Large Duct)	Involves both large and small bile ducts	• Cholestasis labs (elevated ALP/GGT) with typical cholangiogram on MRCP (ERCP for diagnosis occasionally)	• Liver biopsy not needed • IBD in 70% to 80% of patients
Small Duct	Only small bile ducts involved	• Liver biopsy needed to confirm the diagnosis • Cholangiogram normal • Cholestasis labs (elevated ALP/GGT)	• Survival better than classic subtype and less chance of cholangiocarcinoma • May progress to classic PSC
PSC With Features of Autoimmune Hepatitis (PSC-AIH Overlap)	Involves both large and small bile ducts	• Features of AIH (ALT/AST elevation with positive ANA, ASMA and IgG) with cholangiogram consistent with PSC • Liver biopsy needed	• Depending on pattern may need steroids • Prognosis better than classic subtype
PSC with Elevated IgG4	Involves both large and small bile ducts	• Elevated IgG4 with typical cholangiogram of PSC • IgG4 staining of relevant biopsy	• 10% of patients with PSC • Patients with elevated IgG4 in PSC have poorer outcomes than those with normal IgG4

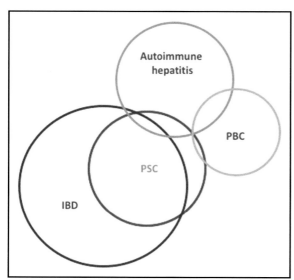

Figure 31-1. PSC-associated immune diseases. The most common immune-mediated disease associated with PSC is IBD (UC > CD), with 70% of PSC patients typically having IBD. The frequency of this association is the rationale for baseline colonoscopy in every patient diagnosed with PSC, even in the absence of symptoms. Less frequently, PSC and autoimmune hepatitis can be present in the same patients, but rarely PSC and PBC.

likely as the disease progresses. Fevers and rigors raise the concern for bacterial cholangitis related to strictures. Jaundice can develop because of dominant stricture/advance stricturing (mainly extrahepatic) or late-stage liver disease. Ascites, variceal bleed, or hepatic encephalopathy develop with end-stage liver disease and cirrhosis. Rapid worsening of symptoms, including pruritus, jaundice, or weight loss, should raise concern for dominant stricture or cholangiocarcinoma. Poor prognostic indicators in PSC include male sex, UC (vs Crohn's disease [CD]), and large (vs small) duct PSC, and conditions associated with worse outcome are dominant strictures and recurrent cholangitis. Since liver disease progression is expected and there is an elevated risk of malignancies in patients with PSC, there is a need for regular follow-up labs and imaging (see Table 31-1).

Hepatobiliary malignancies, including cholangiocarcinoma and gallbladder carcinoma, are more common in patients with PSC than patients without PSC and are associated with high mortality. Cholangiocarcinoma may be the presenting feature of PSC or be diagnosed within the first year of presentation in 30% to 50% of patients. The lifetime risk of developing cholangiocarcinoma in patients with PSC is 10% to 20%.[4] Older age at PSC diagnosis, smoking, alcohol use, elevated bilirubin, a longer duration of IBD, and dominant stricture are associated with a risk of cholangiocarcinoma. Although guidelines do not have specific recommendations for screening for cholangiocarcinoma, most experts recommend MRCP with contrast magnetic resonance imaging and CA19-9 yearly. PSC patients are also at risk of developing gallbladder polyps, which can lead to cancer in 3% of patients. Ultrasound surveillance of the gallbladder is recommended every year. Cholecystectomy if polyps are > 0.8 cm should be considered.

Patients with PSC and IBD have a 4-fold increased risk of developing colon cancer as compared to those with IBD alone.[12] Colonoscopy with biopsies for colon cancer surveillance is recommended every year even after liver transplantation.

Approach to Managing Primary Sclerosing Cholangitis

Management of PSC is complicated and has unique challenges. Because of the progressive nature of the disease, treatment is not only focused on primary liver disease but also on coexisting conditions and management of complications of end-stage liver disease (Figure 31-2).

Table 31-4

Complications of Primary Sclerosing Cholangitis

Complications	*General Approach to Management*
Biliary cirrhosis, portal hypertension	• Referral for liver transplant evaluation • Screening for varices • Surveillance for HCC (in addition to CCA and gallbladder cancer)
Biliary ductal stone formation	• ERCP for removal • UDCA for prevention of recurrent stones
Recurrent bacterial cholangitis	• Antibiotics • Evaluation for dominant stricture as contributing cause • Indication to refer for liver transplantation
Cholangiocarcinoma and gallbladder carcinoma	• Surveillance with CA19-9 and MRCP/MRI annually
Nutritional failure, metabolic bone disease	• Nutritionist consultation • Evaluation for fat-soluble vitamin deficiencies annually; replete if low • Bone density assessment at baseline and every 2 to 3 years depending on age and other cofactors
Increase risk of colon cancer (IBD patients)	• Colonoscopy annually
Pruritus	• Moisturizers • Medications: Antihistamines, doxepin, cholestyramine, rifampin, naltrexone, UDCA

Medical Treatment

There is no established medical therapy for PSC, and no treatment has shown to improve survival or reduce the need for liver transplantation. Ursodeoxycholic acid (UDCA), a hydrophilic bile acid, is the most extensively studied agent in PSC, and its use is controversial. Studies using UCDA in lower doses (10 to 15 mg/kg) showed improvement in biochemical profile but no survival benefit. In modestly higher doses of UDCA (17 to 23 mg/kg), improved biochemical profiles and a trend toward improved survival were seen.[13] However, a large multicenter study of high dose UDCA (28 to 30 mg/kg) vs placebo in patients with PSC was terminated early due to an increased rate of treatment failure and poorer outcome in the UDCA group.[14] Based on these studies, high-dose UDCA is not recommended for the treatment of PSC. While low-medium dose UDCA was not harmful, there is no beneficial effect on progression of PSC. Experts and guidelines differ in their recommendations. The American Association for the Study of Liver Diseases and the American College of Gastroenterology do not recommend starting UDCA, whereas the European Association for the Study of the Liver recommended moderate doses of

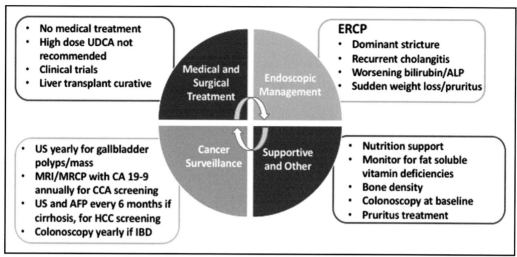

Figure 31-2. Management options for PSC. There are no curative medical therapies for PSC, though liver transplantation is effective for those with complications of biliary cirrhosis. MRCP/ERCP are used selectively to manage and evaluate dominant strictures or acute changes in liver tests. Nutrition support, including fat-soluble vitamins, is important, as well as treatment of pruritus, a common troublesome symptom. Finally, surveillance for cancer—both gallbladder and cholangiocarcinoma—is warranted annually. If cirrhosis is present, surveillance of hepatocellular carcinoma is also warranted with abdominal imaging and AFP every 6 months.

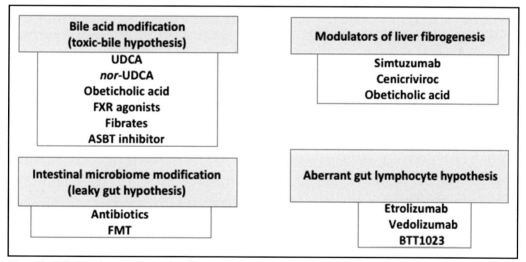

Figure 31-3. Potential mechanisms of PSC pathogenesis and targets for treatment. Medical therapies being evaluated as therapies for PSC can be largely grouped into 4 categories: bile acid modification, modulators of liver fibrogenesis, intestinal microbiome modification, and modulation of aberrant gut lymphocytes.

UDCA (13 to 15 mg/kg). Our approach is to use UDCA at doses of 13 to 15 mg/kg for 6 months and follow-up labs. If there is no improvement in alkaline phosphatase, then stop, but if improvement is seen, continue UDCA.

There are many newer drugs being evaluated in clinical trials that look promising (Figure 31-3). Because of a lack of clear understanding of pathogenesis in PSC, there have been challenges in identifying the correct targets for developing therapies.

Table 31-5
Indications for Liver Transplant in Primary Sclerosing Cholangitis

Complications of portal hypertension (ascites, variceal bleed, HE)
Severe cholestasis with cirrhosis (pruritus, jaundice)
Worsening hepatic synthetic function
Recurrent bacterial cholangitis*
Cholangiocarcinoma*
*Can be eligible for MELD exception points for liver transplant.

Endoscopic Management

Dominant strictures, defined as stenosis of < 1.5 mm in the common bile duct or < 1 mm in the hepatic ducts, are seen in about 50% of patients with PSC. Sudden jaundice, recurrent cholangitis, or onset of or worsening pruritus should raise suspicion for dominant stricture. Cholangiocarcinoma needs to be ruled out in every patient with PSC developing a dominant stricture. A careful evaluation of dominant strictures with ERCP with brushing cytology and FISH (fluorescence in situ hybridization, if available) is recommended. Dominant strictures are associated with poor outcomes in patients with PSC. A single-center study from the United Kingdom showed mean survival of those with dominant strictures was 13.7 years worse than for those without (23 years).[15] Balloon dilatation is preferred for management of dominant stricture; short-term stenting is not superior and is associated with higher rates of complications.

In patients with PSC, there is an increased risk of complications after ERCP, so this test should be restricted to specific indications. Cholangitis is seen in up to 8% procedures and pancreatitis in 7%. ERCP should be considered if worsening symptoms (pruritus, jaundice, recurrent cholangitis), labs (increasing bilirubin or cholestasis labs), or progressive biliary dilatation on imaging studies (ultrasound or MRC) are seen. Patients with PSC before ERCP should receive antibiotics for prophylaxis.

Liver Transplantation

Liver transplantation is the only curative option for patients with PSC. The indications for liver transplant include hepatic decompensation, worsening liver disease, MELD score > 14, recurrent cholangitis, as well as cholangiocarcinoma in select patients (Table 31-5). Early referral to the transplant center is the key. Overall, 5-year survival after liver transplant in patients with PSC is 80% to 85%.[16] Risk of PSC recurrence post–liver transplant is about 20% to 25%. There is also a higher frequency of acute cellular rejections and IBD exacerbations post–liver transplant.

Conclusion

PSC is a progressive cholestatic liver disease leading to fibrosis and cirrhosis in majority of the patients with no effective medical treatment. Diagnosis of PSC is based on a combination of clinical manifestations, laboratory, and imaging. PSC diagnosis should be suspected in all patients with IBD and elevated alkaline phosphatase and/or gamma glutamyl transferase values. MRCP is the modality of choice for the diagnosis of PSC. PSC is strongly associated with IBD (70% to 80%) and increased risk of developing colon, bile duct, and gallbladder cancers, and regular surveillance for these malignancies is warranted. There are no effective therapies, though new drug therapies are being actively sought. Liver transplantation should be considered for those with liver complications.

References

1. Bambha K, Kim WR, Talwalkar J, et al. Incidence, clinical spectrum, and outcomes of primary sclerosing cholangitis in a United States community. *Gastroenterology.* 2003;125(5):1364-1369.
2. Hirschfield GM, Karlsen TH, Lindor KD, Adams DH. Primary sclerosing cholangitis. *Lancet.* 2013;382(10139): 1587-1599.
3. Molodecky NA, Kareemi H, Parab R, et al. Incidence of primary sclerosing cholangitis: a systematic review and meta-analysis. *Hepatology.* 2011;53(5):1590-1599.
4. Boonstra K, Weersma RK, van Erpecum KJ, et al. Population-based epidemiology, malignancy risk, and outcome of primary sclerosing cholangitis. *Hepatology.* 2013;58(6):2045-2055.
5. Hov JR, Boberg KM, Karlsen TH. Autoantibodies in primary sclerosing cholangitis. *World J Gastroenterol.* 2008;14(24):3781-3791.
6. Angulo P, Pearce DH, Johnson CD, et al. Magnetic resonance cholangiography in patients with biliary disease: its role in primary sclerosing cholangitis. *J Hepatol.* 2000;33(4):520-527.
7. Dave M, Elmunzer BJ, Dwamena BA, Higgins PD. Primary sclerosing cholangitis: meta-analysis of diagnostic performance of MR cholangiopancreatography. *Radiology.* 2010;256(2):387-396.
8. Kaya M, Angulo P, Lindor KD. Overlap of autoimmune hepatitis and primary sclerosing cholangitis: an evaluation of a modified scoring system. *J Hepatol.* 2000;33(4):537-542.
9. Webster GJ, Pereira SP, Chapman RW. Autoimmune pancreatitis/IgG4-associated cholangitis and primary sclerosing cholangitis—overlapping or separate diseases? *J Hepatol.* 2009;51(2):398-402.
10. Loftus EV Jr, Harewood GC, Loftus CG, et al. PSC-IBD: a unique form of inflammatory bowel disease associated with primary sclerosing cholangitis. *Gut.* 2005;54:91-96.
11. Kaplan GG, Laupland KB, Butzner D, Urbanski SJ, Lee SS. The burden of large and small duct primary sclerosing cholangitis in adults and children: a population-based analysis. *Am J Gastroenterol.* 2007;102(5):1042-1049.
12. Khaderi SA, Sussman NL. Screening for malignancy in primary sclerosing cholangitis (PSC). *Curr Gastroenterol Rep.* 2015;17(4):17.
13. Lindor KD. Ursodiol for primary sclerosing cholangitis. *N Engl J Med.* 1997;336:691-695.
14. Lindor KD, Kowdley KV, Luketic VA, et al. High-dose ursodeoxycholic acid for the treatment of primary sclerosing cholangitis. *Hepatology.* 2009;50(3):808-814.
15. Chapman MH, Webster GJ, Bannoo S, Johnson GJ, Wittmann J, Pereira SP. *Eur J Gastroenterol Hepatol.* 2012;24(9): 1051-1058.
16. Graziadei IW, Wiesner RH, Marotta PJ, et al. Long-term results of patients undergoing liver transplantation for primary sclerosing cholangitis. *Hepatology.* 1999;30(5):1121-1127.

QUESTION 32

WHAT IS THE BEST MEDICAL THERAPY FOR IBD IN OLDER PATIENTS?

Seymour Katz, MD

Before embarking on choices of therapy, the diagnosis must be verified, especially in older adults with the potential for confounding multiple diagnoses (ie, ischemia, radiation, segmental colitis with colonic diverticular disease, secondary gastrointestinal infections, or nonsteroidal anti-inflammatory drug use).

A distinction of "fit vs frail" older patient impacts the choice of medication and how far to push more toxic options. Clinical symptom implementation takes precedence over "deep remission" (ie, endoscopic, histologic, biomarker remission).

Combined oral and topical mesalamine remains the standard of care for mild to moderate ulcerative colitis provided the patient has the manual dexterity to administer rectal therapy. Caution is required for potential nephrotoxicity with mesalamines, especially in patients with preexisting renal diseases (ie, renal stones, diabetes, or extensive vascular disease). Interstitial nephritis is rare but always lurks in the background.[1] There is little to no value of 5-aminosalicylic acid (5-ASA) in Crohn's disease except very mild Crohn's colitis. Corticosteroids are to be avoided except for a very limited exposure. Too often older patients are on a "maintenance" corticosteroid due to fear of advancing to other immunosuppressive therapies. The risks of corticosteroids are well known but may be disguised as depression or dementia in older adults. Any corticosteroid use requires an exit strategy.[2]

First pass metabolism corticosteroids (eg, budesonide) have a role in ileal or ileal right-sided colonic disease. Even with limited bioavailability, the risk for corticoid excess–induced "Cushing" still exists. Immunomodulators should be avoided in older adults because of greater risk of infection, skin cancers, or lymphoproliferative disease compared to the younger patient with inflammatory bowel disease (IBD), except in circumstances where alternatives are unavoidable.[3] If used,

Rubin DT, Friedman S, Farraye FA, eds. *Curbside Consultation in IBD: 49 Clinical Questions, Third Edition* (pp 211-213).
© 2022 Taylor & Francis Group.

the thiopurine methyltransferase enzyme must be determined, and metabolites (6TGN) must be followed, but this still requires vigilance for myelosuppression. Thiopurine use in combination therapy with biologics to limit antibody formation and increase drug levels, if used, can be discontinued after 6 months. There is evidence that adequate drug levels would negate need for thiopurine coadministration.

Biologics (anti-TNF, anti-integrin, interleukin [IL] 12/IL-23 inhibitors) are shamefully underutilized in older adults due to fear of greater opportunistic infection, neoplasia, cost, altered compliance, and early termination. Nevertheless, the benefits often overweigh the risks by permitting lesser hospitalizations and surgical intervention. Extraintestinal manifestations of IBD often herald more severe disease and warrant earlier use of biologics.[4] Data from Janus kinase inhibitors remain scant in older adults and must await post-marketing experience. Therapeutic drug monitoring is the standard of care with biologic therapy.

Key points of care:
- Fibrostenotic diseases (strictures) require surgery. Do not waste precious time or medical resources and include surgical consultations early.
- Older adult patients have a different biology (ie, less total body), and intravascular water can create toxic drug levels when given conventional doses, so "start low and go slow" with dosing.
- Drug-drug interactions are common with the polypharmacy of older adults, with an average number of medications often exceeding 10 per day. Be sure to review the patient's drug list at **each visit**. For example, 5-ASA interferes with anticoagulants so careful INR/pro-time monitoring is essential in this population with atrial fibrillation and extensive thromboembolic disease; avoid anticholinergics, opiates, and sedatives.
- Multiple comorbidities (ie, cardiovascular, chronic obstructive pulmonary disease, diabetes) directly impact IBD morbidity and mortality.[5]
- Concomitant therapy of biologics with chemotherapeutic regimens is not contraindicated and opens the opportunity for treating aggressive IBD in the presence of cancer. Such decisions must be coordinated with the chemotherapist.[6,7]
- Always test for *Clostridioides difficile* even when in remission.
- Vaccinations are to be updated, particularly if therapy with an immunosuppressive is contemplated. Pneumonia and herpes zoster are greater threats and are preventable.
- Malnutrition, dehydration, and electrolyte depletion are common and underdiagnosed.[8,9]
- A second observer should be present for all communications. Written instructions increase quality and effectiveness of care.[10]
- Challenge transfer of information from clinical trials since older adults are often excluded.
- Face-to-face visits with the treating MD permits review of the points covered.
- Primum non nocere: First do no harm.

Management strategies:
- Update list of providers: Laminated card, *not* iPhone/iPad, telephone/email.
- Maintain updated medication (lists of all prescription and over-the-counter medications).
- Schedule routine office visits and always with a second listener.
- Confirm updated health care maintenance, including vaccinations, dental, vision, and cancer screening.
- Provide clearly written instructions reviewed by staff and/or a companion at the end of the visit.

Goals of treatment for older patients with IBD:

- Restore normal bowel function.
- Improve quality of life.
- Induce and maintain steroid-free remission.
- Modify natural history of IBD
  ○ Avoid hospitalization and decrease risk of surgery.
  ○ Eliminate disability, maintain independence, lower costs of care.
  ○ Evaluate therapy choices based on risk vs benefits.

References

1. Gisbert, JP, Gonzalez-Lama Y, Mate J. 5-aminosalicylates and renal function in inflammatory bowel disease: a systematic review. *Inflamm Bowel Dis.* 2007;13(5):629-638.
2. Geisz M, Ha C, Kappelman MD, Martin CF, et al. Medication utilization and the impact of continued corticosteroid use on patient-reported outcomes in older patients with inflammatory bowel disease. *Inflamm Bowel Dis.* 2016;22(6):1435-41.
3. Kotlyar DS, Lewis JD, Beaugerie L, et al. Risk of lymphoma in patients with inflammatory bowel disease treated with azathioprine and 6-mercaptopurine: a meta-analysis. *Clin Gastroenterol Hepatol.* 2015;13(5):847-858 e4; quiz e48-50.
4. Duricova D, Leroyer A, Savoye G, et al. Extra-intestinal manifestations at diagnosis at paediatric- and elderly-onset ulcerative colitis are associated with a more severe disease outcome: a population-based study. *J Crohns Colitis.* 2017;11(11):1326-1334.
5. Juneja M, Baidoo L, Schwartz MB et al. Geriatric inflammatory bowel disease: phenotypic presentation, treatment patterns, nutritional status, outcomes, and comorbidity. *Dig Dis Sci.* 2012;57(9):2408-2415.
6. Nyboe Andersen N, Pasternak B, Basit S. Association between tumor necrosis factor-alpha antagonists and risk of cancer patients with inflammatory bowel disease. *JAMA.* 2014;311(23):2406-2413.
7. Axelrad J, Bernheim O, Colombel J-F, et al. Risk of new or recurrent cancer in patients with inflammatory bowel disease and previous cancer exposed to immunosuppressive and anti-TNF necrosis factor agents. *Clin Gastroenterol Hepatol.* 2016;14(1):58-64.
8. Ananthakrishnan AN, McGinley EL, Binion DG. Inflammatory bowel disease in the elderly is associated with worse outcomes: a national study of hospitalizations. *Inflamm Bowel Dis.* 2009;15(2):182-189.
9. Calder PC. Feeding the immune system. *Proc Nutr Soc.* 2013;72(3): 299-309.
10. Boyt C, Green AF, Boult LB, Pacala JT, Snyder C, Leff, B. Successful models of comprehensive care for older adults with chronic conditions: evidence for the Institute of Medicine's "retooling for an aging America" report. *J Am Geriatr Soc.* 2009;57(12):2328-2337.

HOW SHOULD CLINICIANS TREAT MEN WITH IBD? WHAT ARE THE UNIQUE CONCERNS?

Aoibhlinn O'Toole, MD and Sonia Friedman, MD

The majority of patients with Crohn's disease (CD) and ulcerative colitis (UC) are diagnosed between the ages of 15 and 35 years during the peak years of fertility and reproduction. While there are multiple research studies examining pregnancy and birth outcomes in women with inflammatory bowel disease (IBD), there is less attention paid to the reproductive health of men with IBD. Specific concerns for men with IBD discussed in this chapter are sperm quality, fertility, the effect of medications taken at conception on birth outcomes, and testosterone replacement therapy. Sexual function is discussed in Question 49.

Sperm Quality

Spermatogenesis takes 70 to 90 days in humans, and a 3-month cutoff is used in studies looking at the toxic effects of a drug on sperm development and thus potential effect on the offspring. Potential mechanisms for a paternal drug effect include (1) a direct effect on spermatocytes, (2) an impact on the mother by systemic effect of the drug or metabolites or absorption through the vaginal mucosa, and/or (3) drugs or metabolites in seminal fluid that might have an impact on sperm maturation and/or a direct effect on the uterus.

Sperm DNA damage or fragmentation may result from various endogenous and exogenous exposures, including effects of medications and inflammation. In most studies, sperm quality has been assessed by World Health Organization (WHO) criteria, which is a conventional light microscopic analysis of semen volume, sperm concentration, motility, and morphology. WHO semen evaluation correlates poorly with fertility and does not evaluate the genomic integrity of

Rubin DT, Friedman S, Farraye FA, eds. *Curbside Consultation in IBD: 49 Clinical Questions, Third Edition* (pp 215-220).
© 2022 Taylor & Francis Group.

the spermatozoa. The need for a marker that can better discriminate infertile men from fertile men and predict pregnancy outcome as well as give information about sperm genomic integrity has driven the search for methods to evaluate sperm quality and DNA integrity to complement basic WHO analysis. Normal sperm chromatin structure is essential for the correct transmission of genetic information, and there is fair evidence that there is a negative correlation between sperm DNA fragmentation and male fertility.

There have been several papers that measured sperm DNA integrity in men with IBD. Ley et al studied 6 men with IBD on methotrexate and found reduced sperm integrity based on significant increases in levels of DNA fragmentation and damage from oxidative stress compared to controls. WHO semen criteria were normal.[1] In more comprehensive studies, Grosen et al examined sperm DNA integrity in men on thiopurines, anti–tumor necrosis factor (TNF) medications, vedolizumab, and in men with active IBD.[2,3] They found that DNA integrity was not affected by thiopurines, vedolizumab, or increased disease activity and was affected in a clinically insignificant way by anti-TNF medications. This new information suggests that thiopurines, anti-TNF medications, vedolizumab, and increased disease activity do not impact fertility.

Fertility

Only a large prospective study of men with IBD and controls can adequately measure fertility, and this is very difficult to accomplish. Measuring sperm DNA integrity is one way to assess potential fertility, as are population-based studies with adequate control groups. A recent population-based study from Utah found no differences in paternity rate or birth outcomes in men with CD (n = 421) or UC (n = 473) compared with their age-matched siblings (n = 1851).[4] The same authors found no difference in WHO semen parameters or number of offspring in men with IBD (n = 55) compared with age-matched unrelated controls (n = 47).[5] Medication use and disease activity were unavailable for the cohort. There were no available data on early pregnancy outcomes (miscarriages, stillbirths, or ectopic pregnancies). Significantly, the mean interval between births was equal between the children of affected and unaffected fathers, so there was likely no difference in the difficulty of achieving a pregnancy.

VOLUNTARY CHILDLESSNESS

Voluntary childlessness, or the decision not to have children, is often confused with infertility, which is involuntary. A systematic review on fertility in nonsurgically treated IBD showed that in men with CD (493 men in 2 population-based studies and 1 referral center study), there was an 18% to 50% reduction in fertility compared with controls, although the authors suggest that this is due to voluntary childlessness as opposed to involuntary infertility. There was no evidence of reduced fertility in men with UC.[6]

INHERITANCE

A recent study from Denmark estimated the risk of IBD in the offspring of fathers with IBD. The authors found that the adjusted incidence rate ratio (IRR) for CD in the offspring of fathers with CD was 7.53 (95% CI, 6.36 to 8.91). For fathers with UC, the IRR for having a child with UC was 4.25 (95% CI, 3.70 to 4.87).[7] A second study from Sweden examined parents with 1 of 34 autoimmune diseases but did not separate the risk in mothers and fathers. The authors found that the IRR for UC in the offspring of a parent diagnosed with UC was 3.9 (95% CI, 3.5 to 4.3) and 6.0 (95% CI, 5.4 to 6.7) for CD in the offspring of a parent diagnosed with CD.

Paternal Medications Taken Within 3 Months Prior to Conception and Birth Outcomes

5-Aminosalicylates

In men, sulfasalazine therapy causes a reversible decrease in sperm motility and count.[8] The effect is dose related and unaffected by supplemental folic acid. Men should stop sulfasalazine 3 months prior to conception, and if this is not possible consider semen analysis. Phthalates were utilized in certain mesalamine products (Asacol HD) due to their ability to localize medication release. Experimental studies in animals have shown that dibutyl phthalate and di-(2-ethylhexyl) phthalate have the potential to alter or inhibit reproductive biology and in utero development. Asacol HD has been dibutyl phthalate free since 2016.

Corticosteroids

In men, corticosteroid excess may be associated with suppressed levels of plasma and urinary testosterone, decreased libido, and impaired spermatogenesis. Paternal corticosteroid use and birth outcomes were studied in 2380 men who received prescriptions for steroids within 3 months of conception and no significant increased risk of adverse birth outcomes was reported.[9]

Thiopurines

No increase in major malformations was found (3% vs 2.2%) in offspring from 115 pregnancies where the fathers were exposed to thiopurines at the time of conception.[10] Studies from the Danish national registries report no negative impact of paternal preconception use of azathioprine, 6-mercaptopurine (n = 735 children) or methotrexate (n = 209 children) on selected long-term childhood health outcomes when compared to children of controls.[11] There was no significantly increased risk of congenital abnormalities or preterm birth in the children of 699 fathers who took azathioprine/6-mercaptopurine within 3 months of conception, compared with men who did not take azathioprine/6-mercaptopurine within 3 months of conception.[12]

Methotrexate

The European Crohn's and Colitis Organization guidelines state that methotrexate is contraindicated for men aiming to father a child and should be stopped 3 to 6 months prior to conception. However, recent studies suggest that methotrexate use in males around the time of conception is safe. Eck et al used the Danish population databases to assess for adverse birth outcomes in 127 births where the fathers were exposed to methotrexate and found no association between paternal exposure to methotrexate within 90 days before pregnancy and congenital malformations, stillbirths, or preterm birth.[13] This finding is supported by a further Danish population-based study of 193 exposed children whose fathers took methotrexate within 3 months before conception that revealed no adverse effects of congenital abnormalities, small for gestational age, or preterm birth.[14]

Biologics

A nationwide Danish study on the safety of paternal use of anti–tumor necrosis factor-α (TNF-α) agents in fathers with IBD found no increased risk of congenital abnormalities, small for gestational age, or preterm birth.[15] Analysis of 15 pregnancies fathered by patients receiving vedolizumab identified no specific safety concerns.[16] We have no data on the effect of ustekinumab on male reproduction.

Testosterone in IBD

Testosterone is central to male sexual performance and directly influences erection, arousal, and ejaculatory function. Steroid and opiate use, as well as chronic inflammation, contribute to depression of circulating testosterone levels.[17] Hypogonadism has been reported in up to 40% of male patients with IBD and contributes to metabolic bone disease.[18] Testosterone replacement therapy has been successfully used to treat erectile and arousal disorders. Delayed puberty frequently complicates the clinical course of young patients with IBD, more often in CD than UC. Serum androgens are consistently reported to be reduced in patients with delayed puberty and IBD. Pubertal delay in adolescent males can be treated with parenteral testosterone, particularly if causing psychological distress. Furthermore, infliximab use in adolescents with CD has been shown to increase sex hormone and gonadotrophin levels, with improvements in disease activity and reduced measures of inflammation.[19] Others have explored the therapeutic benefit of testosterone as a treatment for CD, and in a prospective German and Syrian study of 92 hypogonadal men receiving testosterone therapy there was a significant decrease in the Crohn's Disease Activity Index.[20] The therapeutic benefit of testosterone supplementation to treat IBD requires further study.

We recommend that IBD and primary care providers screen for hypogonadism in patients who present with sexual dysfunction and with metabolic bone disease. The normal range for early morning testosterone in a male is between 300 ng/dL to 1000 ng/dL. Hypogonadism is diagnosed when the morning serum total testosterone level is less than 300 ng/d. In the presence of low testosterone levels, sex hormone-binding globulin should be measured to calculate the free bioavailable testosterone. Long-acting injectable testosterone undecanoate and transdermal gel preparations are preferable to short-acting injections and oral testosterone due to better efficacy and safety profiles; the choice of testosterone replacement therapy should be discussed with the patient and his endocrinologist or urologist (Figure 33-1).

Conclusion

Men's health is an understudied area in IBD. While sperm quality does not seem to be affected by IBD activity, thiopurines, anti-TNF medications, or vedolizumab, only 3 IBD studies have measured it properly by assessing sperm DNA fragmentation. Although we know that sperm quality can have a significant impact on fertility and birth outcomes, there are little data on the effects of other IBD medications such as corticosteroids or methotrexate on sperm. Male fertility rates can be measured accurately only in large prospective studies, and an estimate can be confounded by voluntary childlessness. Male fertility in IBD needs to be additionally investigated with studies examining time to pregnancy and early pregnancy outcomes. We recently gained more knowledge regarding the short-term safety of paternal medications taken within 3 months of conception, with large population-based studies demonstrating the safety of infliximab, adalimumab, azathioprine, 6-mercaptopurine, methotrexate, and steroids. There is a lack of data,

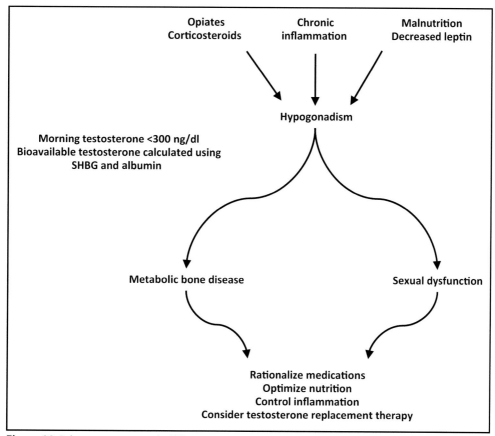

Figure 33-1. Low testosterone in IBD.

however, on the long-term outcomes of children exposed to periconceptual paternal medications. Screening for hypogonadism is recommended in patients who present with sexual dysfunction or with metabolic bone disease, and testosterone replacement therapy can be considered. Close collaboration between the gastroenterology health care provider and the patient is recommended for the best management of these relevant, often neglected aspects in men with IBD.

References

1. Ley D, Jones J, Parrish J, et al. Methotrexate reduces DNA integrity in sperm from men with inflammatory bowel disease. *Gastroenterology.* 2018;154(8):2064-2067.e3.
2. Grosen A, Nursting J, Bungum M, et al. Sperm DNA integrity is unaffected by thiopurine treatment in men with inflammatory bowel disease. *J Crohns Colitis.* 2019;13(1):3-11.
3. Grosen A, Bungun M, Christensen LA, et al. Semen quality and sperm DNA integrity in patients with severe active inflammatory bowel disease and effects of tumor necrosis factor-alpha inhibitors. *J Crohns Colitis.* 2019;13(5): 564-571.
4. Martin L, Peche W, Peterson K, et al. Population-based paternity rate and partner birth outcomes among Utah men with inflammatory bowel disease. *Am J Gastroenterol.* 2017;112(11):1722-1727.
5. Martin L, Mullaney S, Peche W, et al. Population-based semen analysis results and fertility among patients with inflammatory bowel disease: results from Subfertility Health Assisted Reproduction and the Environment (SHARE) study. *Urology.* 2017;107:114-119.
6. Tavernier N, Fumery M, Peyrin-Biroulet L, Colombel J-F, Gower-Rosseau C. Systematic review: fertility in non-surgically treated inflammatory bowel disease. *Aliment Pharmacol Ther.* 2013;38(8):847-853.

7. Moller FT, Andersen V, Wohlfahrt J, Jess T. Familial risk of inflammatory bowel disease: a population-based cohort study 1977-2011. *Am J Gastroenterol.* 2015;110(4):564-571.

8. O'Moráin C, Smethurst P, Doré CJ, Levi AJ. Reversible male infertility due to sulphasalazine: studies in man and rat. *Gut.* 1984;25(10):1078-1084.

9. Larsen MD, Smethurst P, Doré CJ, Levi AJ. Birth outcome of children fathered by men treated with systemic corti-costeroids during the conception period—a cohort study based on nationwide data. *Basic Clin Pharmacol Toxicol.* 2018;122(1):133-138.

10. Teruel C, López-San Román A, Bermejo F, et al. Outcomes of pregnancies fathered by inflammatory bowel disease patients exposed to thiopurines. *Am J Gastroenterol.* 2010;105(9):2003-2008.

11. Friedman S, Larsen MD, Magnussen B, Jølving LR, de Silva P, Nørgård BM. Paternal use of azathioprine/6-mercaptopurine or methotrexate within 3 months before conception and long-term health outcomes in the offspring-A nationwide cohort study. *Reprod Toxicol.* 2017;73:196-200.

12. Nørgård BM, Magnussen B, Larsen MD, Friedman S. Reassuring results on birth outcomes in children fathered by men treated with azathioprine/6-mercaptopurine within 3 months before conception: a nationwide cohort study. *Gut.* 2017;66(10):1761-1766.

13. Eck LK, Jensen TB, Mastrogiannis D, Torp-Pedersen A. Risk of adverse pregnancy outcome after paternal exposure to methotrexate within 90 days before pregnancy. *Obstet Gynecol.* 2017;129(4):707-714.

14. Winter RW, Larsen MD, Magnussen B, Friedman S, Kammerlander H, Nørgård BM. Birth outcomes after precon-ception paternal exposure to methotrexate: a nationwide cohort study. *Reprod Toxicol.* 2017;74:219-223.

15. Larsen MD, Friedman S, Magnussen B, Nørgård BM. Birth outcomes in children fathered by men treated with anti-TNF-alpha agents before conception. *Am J Gastroenterol.* 2016;111(11):1608-1613.

16. Mahadevan U, Vermeire S, Lasch K et al. Vedolizumab exposure in pregnancy: outcomes from clinical studies in inflammatory bowel disease. *Aliment Pharmacol Ther.* 2017;45(7):941-950.

17. Reid IR, Wattie DJ, Evans MC, Stapleton JP. Testosterone therapy in glucocorticoid-treated men. *Arch Intern Med.* 1996;156(11):1173-1177.

18. Szathmári M, Vásárhelyi B, Treszl A, Tulassay T, Tulassay Z. Association of dehydroepiandrosterone sulfate and testosterone deficiency with bone turnover in men with inflammatory bowel disease. *Int J Colorectal Dis.* 2002;17(2):63-66.

19. DeBoer MD, Thayu M, Griffin LM, et al. Increases in sex hormones during anti-tumor necrosis factor alpha therapy in adolescents with Crohn's disease. *J Pediatr.* 2016;171:146-52.e1-2.

20. Nasser M, Haider A, Saad F, et al. Testosterone therapy in men with Crohn's disease improves the clinical course of the disease: data from long-term observational registry study. *Horm Mol Biol Clin Investig.* 2015;22(3):111-117.

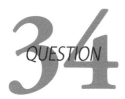

QUESTION 34

WHAT IS THE UPDATED APPROACH TO IBD MEDICAL THERAPY IN PREGNANCY AND WHAT IS KNOWN ABOUT NEONATAL OUTCOMES IN BABIES BORN TO MOTHERS WITH IBD?

Muhammad Bader Hammami, MD and Uma Mahadevan, MD

The choice of therapy for patients with inflammatory bowel disease (IBD) before, during, and after pregnancy should be based on known medication safety, individual patient disease characteristics, and risk for relapse. Active IBD itself is one of the strongest predictors of poor pregnancy outcomes[1,2]; therefore, the risks associated with discontinuing medications must be weighed against any risks of the medications themselves.

Management During Preconception

The path to a healthy pregnancy starts with preconception planning. Patient care should ideally be provided by a multidisciplinary team, which includes a gastroenterologist, obstetrician, maternal-fetal medicine specialist, and colorectal surgeon if needed. Patients should be up-to-date with their health care maintenance, vaccinations, and surveillance colonoscopy. Their disease activity should be assessed with either endoscopy, fecal calprotectin, or imaging, as appropriate. Disease control should be optimized, and medications should be adjusted to achieve steroid-free remission for at least 3 months prior to conception. Teratogenic medications should be discontinued, and folic acid supplementation should be initiated.

Methotrexate is an abortifacient, teratogenic antimetabolite that blocks thymidine synthesis. It has a long half-life, and its use is contraindicated during pregnancy. Women on methotrexate should be counseled to avoid conception within 3 months of its use. Women on combination biologic and thiopurine therapy in sustained remission and with adequate trough levels may consider stopping thiopurines due to a possible association with increased infant infections.[3] Monoclonal

Rubin DT, Friedman S, Farraye FA, eds. *Curbside Consultation in IBD: 49 Clinical Questions, Third Edition* (pp 221-225).
© 2022 Taylor & Francis Group.

antibody therapy does not need to be discontinued but should be adjusted to achieve preconception treatment goals. A study from the French GETAID (Groupe d'Etude Thérapeutique des Affections Inflammatoires du Tube Digestif) group reported an 32% rate of postpartum disease activity in women who preventively stopped anti–tumor necrosis factor (TNF) therapy during pregnancy.[4] Finally, human pregnancy outcomes with Janus kinase inhibitors (tofacitinib) are sparse and confounded by frequent concomitant methotrexate use. Since Janus kinase inhibitors have been shown to be teratogenic in animal models, if possible they should be discontinued or transitioned to other drugs prior to conception until better safety data are available.

Continuing Treatment During Pregnancy

All mesalamine (sulfasalazine and 5-aminosalicylate) formulations, including enema and suppository, may be continued during pregnancy without any known increased risk.[5] Sulfasalazine should be given with at least 2 mg of folic acid per day. Thiopurines (6-mercaptopurine and its prodrug azathioprine) disrupt nucleic acid synthesis, cause chromosomal damage, and are teratogenic in animal models at doses equal to or greater than human therapeutic doses.[6] However, animal studies used parenteral or intraperitoneal routes of administration (which have much higher bioavailability than the oral route). Thiopurine metabolites cross the human placenta[7]; however, a multicenter, retrospective study comparing 187 patients with IBD treated with thiopurines, 66 treated with anti-TNF agents, and 318 unexposed found no difference in pregnancy complications among the groups.[8] Further, in multivariate analysis, thiopurine treatment was also associated with favorable global pregnancy outcomes, defined as a decreased rate of spontaneous abortion and lack of obstetric complications. In the PIANO (Pregnancy in IBD and Neonatal Outcomes) registry, among the > 469 thiopurine-exposed pregnancies, there was no increased risk of congenital anomalies or pregnancy complications compared to infants of unexposed mothers.[3] Thus, it is reasonable to continue thiopurine monotherapy during pregnancy to maintain remission, as the risks of active disease likely outweigh the risks associated with thiopurine use. However, thiopurines should not be started for the first time during pregnancy due to their slow onset of action and the small risk of bone marrow suppression and pancreatitis.

Of the 4 anti-TNF medications US Food and Drug Administration–approved for IBD, infliximab and adalimumab have the most available pregnancy safety data and are low risk for use through pregnancy.[9] In the PIANO registry, 846 women have been exposed to anti-TNF medications during pregnancy: 421 infliximab, 279 adalimumab, 135 certolizumab pegol, and 11 golimumab; to date, no increased risk of congenital anomalies was found compared to the unexposed IBD cohort.[3] Other series with > 100 IBD pregnancies, each exposed to adalimumab,[10] infliximab,[11] and certolizumab pegol,[12] showed similar results. A systematic review, including > 1500 IBD pregnancies exposed to anti-TNF antibodies, also revealed no evidence of increased rate of adverse pregnancy outcomes or congenital anomalies.[13]

There are limited safety data on vedolizumab (a humanized monoclonal immunoglobulin G1 antibody against $\alpha_4\beta_7$ integrin), natalizumab (a humanized IgG4 monoclonal antibody against the a4-integrin cell adhesion molecule), and ustekinumab (an IgG1 monoclonal anti–interleukin [IL] 12/IL-23 antibody). Most of the limited data on natalizumab-exposed pregnancies come from multiple sclerosis patients. A global, observational, exposure registration follow-up study of 362 natalizumab-exposed pregnancies found no increased risk of congenital anomalies.[14] A series of 24 women (23 with IBD) treated with vedolizumab reported 10 live births, 5 elective abortions, 4 spontaneous abortions, and 1 congenital anomaly.[15] Finally, a series of 26 ustekinumab-exposed pregnancies reported 5 spontaneous abortions (19%), a rate similar to the general population rate.[16]

Management of Flares

The management of flares in pregnant patients is similar to that of nonpregnant patients with the following exceptions: Traditional serum markers of disease activity, such as hemoglobin, sedimentation rate, and albumin are altered by pregnancy. A nonsedated flexible sigmoidoscopy can be performed in any trimester, but colonoscopies should be done with obstetric anesthesia monitoring. Appropriate imaging studies include magnetic resonance imaging (without gadolinium, particularly in the first trimester) and ultrasound, but computed tomography should be limited to urgent situations or when access is limited. Indications for surgery are the same as in nonpregnant patients with IBD; surgery has not been associated with high infant or maternal mortality in this setting.[17]

Similarly, indications for glucocorticoids are the same as in nonpregnant patients; the lowest possible dose should be used, and they should not be considered an alternative to standard maintenance therapy. Glucocorticoids have the potential for exacerbating pregnancy-induced hypertension, gestational diabetes, and preterm delivery due to premature rupture of membranes.[18] In the PIANO registry, glucocorticoids were significantly associated with gestational diabetes (OR, 2.8; 95% CI, 1.3 to 6.0), low birth weight (OR, 2.8; 95% CI, 1.3 to 6.1), and preterm birth (OR, 1.8; 95% CI, 1.0 to 3.1).[19] Therefore, pregnant women on glucocorticoids should be appropriately monitored for these complications. Though older studies raised concerns for an increased risk of cleft palate, a recent Danish cohort study of 51,973 pregnancies with first-trimester exposure to glucocorticoids showed no elevated risk (OR, 1.05; 95% CI, 0.80 to 1.38).[20] Finally, there may be a role for cyclosporine, a calcineurin inhibitor, as a salvage therapy to avert colectomy in pregnant patients with a fulminant ulcerative colitis flare refractory to conventional treatment.[21]

Management During the Perinatal Period

Given the reassuring data on biologic safety and data suggesting discontinuation leads to flares and worse pregnancy outcomes,[22] biologic therapies should be continued throughout pregnancy and lactation. When possible, one can time the last dose in pregnancy so that trough is achieved near the estimated date of confinement (ie, an every-6-week drug is last given 5 to 6 weeks prior to delivery). After delivery, dosing should be resumed based on schedule and can be given as soon as 24 hours after vaginal delivery and 48 hours after cesarean section, provided absence of maternal infections. Due to potential immune suppression, infants exposed to biologics in utero should not receive live vaccines (such as rotavirus) for the first 6 months of life unless drug levels are undetectable.[23] This recommendation does not apply to infants with prenatal certolizumab exposure, due to its minimal transplacental transfer. All other childhood vaccinations can and should be given on schedule and achieve good response.[24] Mesalamine and thiopurine therapy may be continued through lactation. A recent study of biologics during breastfeeding showed minimal transfer and no increased adverse events to the infant compared to nonexposed breastfed and nonbreastfed infants.[25]

In conclusion, mesalamine formulations, thiopurines, and biologics are low risk during pregnancy and lactation. As there is a great deal of concern about their use on the part of mothers as well as the managing multidisciplinary team, education and preconception planning are paramount. Education will not only reduce stress but also prevent unnecessary discontinuation of medications and subsequent flares. As always, a healthy mother is the best recipe for a healthy pregnancy. The American Gastroenterological Association recently published a clinical care pathway for the management of pregnant women with IBD[26] and an accompanying patient website (https://ibdparenthoodproject.gastro.org/), which is an excellent resource for patient education.

What Is Known About Neonatal Outcomes in Babies Born to Mothers With IBD?

Based on the reassuring pregnancy safety data discussed earlier, women continue biologic and thiopurine therapies during pregnancy. Thiopurine metabolites are cleared rapidly (within 1 month of birth), but biologic therapy may be present in infants for over 9 months. In the prospective PIANO registry, using the validated Ages and Stages Questionnaire, infants with in utero exposure to immunomodulators, anti-TNF inhibitors (infliximab, adalimumab, or certolizumab), or a combination of both achieved equivalent or superior developmental scores compared to infants not exposed to these agents. These results were unchanged when controlled for maternal income and education level.[3] In the PIANO registry, third trimester anti-TNF exposure did not detrimentally affect infant growth rate, immune development up to 1 year of age, or number of infections.[27] In an uncontrolled study of 25 anti-TNF–exposed children followed for a median of 34 months (range, 14 to 70 months), Bortlik et al found normal psychomotor development in all but 1 child, detectable serologic response to vaccination in all children, normal cellular immunity in the 17 children evaluated, and a clinically insignificant decrease in IgA or IgG levels in 7 children.[28] In another Czech cohort of children born to mothers with IBD on anti-TNF-α during pregnancy, in utero anti-TNF-α exposure did not have a negative impact on postnatal development with regard to infectious complications, allergies, or psychomotor development when compared to unexposed children of non-IBD women.[29] Though these childhood outcomes are reassuring, more long-term neonatal safety data for in utero exposure to these therapies are warranted.

References

1. Cornish J, Tan E, Teare J, et al. A meta-analysis on the influence of inflammatory bowel disease on pregnancy. *Gut.* 2007;56(6):830-837.
2. O'Toole A, Nwanne O, Tomlinson T. Inflammatory bowel disease increases risk of adverse pregnancy outcomes: a meta-analysis. *Dig Dis Sci.* 2015;60(9):2750-2761.
3. Mahadevan U, Long M, Kane S, et al. Pregnancy and neonatal outcomes after fetal exposure to biologics and thiopurines among women with inflammatory bowel disease. *Gastroenterology.* 2021;160:1131-1139.
4. Seirafi M, de Vroey B, Amiot A, et al. Factors associated with pregnancy outcome in anti-TNF treated women with inflammatory bowel disease. *Aliment Pharmacol Ther.* 2014;40(4):363-373.
5. Mogadam M, Dobbins WO III, Korelitz BI, Ahmed SW. Pregnancy in inflammatory bowel disease: effect of sulfasalazine and corticosteroids on fetal outcome. *Gastroenterology.* 1981;80(1):72.
6. Polifka JE, Friedman JM. Teratogen update: azathioprine and 6-mercaptopurine. *Teratology.* 2002;65(5):240-261.
7. Saarikoski S, Seppala M. Immunosuppression during pregnancy: transmission of azathioprine and its metabolites from the mother to the fetus. *Am J Obstet Gynecol.* 1973;115(8):1100-1106.
8. Casanova MJ, Chaparro M, Domenech E, et al. Safety of thiopurines and anti-TNF-alpha drugs during pregnancy in patients with inflammatory bowel disease. *Am J Gastroenterol.* 2013;108(3):433-440.
9. McConnell RA, Mahadevan U. Use of immunomodulators and biologics before, during, and after pregnancy. *Inflamm Bowel Dis.* 2015;22(1):213-223.
10. Jurgens M, Brand S, Filik L, et al. Safety of adalimumab in Crohn's disease during pregnancy: case report and review of the literature. *Inflamm Bowel Dis.* 2010;16(10):1634-1636.
11. Lichtenstein GR, Feagan BG, Cohen RD, et al. Serious infection and mortality in patients with Crohn's disease: more than 5 years of follow-up in the TREAT registry. *Am J Gastroenterol.* 2012;107(9):1409-1422.
12. Mahadevan U, Vermeire S, Wolf DC, et al. Pregnancy outcomes after exposure to certolizumab pegol: updated results from safety surveillance. *Gastroenterology.* 2015;148:S-858-S-859.
13. Nielsen OH, Loftus EV Jr, Jess T. Safety of TNF-alpha inhibitors during IBD pregnancy: a systematic review. *BMC Med.* 2013;11:174.
14. Cristiano L, Friend S, Bozic C, et al. Evaluation of pregnancy outcomes from the Tysabri (natalizumab) pregnancy exposure registry. *Neurology.* 2013;80:P02.127.
15. Dubinsky M, Mahadevan U, Vermeire S, et al. Vedolizumab exposure in pregnancy: outcomes from clinical studies in inflammatory bowel disease. *J Crohns Colitis.* 2015;9:S361-S362.

16. Schaufelberg BW, Horn E, Cather JC, et al. Pregnancy outcomes in women exposed to ustekinumab in the psoriasis clinical development program. *J Am Acad Dermatol.* 2014;70:AB178.

17. Dozois EJ, Wolff BG, Tremaine WJ, et al. Maternal and fetal outcome after colectomy for fulminant ulcerative colitis during pregnancy: case series and literature review. *Dis Colon Rectum.* 2006;49(1):64-73.

18. Cowchock FS, Reece EA, Balaban D, et al. Repeated fetal losses associated with antiphospholipid antibodies: a collaborative randomized trial comparing prednisone with low-dose heparin treatment. *Am J Obstet Gynecol.* 1992;166(5):1318.

19. Lin K, Martin CF, Dassopoulos T, et al. Pregnancy outcomes amongst mothers with inflammatory bowel disease exposed to systemic corticosteroids: results of the PIANO registry. *Gastroenterology.* 2014;146:S1.

20. Hviid A, Molgaard-Nielsen D. Corticosteroid use during pregnancy and risk of orofacial clefts. *CMAJ.* 2011;183: 796-804.

21. Paziana K, Del Monaco M, Cardonick E, et al. Ciclosporin use during pregnancy. *Drug Saf.* 2013;36(5):279-294.

22. Luu M, Benzenine E, Doret M, et al. Continuous anti-TNF use throughout pregnancy: possible complications for the mother but not for the fetus. A retrospective cohort on the French national health insurance database (EVASION). *Am J Gastroenterol.* 2018;113(11):1669-1677.

23. Julsgaard M, Christensen LA, Gibson PR, et al. Concentrations of adalimumab and infliximab in mothers and newborns, and effects on infection. *Gastroenterology.* 2016;151(1):110-119.

24. Beaulieu DB, Ananthakrishnan AN, Martin C, et al. Use of biologic therapy by pregnant women with inflammatory bowel disease does not affect infant response to vaccines. *Clin Gastroenterol Hepatol.* 2018;16(1):99-105.

25. Matro R, Martin CF, Wolf D, et al. Exposure concentrations of infants breastfed by women receiving biologic therapies for inflammatory bowel diseases and effects of breastfeeding on infections and development. *Gastroenterology.* 2018;155(3):696-704.

26. Mahadevan U, Robinson C, Bernasko N, et al. Inflammatory bowel disease (IBD) in pregnancy clinical care pathway: a report from the American Gastroenterological Association IBD Parenthood Project Working Group. *Gastroenterology.* 2019;156(5):1508-1524.

27. Mahadevan U, Martin CF, Dubinsky M, et al. Exposure to anti-TNFa therapy in the third trimester of pregnancy is not associated with increased adverse outcomes: results from the PIANO registry. *Gastroenterology.* 2014;146(5):S170.

28. Bortlik M, Duricova D, Machkova N, et al. Impact of antitumor necrosis factor alpha antibodies administered to pregnant women with inflammatory bowel disease on long-term outcome of exposed children. *Inflamm Bowel Dis.* 2014;20(3):495-501.

29. Duricova D, Dvorakova E, Hradsky O, et al. Safety of anti-TNF-alpha therapy during pregnancy on long-term outcome of exposed children: a controlled, multicenter observation. *Inflamm Bowel Dis.* 2019;25(4):789-796.

SECTION V

INFECTION AND MALIGNANCY PREVENTION

HOW DO YOU HANDLE A PATIENT WITH IBD WITH CLOSTRIDIOIDES DIFFICILE INFECTION?

Alexander N. Levy, MD and Jessica R. Allegretti, MD, MPH

Scope of the Problem

Clostridioides difficile, a gram-positive, spore-forming, toxin-producing anaerobic bacillus first identified in the 1970s, was initially thought of as a rare cause of infectious diarrhea. *C difficile* infection (CDI) has since become the most common cause of health care–associated infection in the United States, with nearly 450,000 cases and 35,000 deaths annually.[1] The rising burden of CDI is even more pronounced in inflammatory bowel disease (IBD), with an overall 10% lifetime risk of getting CDI. Notably, CDI incidence has doubled in Crohn's disease (CD) and tripled in ulcerative colitis (UC).[2] Compounding this problem, patients with IBD have 4.5-fold higher risk of CDI recurrence.

The impact of CDI in patients with IBD cannot be overstated. Patients with IBD with CDI are at increased risk for fulminant colitis and colectomy. They have higher mortality rates and require longer hospitalizations than the general population, all contributing to increased health care costs. CDI can also precipitate exacerbations of underlying IBD, requiring escalation of therapy.[3]

Clinical differentiation of IBD flare vs CDI coinfection can be challenging, in part due to overlapping symptoms and the rising prevalence of *C difficile* colonization in IBD. Furthermore, CDI in IBD is more likely to present at younger age, in the community setting, and without recent antibiotic use, contrary to traditional risk factors for CDI in the general population.[4] IBD itself seems to be an independent risk factor for developing CDI, with colitis conferring the greatest risk.[2] Chronic immunosuppression and intestinal dysbiosis, characterized by reduced biodiversity and disrupted microbial function, may also help explain increased susceptibility to CDI, even in

Rubin DT, Friedman S, Farraye FA, eds. *Curbside Consultation in IBD: 49 Clinical Questions, Third Edition* (pp 229-233).
© 2022 Taylor & Francis Group.

the absence of traditional risk factors.[5] Given the clinical ramifications, it remains crucial that clinicians accurately identify infection and treat aggressively.

Clinical Presentation of C difficile *Infection*

The spectrum of *C difficile* illness in IBD ranges from mild diarrhea to fulminant colitis. Endoscopically, mucosa can appear diffusely ulcerated, mimicking that seen in active IBD colitis; however, pseudomembranes are uncommon. Severe CDI can manifest as fevers, leukocytosis, acute renal failure, or shock.[2] Patients with IBD with CDI are also at increased risk for ileus and toxic megacolon. Patients at high risk for bowel perforation carry significant morbidity and mortality and should ideally be managed in an intensive care unit.[6] However, colectomy in this population is typically due to worsening of IBD and not from fulminant CDI.

C difficile *Infection Recurrence in IBD*

CDI recurrence, defined by reoccurrence within 8 weeks following symptom resolution, occurs primarily via endogenous persistence of *C difficile* spores, although acquisition of new strains is seen in about 20% of cases.[7] Recurrence occurs in 20% to 30% of all patients regardless of initial therapy, and notably these rates are even higher in patients with IBD.[6] Following an initial course of anti-CDI therapy, the CDI recurrence rate is 4.5-fold higher, and the prevalence of toxigenic *C difficile* carrier state is 8-fold greater in IBD patients compared to non-IBD, which may be an indicator of disease severity.[5] Risk factors for recurrent CDI include advanced age, prior recurrence, recurrent antibiotic exposure, and infection with hypervirulent strains. Reduced intestinal biodiversity has also been implicated as a risk factor for recurrent CDI in IBD. Chang et al demonstrated reduced levels of *Bacteroidetes* and *Firmicutes* in fecal samples of patients with recurrent CDI but not in patients with only a single episode of CDI.[8] Given that biodiversity is reduced in recurrent CDI, and is characteristically low in IBD, it is likely to be low in recurrent CDI in patients with IBD.

Diagnosis of C difficile *Infection in Patients With IBD*

Diagnosis of CDI requires a positive stool test indicating the presence of bacterial toxin A and/or B in a patient with diarrhea. Up until the early 2000s the most commonly used stool test to identify the presence of toxigenic *C difficile* was enzyme immunoassay (EIA) toxin (TcdA and/or TcdB). This assay is highly specific for infection, but used in isolation had limited sensitivity, so detection often required multiple samples. Given concern for false negatives, there was wide adoption of a polymerase chain reaction (PCR) test, which tests for the presence of the TcdB gene. This test is highly sensitive. However, given it is detecting a gene for toxin and not toxin itself, it cannot distinguish between infection and colonization. As PCR testing became more widely available there was a notably disproportionate rise in incidence of CDI in the IBD population.[1]

A large cohort study in 2015 demonstrated that patients testing positive for CDI by toxin EIA had worse outcomes than those who tested positive by PCR. Patients who tested positive by PCR alone had similar outcomes to patients who tested negative by both tests.[9] The prevalence of toxigenic *C difficile* carrier state is 8-fold greater in patients with IBD compared with non-IBD controls, although the mechanism and clinical implications are not well understood.[10] Patients positive via PCR may be only colonized and not have an active infection, and this limitation of

PCR-based CDI testing has significant implications in IBD, as it is commonly difficult to clinically distinguish IBD flare from CDI. In the setting of active IBD, withholding immunosuppression while treating *C difficile* colonization suspected to be CDI can lead to disease deterioration.

Largely due to the limitations of molecular testing, our institution recently discontinued PCR-based testing, adopting a 2-step diagnostic approach supported by the European Society of Clinical Microbiology and Infectious Diseases (ESCMID).[11] This incorporates the highly sensitive glutamate dehydrogenase (GDH) immunoassay followed by highly specific toxin A/B immunoassay. We primarily use PCR testing when suspicion for CDI remains high despite negative immunoassay tests and patients are not responding to immunosuppression. We recommend always using a 2-step method when possible to confirm infection with either GDH or PCR followed by the EIA toxin test.

Treatment of C difficile Infection in IBD

INITIAL EPISODE

IBD should be considered a marker of CDI severity given the high risk of adverse outcomes. As such our institution maintains an aggressive treatment strategy. Although prospective data are limited due to most CDI trials excluding patients with IBD, our group uses oral vancomycin as a first-line treatment of an initial episode of CDI. This is supported by the new Infectious Diseases Society of America (IDSA) guidelines.[12] This practice is additionally supported by studies demonstrating lower colectomy rate, readmission, and shorter hospitalizations with vancomycin treatment. Metronidazole should not be used as a first-line agent in these patients given the increase failure rates, in addition to its gastrointestinal side effects. Fidaxomicin, by virtue of its minimal gut absorption, narrow antimicrobial spectrum, and bactericidal properties, is another appropriate option for first-line management for CDI in patients with IBD and is also supported by the IDSA guidelines. When compared to vancomycin it was superior at preventing recurrent CDI.[13] Higher cost and difficulty with payer approval has limited its adoption into our treatment algorithm.

In cases where it is difficult to clinically distinguish IBD flare from CDI, especially if you only have PCR testing available, our practice is to treat CDI and monitor closely for 48 hours. If we do not observe clinical improvement, we will start or escalate immunosuppression with intravenous corticosteroids or biologic therapy in an effort to prevent escalation of the underlying IBD. CDI should respond to vancomycin, so if no symptom improvement is noted symptoms are likely from IBD or other reasons.

We do not recommend treating asymptomatic carriers of *C difficile* with antimicrobials as there is insufficient evidence that it will alter future CDI risk, and may even trigger increased spore shedding.[14]

RECURRENT C DIFFICILE INFECTION IN IBD

For first-time recurrence, it is important to not use the same treatment you used for the first episode.[12] Therefore, we recommend treating a first recurrence with fidaxomicin or a prolonged taper if a standard course of vancomycin was used initially.

Recently, *C difficile* vaccines have demonstrated promise in treatment of primary and recurrent CDI but are still under investigation.[15] Bezlotoxumab, a human monoclonal antibody against toxin B, has been shown to reduce CDI recurrence in patients with IBD in post hoc analysis of MODIFY trials.[16] The early outcome data on CDI immunotherapy are encouraging. It is important to note that bezlotoxumab is approved for prevention of recurrence and not treatment of CDI. It should be used after a course of antibiotics.

Probiotics are live microorganism preparations consisting of bacterial strains and yeast that have been used to reconstitute normal microbial homeostasis. However, data do not support the use of probiotics for preventing recurrent CDI. Interestingly though, recent studies may show benefit in their use at preventing initial CDI in high-risk patients.[17] Notably patients with IBD are excluded from most studies.

FECAL MICROBIOTA TRANSPLANTATION FOR RECURRENT *C DIFFICILE* INFECTION

Fecal microbiota transplantation (FMT), the instillation of minimally manipulated microbiota from healthy donors to affected patients, has emerged as a highly effective treatment for recurrent CDI. In the general population, multiple meta-analyses and systematic reviews have shown efficacy of FMT for CDI approaching 90%.[18] The available data on FMT in IBD associated with CDI are less robust; however, recent advances in FMT support an expanded role for combating CDI in this at-risk population. In the largest multicenter series to date, our group observed a 79% cure rate after initial FMT and an overall CDI cure rate of 90%. Post-FMT IBD flare occurred in a minority (13%) of patients, and no severe adverse effects directly attributable to FMT were found, supporting its safety in IBD.[5]

Given the potential for poor outcomes in IBD, we believe FMT should be considered early in recurrent CDI. The 2013 American College of Gastroenterology CDI practice guidelines suggest FMT after 3 recurrences; however, this recommendation does not specifically mention patients with IBD.[19] Our group currently has a trial investigating earlier use of FMT for CDI specifically in patients with IBD to understand the role of early eradication of CDI as well as IBD outcomes post FMT.

Clinicians considering starting a fecal transplant program at their institution should be aware that FMT is not currently US Food and Drug Administration–approved for any indication. However, it can be used for recurrent CDI under enforcement discretion currently, though this is subject to change.

In an effort to create a practical framework for providers interested in performing FMT, our group published the 5D framework for FMT.[20] First is *decision*, which concerns if the candidate is appropriate and if they meet criteria for FMT. Second is *donor* acquisition, which can be patient directed vs using a sample from a stool bank. Third is *discussion,* involving informed consent, which should include a discussion of both real and theoretical risks and benefits of FMT. Fourth is *delivery*, the mode in which you deliver the material. Colonoscopy and sigmoidoscopy remain the most common delivery modes in adults; however, FMT capsules are available and gaining popularity. The fifth is *discharge*. From our experience, risk of FMT failure is greatest within the first 4 weeks, though patients should be followed for 8 weeks to assess for FMT failure. If they experience failure within 8 weeks we repeat FMT. Post-FMT we counsel our patients to avoid unnecessary antibiotics.

Conclusion

Patients with IBD are at increased risk of CDI and its negative sequelae, including fulminant colitis, colectomy, and mortality. Patients with IBD with CDI are also at increased risk for exacerbation of underlying IBD. In an effort to reduce adverse outcomes it is critical that early diagnosis of CDI be made and an aggressive treatment strategy be implemented. Patients should be monitored closely after initiating antimicrobials, and lack of clinical response within 48 hours should prompt escalation of immunosuppression. Novel therapeutics such as FMT and immunotherapy may prove to be the future of CDI treatment in IBD, but additional research is needed.

References

1. Lessa FC, Winston LG, McDonald LC, Emerging Infections Program. Burden of *Clostridium difficile* infection in the United States. *N Engl J Med.* 2015;372(24):825-834.

2. Issa M, Vijayapal A, Graham MB, et al. Impact of *Clostridium difficile* on inflammatory bowel disease. *Clin Gastroenterol Hepatol.* 2007;5(3):345–351 (2007).

3. Navaneethan U, Mukewar S, Venkatesh PGK, Lopez R, Shen B. *Clostridium difficile* infection is associated with worse long-term outcome in patients with ulcerative colitis. *J Crohns Colitis.* 2012;6(3):330-336.

4. Issa M, Ananthakrishnan AN, Binion DG. *Clostridium difficile* and inflammatory bowel disease. *Inflamm Bowel Dis.* 2008;14(10):1432-1442.

5. Fischer M, Kao D, Kelly C, et al. Fecal microbiota transplantation is safe and efficacious for recurrent or refractory *Clostridium difficile* infection in patients with inflammatory bowel disease. *Inflamm Bowel Dis.* 2016;22(10): 2402-2409.

6. Rao K, Higgins PDR. Epidemiology, diagnosis, and management of *Clostridium difficile* infection in patients with inflammatory bowel disease. *Inflamm Bowel Dis.* 2016;22(7):1744-1754.

7. Barbut F, Richard A, Hamadi K, Chomette B, Burghoffer B, Petit JC. Epidemiology of recurrences or reinfections of *Clostridium difficile*-associated diarrhea. *J Clin Microbiol.* 2000;38(6):2386-2388.

8. Chang JY, Antonopoulos DA, Kalra A et al. Decreased diversity of the fecal microbiome in recurrent *Clostridium difficile*-associated diarrhea. *J Infect Dis.* 2008;197(3):435-438.

9. Polage CR, Gyorke CE, Kennedy MA, et al. Overdiagnosis of *Clostridium difficile* infection in the molecular test era. *JAMA Intern Med.* 2015;175(11):1792-1801.

10. Clayton EM, Raya MC, Shanahan F et al. The vexed relationship between *Clostridium difficile* and inflammatory bowel disease: an assessment of carriage in an outpatient setting among patients in remission. *Am J Gastroenterol.* 2009;104:1162:1169.

11. Crobach MJT, Bauer MP, Kuijper EJ, European Society of Clinical Microbiology and Infections Diseases. European Society of Clinical Microbiology and Infectious Diseases: update of the diagnostic guidance document for *Clostridium difficile* infection. *Clin Microbiol Infect.* 2016;22(4):S63-S81.

12. McDonald LC, Gerding DM, Johnson S, et al. Clinical practice guidelines for *Clostridium difficile* infection in adults and children: 2017 update by the Infectious Diseases Society of America (IDSA) and Society for Healthcare Epidemiology of America (SHEA). *Clin Infect Dis.* 2018;66(7):987-994.

13. Crook DW, Walker AS, Kean Y, et al. Fidaxomicin versus vancomycin for *Clostridium difficile* infection: meta-analysis of pivotal randomized controlled trials. *Clin Infect Dis.* 2012;55(2):S93-S103.

14. Johnson S, Homann SR, Betin KM, Quick JN, Peterson LR, Gerding DN. Treatment of asymptomatic *Clostridium difficile* carriers (fecal excretors) with vancomycin or metronidazole. A randomized, placebo-controlled trial. *Ann Intern Med.* 1992;117(4):297-302.

15. Legenza LM, Barnett SG, Rose WE. Vaccines in development for the primary prevention of *Clostridium difficile* infection. *J Am Pharm Assoc.* 2017;57(4):547-549.

16. Kelly CP, Wilcox M, Glerup H, Aboo N. Characteristics and outcomes in patients with *C. difficile* infection (CDI) and inflammatory bowel disease: bezlotoxumab versus placebo. *Gastroenterology.* 2017;152(5):S340.

17. Goldenberg JZ, Yap C, Lytvyn L et al. Probiotics for the prevention of *Clostridium difficile*-associated diarrhea in adults and children. *Cochrane Database Syst Rev.* 2017;12(12):CD006095.

18. Drekonja D, Reich J, Gezahegn S, et al. Fecal microbiota transplantation for *Clostridium difficile* infection: a systematic review. *Ann Intern Med.* 2015;162(9):630-638.

19. Surawicz CM, Brandt LJ, Binion DJ, et al. Guidelines for diagnosis, treatment, and prevention of *Clostridium difficile* infections. *Am J Gastroenterol.* 2013;108(4):478-498; quiz 499.

20. Allegretti JR, Kassam Z, Osman M, Budree S, Fischer M, Kelly CR. The 5D framework: a clinical primer for fecal microbiota transplantation to treat *Clostridium difficile* infection. *Gastrointest Endosc.* 2018;87(1):18-29.

HOW DO YOU TREAT IBD IN THE SETTING OF CURRENT OR PREVIOUS CANCER?

Steven H. Itzkowitz, MD and Jordan E. Axelrad, MD, MPH

The Risk of Cancer in Patients With IBD

Chronic intestinal inflammation is the primary risk factor for developing gastrointestinal malignancy in the setting of inflammatory bowel disease (IBD). Indeed, chronic inflammation predisposes to colorectal cancer, small bowel adenocarcinoma, cholangiocarcinoma, and anal cancer (Table 36-1).[1]

Given that chronic inflammation underlies the disease state of IBD, medications that staunch inflammation by suppressing the immune system represent the foundation of IBD treatment. Theoretically, if a medication reduces inflammation, it might be expected to reduce the incidence of inflammation-associated cancer. To some extent, this has been suggested for mesalamine and thiopurines. Less is known about whether this also applies to newer agents such as small molecules (Janus kinase [JAK] inhibitors) and biologic agents (tumor necrosis factor–α [TNF-α] antagonists, anti-integrins, or anti–interleukin [IL] 12/IL-23). On the other hand, because immunosuppressive agents act on the immune system, they might also conceivably promote carcinogenesis (therapy-associated malignancies).

Several population-based studies have reported a risk of therapy-associated malignancies in patients with IBD. The majority of these studies focused on exposure to thiopurines, TNF-α antagonists, or their combination. Specific cancers thought to be due to long-standing immunosuppression in the setting of IBD include lymphomas, acute myeloid leukemia, myelodysplastic syndromes, skin cancers (melanoma, squamous cell carcinoma, basal cell carcinoma), oral cancers, and urinary tract cancers (Table 36-2).[1] Data are limited regarding the risk of malignancy second-

Rubin DT, Friedman S, Farraye FA, eds. *Curbside Consultation in IBD: 49 Clinical Questions, Third Edition* (pp 235-240).
© 2022 Taylor & Francis Group.

Table 36-1

Cancer Secondary to Chronic Intestinal Inflammation

Cancer Type	Standardized Incidence Ratio (95% CI)
Colorectal cancer	1.7 (1.2-2.2) in colonic disease
Small bowel adenocarcinoma	14.4 (8.78-22.2) in small bowel Crohn's disease
Anal cancer	Rare (data not available)
Cholangiocarcinoma	917 (298-2141) in ulcerative colitis with primary sclerosing cholangitis

Table 36-2

Cancer Secondary to Immunosuppression

Increased Under Thiopurines	Increased Under Anti-TNF-α	Increased Risk Under Anti-Metabolite With Anti-TNF-α
Non-Hodgkin lymphoma Acute myeloid leukemia and myelodysplastic syndromes Nonmelanoma skin cancer (squamous cell carcinoma, basal cell carcinoma) Oral cancer Urinary tract cancer	Melanoma	Hepatosplenic T-cell lymphoma

ary to newly approved therapies, including anti–IL-12/IL-23 agents, JAK inhibitors, and anti-integrins. Safety data from the psoriasis literature suggest that anti–IL-12/IL-23 is not associated with an increased risk of cancer; however, cumulative dose exposure may not be comparable to patients with IBD.[2] Safety data from rheumatoid arthritis literature suggest that JAK inhibition is not associated with excess cancers, but again cumulative dose exposure may not be comparable to patients with IBD.[3] Recent data on anti-integrins in IBD have suggested no association with malignancy.[4]

The Risk of Cancer in Patients With IBD Who Have a History of Cancer

Given the evidence-based and theoretical risks of therapy-associated malignancy, patients with a history of cancer have usually been excluded from clinical trials of newer IBD medications. Moreover, there is substantial evidence in the solid organ transplant literature that immunosuppression, specifically thiopurines and calcineurin inhibitors, increases the risk of new and recurrent malignancies in patients with a history of cancer. Pretransplant malignancy has been associated with an increased risk of all-cause mortality, cancer-specific mortality, and of developing de novo malignancies after transplantation compared with those without a history of malignancy. This risk seems directly correlated with time from cancer diagnosis, where transplantation less than 5 years from a cancer diagnosis is associated with a nearly 3-fold greater risk of cancer recurrence compared to transplantation more than 5 years from a cancer diagnosis.[5]

As such, oncologists and gastroenterologists generally suspend immunosuppression for IBD after a diagnosis of cancer, both while undergoing cancer treatment and even during remission from cancer. This approach may worsen IBD and complicate appropriate cancer management. So, what is known about the safety of using IBD medications in patients with IBD who have a history of cancer but are in remission?

A French prospective observational cohort found that exposure to immunosuppression among patients with IBD in general was indeed associated with the development of cancer with an adjusted hazard ratio (aHR) of 1.9 (95% CI, 1.2 to 3.0). However, in those patients with a history of cancer, exposure to immunosuppression did not increase the risk of new or recurrent cancer. Given the limited number of patients with IBD and a history of cancer with subsequent exposure to immunosuppression in that cohort, this conclusion only applied to thiopurine exposure; no conclusions could be drawn regarding anti-TNF-α therapies.[6]

An observational study in the United States found that nearly 30% of patients with IBD and a history of cancer developed new or recurrent cancer.[7] However, exposure to TNF-α antagonists, thiopurines, or their combination was not associated with an increased risk of new or recurrent cancer within 5 years following a diagnosis of cancer compared to patients with IBD who never received these immune modifying agents (log-rank P = .14). In addition, duration of TNF-α antagonists after a diagnosis of cancer was not associated with the risk or type of new or recurrent cancer.[7] More recently, in a population-based cohort study of 25,738 patients with immune-mediated disease, including IBD, and a history of cancer, the incidence of new or recurrent cancer was 30 cases (95% CI, 24.0 to 38.2) per 1000 person years in the TNF-α antagonist treatment group and 34.4 cases (31.7 to 37.3) per 1000 person years an unexposed control group, yielding an aHR of 0.82 (95% CI, 0.61 to 1.11).[8] While these exploratory data are reassuring, further prospective study is required.

In a meta-analysis of 16 studies comprising 11,702 persons with immune-mediated diseases, contributing 31,258 person years of follow-up evaluation after a diagnosis of cancer, there were similar rates of cancer recurrence among individuals with prior cancer who received no immunosuppression, anti-TNF therapy, immune-modulator therapy, or combination treatments.[9]

Cancer Treatment in the Patient With IBD

There are few data regarding the effects of cancer treatment on IBD, and the effect of IBD and IBD therapies on cancer outcomes.

Several studies have demonstrated a major modification in IBD medications after a diagnosis of cancer. In a French observational study, a diagnosis of extraintestinal cancer had a marked impact on the management of IBD, with a lower use of thiopurines (19% vs 25%, $P < .001$) and an increased use of intestinal surgery (4.0% vs 2.5%, $P = .05$), but was not associated with significant modifications in activity of IBD.[10] Moreover, radiation oncologists have generally been reluctant to administer pelvic irradiation in the setting of IBD, as tolerance in these patients is largely unknown. However, limited data suggest safety.[11] In small studies of patients with rectal and prostate cancer, acute gastrointestinal toxicities may be exacerbated in patients with active IBD on therapy, but overall gastrointestinal toxicities were low.[11,12]

In a study of 84 patients with IBD and extraintestinal cancer, 67% of patients with active IBD at their cancer diagnosis experienced remission from IBD thought secondary to cytotoxic chemotherapy, whereas 17% of patients in remission from IBD at their cancer diagnosis experienced a flare during or within 5 years after their cancer treatment.[13] In the IBD remission group, the risk of flare was greatest among patients who received hormone therapies (hormone monotherapy HR = 11.6, 95% CI, 1.4 to 96 or combination cytotoxic chemotherapy with adjuvant hormone therapy HR = 12.3, 95% CI, 1.5 to 99), suggesting that hormone therapies for breast and prostate cancer may increase the risk of IBD reactivation or counter the protective effects of cytotoxic chemotherapy.[13] In a larger study of 447 patients with IBD who had either breast (78%) or prostate (22%) cancer, exposure to hormone therapy for cancer was associated with an increased risk for relapse of IBD and related adverse outcomes.[14] Not all studies, however, suggest a negative impact of hormone therapy. In a recent study examining the impact of prostate cancer treatment in men with IBD, surgery for cancer was more common in patients with IBD, and flare in the year prior to cancer was the only predictor of disease exacerbation in the year following cancer treatment, not exposure to hormone therapy.[15] However, preference for prostate surgery may have reduced the requirement for hormone therapies.

Little is known regarding chemotherapy tolerance and specific cancer outcomes in patients with IBD. It has been postulated that the mere presence of underlying IBD yields gastrointestinal mucosa more vulnerable to the toxic effects of chemotherapy, but this is speculative. In a study of 158 patients with colorectal cancer, patients with IBD experienced more chemotherapy treatment alterations than those without IBD (74% vs 44%, $P = .03$), largely due to a higher frequency of treatment delays.[12] In the same study, there were no significant differences in 5-year overall survival or recurrence-free survival between patients with stage I to III colorectal cancer who did, or did not have, IBD. However, survival was shorter in patients with stage IV with IBD compared with patients without.[12] Several other studies have demonstrated comparable overall survival rates in patients with IBD and colorectal cancer to those without.[16]

There are few data regarding the concomitant use of IBD therapies during active malignancy, mostly limited to small case series or case reports. There is emerging data regarding the intermittent use of TNF antagonists and anti-integrins to treat colitis instigated by immune-checkpoint inhibitors—cancer therapies that are becoming increasingly used for a variety of malignancy types.[17] These limited data suggest that biologics can be safely used during active malignancy and active chemotherapy or immunotherapy; however, robust prospective data in patients with IBD on long-term immunosuppression are lacking.

Conclusion

Given the multitude of cancer types, stages, and overall complexity of care required for the patient with IBD who develops cancer, we recommend a multidisciplinary approach to the treatment of both the cancer and IBD. This should include IBD specialists, pathologists, surgeons, radiologists, medical oncologists, and radiation oncologists. Risk of cancer recurrence will be highly dependent on cancer type, cancer stage, and time since cancer diagnosis. The requirement for IBD therapy will be highly dependent on IBD history and activity at the time of cancer

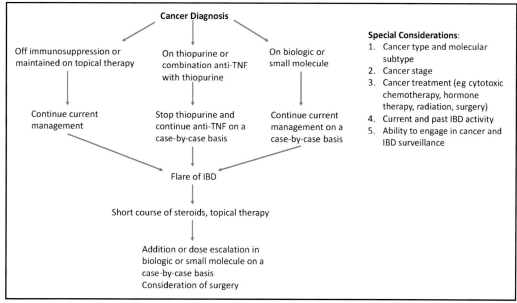

Figure 36-1. Management of IBD after a diagnosis of cancer.

diagnosis. Currently, there are insufficient data to recommend a definitive management strategy for all patients with IBD who develop cancer. Due to the risks of a first malignancy associated with thiopurines, we recommend cessation during and after a diagnosis of cancer (Figure 36-1). For patients who develop cancer while on biologic therapy, we suggest continuing the biologic on a case-by-case basis. For patients with a history of cancer, we recommend the use of biologics as needed for IBD with close surveillance for new or recurrent cancer.

References

1. Beaugerie L, Itzkowitz SH. Cancers complicating inflammatory bowel disease. *N Engl J Med.* 2015;372(15):1441-1452.
2. Papp K, Gottlieb AB, Naldi L, et al. Safety surveillance for ustekinumab and other psoriasis treatments from the psoriasis longitudinal assessment and registry (PSOLAR). *J Drugs Dermatol.* 2015;14(7):706-714.
3. Cohen S, Curtis JR, DeMasi R, et al. Worldwide, 3-year, post-marketing surveillance experience with tofacitinib in rheumatoid arthritis. *Rheumatol Ther.* 2018;5(1):283-291.
4. Colombel J-F, Sands BE, Rutgeerts P, et al. The safety of vedolizumab for ulcerative colitis and Crohn's disease. *Gut.* 2017;66(5):839-851.
5. Acuna SA, Huang JW, Dossa F, et al. Cancer recurrence after solid organ transplantation: A systematic review and meta-analysis. *Transplant Rev.* 2017;31(4):240-248.
6. Beaugerie L, Carrat F, Colombel J-F, et al. Risk of new or recurrent cancer under immunosuppressive therapy in patients with IBD and previous cancer. *Gut.* 2014;63:1416-1423.
7. Axelrad J, Bernheim O, Colombel J-F, et al. Risk of new or recurrent cancer in patients with inflammatory bowel disease and previous cancer exposed to immunosuppressive and anti-tumor necrosis factor agents. *Clin Gastroenterol Hepatol.* 2016;14:58-64.
8. Waljee AK, Higgins PDR, Jensen CB, et al. Anti-tumor necrosis factor-α therapy and recurrent or new primary cancers in patients with inflammatory bowel disease, rheumatoid arthritis, or psoriasis and previous cancer in Denmark: a nationwide, population-based cohort study. *Lancet Gastroenterol Hepatol.* 2019;5(3):276-294.
9. Shelton E, Laharie D, Scott FI, et al. Cancer recurrence following immune-suppressive therapies in patients with immune-mediated diseases: a systematic review and meta-analysis. *Gastroenterology.* 2016;151(1):97-109.e4.
10. Rajca S, Seksik P, Bourrier A, et al. Impact of the diagnosis and treatment of cancer on the course of inflammatory bowel disease. *J Crohns Colitis.* 2014;8(8):819-824.

11. Green S, Stock RG, Greenstein AJ. Rectal cancer and inflammatory bowel disease: natural history and implications for radiation therapy. *Int J. Radiat Oncol Biol Phys*. 1999;44(4):835-840.

12. Axelrad J, Kriplani A, Ozbek U, et al. Chemotherapy tolerance and oncologic outcomes in patients with colorectal cancer with and without inflammatory bowel disease. *Clin Colorectal Cancer*. 2017;16(3):e205-e210.

13. Axelrad JE, Fowler SA, Friedman S, et al. Effects of cancer treatment on inflammatory bowel disease remission and reactivation. *Clin Gastroenterol Hepatol*. 2012;10(9):1021-7.e1.

14. Axelrad JE, Bazarbashi A, Zhou J, et al. Hormone therapy for cancer is a risk factor for relapse of inflammatory bowel diseases. *Clin Gastroenterol Hepatol*. 2019;18(4):872-880.

15. Kirk PS, Govani S, Borza T, et al. Implications of prostate cancer treatment in men with inflammatory bowel disease. *Urology*. 2017;104:131-136.

16. Ali RAR, Dooley C, Comber H, et al. Clinical features, treatment, and survival of patients with colorectal cancer with or without inflammatory bowel disease. *Clin Gastroenterol Hepatol*. 2011;9(7):584-589.e1.

17. Wang Y, Abu-Sbeih H, Mao E, et al. Immune-checkpoint inhibitor-induced diarrhea and colitis in patients with advanced malignancies: retrospective review at MD Anderson. *J Immunother Cancer*. 2018;6(1):37.

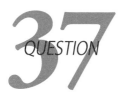

WHAT IS THE UPDATED APPROACH TO SURVEILLANCE AND COLORECTAL CANCER PREVENTION IN IBD?

Jimmy K. Limdi, MBBS and Francis A. Farraye, MD, MSc

Patients with long-standing inflammatory bowel disease (IBD) are at an increased risk of developing colorectal cancer (CRC), accounting for 1% to 2% of CRC cases and 10% to 15% IBD-related mortality.[1] Risk factors for CRC in IBD include extensive colitis, longer disease duration, active endoscopic or histological inflammation, history of dysplasia, anatomical factors such as coexistent primary sclerosing cholangitis (PSC), stricturing disease, inflammatory ("pseudo") polyps, a shortened tubular colon, and a family history of CRC in a first-degree relative diagnosed under 50 years.[1] Of these, colitis-related dysplasia confers the highest risk, prompting gastrointestinal societies to advocate for colon surveillance, no later than 8 years after diagnosis of IBD and at diagnosis in patients with IBD with PSC, to detect dysplasia at an earlier and potentially curable stage.[1,2]

The seminal meta-analysis from 2001 demonstrated considerable risk of CRC from IBD: 2% at 10 years, 8% at 20 years, and 18% at 30 years.[3] A recent population-based study has shown a reassuring decline in CRC incidence at 0.1% in the first decade, 2.9% in the second, 6.7% in the third, and 10% in the fourth, respectively.[4] This is supported by other data demonstrating decrease in the incidence of colectomy for dysplasia.[2,5] This temporal reduction is likely attributable to effective control of inflammation through medications, greater uptake of surveillance permitting earlier detection and resection of dysplasia before CRC develops, and the optimal timing of colectomy when appropriate.[2]

Rubin DT, Friedman S, Farraye FA, eds. *Curbside Consultation in IBD:*
49 Clinical Questions, Third Edition (pp 241-250).
© 2022 Taylor & Francis Group.

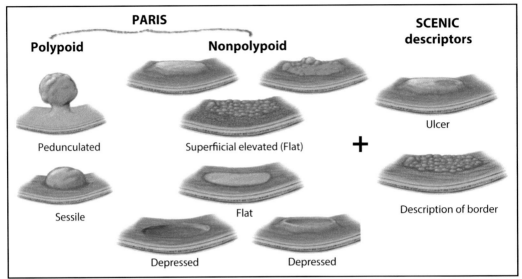

Figure 37-1. SCENIC classification of IBD colorectal neoplasia. (Reproduced with permission from Kaltenbach TR, Soetikno RM, DeVivo R, et al. Optimizing the quality of endoscopy in inflammatory bowel disease: focus on surveillance and management of colorectal dysplasia using interactive image- and video-based teaching. *Gastrointest Endosc.* 2017;86[6]:1107-1117.e1.)

Pathophysiology of IBD-Related Colorectal Cancer

CRC in IBD does not follow the well-recognized adenocarcinoma sequence seen in sporadic CRC and stems from a "field-change" effect, progressing from nondysplastic mucosa to either visible or invisible dysplasia, to carcinoma.[6] The unpredictable sequence of events in IBD-related CRC taken with its potentially aggressive course underpins the need for timely implementation of high-quality surveillance.

Dysplasia in IBD:
Modern Definitions and Terminology

Historically, lesions detected at IBD surveillance colonoscopy were characterized as sporadic adenomas (outside an area of inflammation) or as dysplasia-associated lesion or mass (DALM) if detected within an area of inflammation. DALMs were categorized as "adenoma-like" (if raised or with an endoscopic appearance of sporadic adenoma) or "non-adenoma–like."[7] Adenoma-like DALMs were considered suitable for endoscopic resection with close follow-up, whereas non-adenoma–like DALMs and patients with HGD or multifocal LGD detected by random biopsy were traditionally offered surgery. Modern colonoscopy technology has enabled greater endoscopic identification of dysplasia, and recognition that most dysplasia is visible has led to abandonment of previous terminology with the adoption of new definitions.[8] Thus, the term *visible* dysplasia is used to describe dysplasia within clearly identified lesions and *invisible* dysplasia from random biopsy samples, respectively, with the addition of terms for ulceration and border of the lesion.[2] Visible dysplasia is classified as polypoid (pedunculated or sessile) or non-polypoid (superficial elevated, flat, or depressed) in accordance with the Paris Classification (Figure 37-1). The term *endoscopically resectable* implies that distinct margins of the lesion can be identified, the lesion is completely excised on visual inspection after endoscopic resection, histological assessment is consistent with complete excision, and biopsy specimens taken from mucosa immediately adjacent to the resection margin are free of dysplasia.[2]

Modern IBD Surveillance: A Paradigm Shift in Sampling and Technique

Endoscopic surveillance should be offered to patients with ulcerative colitis (UC) and endoscopic or histologic evidence of inflammation extending proximal to the rectum and to patients with Crohn's disease with inflammation involving more than one-third of the colon. The primary aim of endoscopic surveillance is to reduce mortality and morbidity from IBD-related CRC through the detection and resection of dysplasia or early identification of CRC at a potentially curable stage.[2,8,9] Societal recommendations vary in their surveillance intervals but universally support annual surveillance in those with highest risk of IBD-associated CRC (Table 37-1). US guidelines do not lengthen screening beyond 3 years, whereas European guidelines support a risk stratification approach, increasing the surveillance interval to 5 years in those with low risk.[1,2,7,10]

Historically, surveillance involved taking 32 or more serial colonic biopsies taken every 10 cm from 4 quadrants and from each anatomical segment of the colon to have a 90% probability of detecting the highest grade of dysplasia.[7] Such a strategy might detect 1 case of dysplasia per 1505 biopsies obtained.[11] Modern imaging techniques, including chromoendoscopy (CE), narrow band imaging (NBI), and confocal endomicroscopy, as adjunctive techniques have shown the ability to detect subtle mucosal abnormalities. A growing body of evidence supports CE, which has demonstrated a superior diagnostic yield, therapeutic advantage, and cost-effectiveness when compared with random biopsy and white light endoscopy (WLE) for dysplasia screening and has led to a change in societal recommendations for modern surveillance.[1,2,12-14] The landmark SCENIC (International Consensus Statement on Surveillance and Management of Dysplasia in Inflammatory Bowel Disease) recommends CE over standard WLE, suggests CE over high-definition (HD) colonoscopy for dysplasia surveillance, and has been endorsed by various gastrointestinal societies internationally (Table 37-2).[2]

A number of studies since publication of the SCENIC consensus lend credibility to CE, with targeted biopsies as the preferred technique, albeit not without skepticism and debate.[2,4,6,15-18] Marion and colleagues reported on 68 patients with median disease duration of 21 years followed over a 5-year period.[15] A negative result from CE assessment was the best indicator for a dysplasia-free outcome, and a positive result was associated with earlier referral for colectomy (HR 12.1; 95% CI, 3.2 to 46.2). A 40-year experience with colon surveillance from St Mark's Hospital, London, noted an increase in the incidence rate of dysplasia since the adoption of HD WLE and CE for surveillance but no decrease in the rate of colon cancer. Four characteristics significantly associated with a later diagnosis of HGD or CRC were non-polypoid lesion appearance (Paris type 0-II, visible, slightly elevated or depressed, type 0-III (excavated), or plaque-like) as the strongest risk factor (HR 8.6; 95% CI, 3 to 24.8), and also macroscopically invisible dysplasia (HR 4.1; 95% CI, 1.3 to 13.4), lesion size ≥ 1 cm (HR 3.8; 95% CI, 1.5 to 13.4), and previous history of indefinite dysplasia (HR 2.8; 95% CI, 1.2 to 6.5).[4] A Mayo clinic study also reported an incremental diagnostic yield from CE.[16] A multicenter real-world prospective study reported a 57.4% incremental yield with CE, comparable between SD and HD colonoscopy (51.5% vs 52.3%; $P = .30$) and also comparable dysplasia detection between expert and nonexpert colonoscopists (18.5% vs 13.1%; $P = .20$), with no significant learning curve.[18] In another study of 401 patients, however, there was no difference in dysplasia detection with CE over WLE.[17] A recent systematic review of 18 trials (2638 patients) demonstrated a higher likelihood of detecting patients with dysplasia using CE over SD WLE (OR 0.44; 95% CI, 0.26 to 0.73; high certainty) and iScan (OR 0.47; 95% CI, 0.25 to 0.90; moderate certainty).[13]

Table 37-1

Societal Recommendations With Surveillance

Society	Surveillance Interval	Annual Surveillance
ECCO 2017[2]	Every 5 years if low risk Every 2 to 3 years if intermediate risk (extensive colitis with mild or moderate inflammation OR post-inflammatory polyps OR family history of CRC in first degree relative diagnosed > 50 years of age)	PSC OR stricture or dysplasia diagnosed < 5 years OR family history of CRC in first degree relative diagnosed < 50 years of age OR extensive colitis with severe inflammation
ASGE 2015[1]	Every 1 to 3 years if no risk factors requiring annual surveillance (optimal interval not defined)	Active inflammation OR anatomical abnormality (stricture or dysplasia, multiple pseudopolyps), OR PSC OR family history of CRC in first degree relative diagnosed < 50 years of age
NICE 2011[13]	Every 5 years if low risk (extensive colitis with no active endoscopic or histological inflammation OR left sided colitis OR Crohn's colitis with < 50% involvement) Every 3 years if intermediate risk (extensive colitis with mild or moderate inflammation OR post-inflammatory polyps OR family history of CRC in first degree relative diagnosed > 50 years of age)	PSC OR stricture or dysplasia diagnosed < 5 years OR family history of CRC in first degree relative diagnosed < 50 years of age OR extensive colitis with severe inflammation
BSG 2010[9]	Every 5 years if low risk (extensive colitis with no active endoscopic or histological inflammation OR left sided colitis OR Crohn's colitis with < 50% involvement) Every 3 years if intermediate risk (extensive colitis with mild or moderate inflammation OR post-inflammatory polyps OR family history of CRC in first degree relative diagnosed > 50 years of age)	PSC OR stricture or dysplasia diagnosed < 5 years OR family history of CRC in first degree relative diagnosed < 50 years of age OR extensive colitis with severe inflammation

(continued)

Table 37-1 (continued)
Societal Recommendations With Surveillance

Society	Surveillance Interval	Annual Surveillance
AGA 2010[8]	1 to 2 years after initial screening colonoscopy for extensive or left sided colitis. After 2 negative examinations, surveillance may be performed every 1 to 3 years More frequent surveillance if ongoing extensive colitis with severe inflammation OR family history of CRC in first degree relative OR anatomical abnormality (stricture, inflammatory polyps, "shortened" colon)	PSC

Table 37-2
Recommendations for Surveillance and Management of Dysplasia in Patients With IBD

Detection of Dysplasia on Surveillance Colonoscopy

1. When performing surveillance with white-light colonoscopy, high definition is recommended rather than standard definition (strong recommendation, low-quality evidence).
2. When performing surveillance with standard-definition colonoscopy, chromoendoscopy is recommended rather than white-light colonoscopy (strong recommendation, moderate-quality evidence).
3. When performing surveillance with high-definition colonoscopy, chromoendoscopy is suggested rather than white-light colonoscopy (conditional recommendation, low-quality evidence).
4. When performing surveillance with standard-definition colonoscopy, narrow-band imaging is not suggested in place of white-light colonoscopy (conditional recommendation, low-quality evidence).
5. When performing surveillance with high-definition colonoscopy, narrow-band imaging is not suggested in place of white-light colonoscopy (conditional recommendation, moderate-quality evidence).

(continued)

Table 37-2 (continued)

Recommendations for Surveillance and Management of Dysplasia in Patients With IBD

6. When performing surveillance with image-enhanced high-definition colonoscopy, narrow-band imaging is not suggested in place of chromoendoscopy (conditional recommendation, moderate-quality evidence).

Management of Dysplasia Discovered on Surveillance Colonoscopy

7. After complete removal of endoscopically resectable polypoid dysplastic lesions, surveillance colonoscopy is recommended rather than colectomy (strong recommendation, very low-quality evidence).
8. After complete removal of endoscopically resectable nonpolypoid dysplastic lesions, surveillance colonoscopy is suggested rather than colectomy (conditional recommendation, very low-quality evidence).
9. For patients with endoscopically invisible dysplasia (confirmed by a gastrointestinal pathologist), referral is suggested to an endoscopist with expertise in IBD surveillance using chromoendoscopy with high-definition colonoscopy (conditional recommendation, very low-quality evidence).

Reproduced with permission from Laine L, Kaltenbach T, Barkun A, et al. SCENIC international consensus statement on surveillance and management of dysplasia in inflammatory bowel disease. *Gastrointest Endosc.* 2015;81(3):489-501.e26.

Successful delivery of dysplasia surveillance using CE hinges on myriad factors such as appropriate training and expertise (endoscopist and team), lesion recognition, interobserver variability among pathologists identifying and grading dysplasia, and operational barriers, including availability of dye and equipment and procedural time.[6]

Chromoendoscopy Technique

CE involves application of a contrast agent (0.1% methylene blue or 0.03% to 0.5% indigo carmine) to the colonic mucosal surface. Excellent resources exist to consolidate and enhance skills with CE and lesion recognition.[2,19] Optimal bowel preparation is vital. The colonic mucosa is sprayed segmentally with contrast agent after cecal intubation and upon withdrawal, using a spray catheter or through the forward water-jet channel using an automated pump. Mucosal lesions that disrupt normal surface topography are highlighted by the contrast dye (Figures 37-2 and 37-3).[19] Endoscopically resectable lesions can be resected or tattooed and referred to an endoscopist with expertise in endoscopic mucosal resection or dissection as appropriate. Targeted biopsies should be taken from lesions deemed endoscopically unresectable and from lesions of uncertain significance. At least 2 biopsies from several colonic segments are recommended to determine histological extent and severity of disease, which in turn affect the risk of dysplasia, although random biopsies are no longer recommended.[1,2]

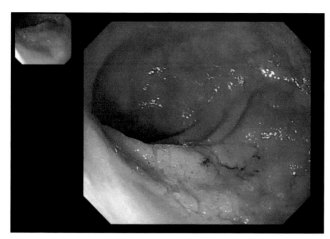

Figure 37-2. Dysplastic lesion at UC surveillance with HD WLE.

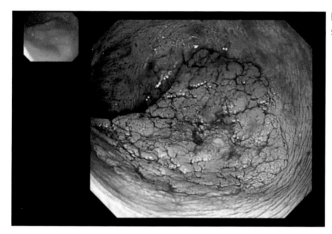

Figure 37-3. Dysplastic lesion at UC surveillance with CE and HD WLE.

Management of Dysplasia

VISIBLE DYSPLASIA

Accurate identification of dysplasia and determination of its resectability is crucial. Lesions should be identified as being within or outside an area of known colitis. Lesions in segments outside an area of known colitis should be treated as sporadic adenomas with standard post-polypectomy surveillance recommendations. Lesions in an area of known colitis should be assessed for endoscopic resectability and completely resected, if possible, by an experienced endoscopist regardless of underlying colitis or grade of dysplasia. Resection may be technically more difficult with inflammation, friability, and scarring. Tattooing and photo documentation may aid subsequent surveillance or resection. Mucosa adjacent to the raised lesion should also be biopsied to evaluate for dysplasia. If completely resected with dysplasia-free margins and no invisible dysplasia elsewhere in the colon, surveillance colonoscopy may be recommended (see Table 37-2). Surveillance with CE is recommended at 3 months and then annually. The SCENIC consensus makes a conditional recommendation for surveillance colonoscopy after complete removal of endoscopically resectable non-polypoid dysplastic lesions, recognizing the higher CRC risk and greater endoscopic difficulty with resectability.

INVISIBLE DYSPLASIA

Invisible dysplasia is dysplasia identified on random (nontargeted) biopsies of colon mucosa without a visible lesion.[2] The SCENIC consensus recommends confirmation of dysplasia by a second gastrointestinal pathologist and referral to an endoscopist with expertise in CE and HD WLE to enable subsequent decisions regarding surveillance vs colectomy.[2] When visible dysplasia is identified in the same area as invisible dysplasia and the lesion is resectable, patients can remain in a surveillance program. If dysplasia is not found, individualized discussions involving surveillance vs colectomy are suggested. When high-grade dysplasia is confirmed by a second specialist pathologist, or incompletely resected raised dysplasia is discovered, colectomy is recommended (see Table 37-2). In older studies not employing CE, the prevalence of synchronous CRC in patients with flat HGD appears to range between 42% to 45%.[4] Of those who deferred colectomy and continued surveillance, 25% developed CRC. Flat nontargeted HGD and endoscopically unresectable lesions or a lesion with dysplasia in the adjacent mucosa are indications for colectomy. It may be difficult to distinguish regeneration and repair from dysplasia in the presence of chronic active inflammation, resulting in a pathological finding that is "indefinite for dysplasia" with a 9% 5-year progression rate to HGD or CRC.[6] Surveillance should take place ideally after "optimal treatment" of underlying inflammation followed by endoscopic reevaluation, probably with CE when the patient is in clinical remission. Given that progression to CRC in patients with dysplasia is higher than those without, a further surveillance examination is advisable within 3 to 6 months.[2,7] The American Society for Gastrointestinal Endoscopy algorithm for the management of lesions detected at surveillance colonoscopy is shown in Figure 37-4.

Newer Imaging Modalities

NBI, confocal laser endomicroscopy, and endocytoscopy are other modalities being studied for the detection of dysplasia in IBD.[6] NBI is an optical CE technology that uses filters to enhance the contrast of the mucosa and vasculature. A recent meta-analysis did not find it to superior to other techniques used in practice.[14] Confocal laser endomicroscopy (CLE) enables real-time histology of lesions, detected at colonoscopy, using intravenous administration of stains such as fluorescein.[20] Following topical or intravenous application of a fluorescence agent, the CLE probe is applied to the mucosal surface, which highlights the extracellular matrix, allowing for in vivo evaluation. Limitations of this technique are increased length of time (approximately 15 to 25 minutes more than WLE with target biopsy and CE with targeted biopsy, respectively), cost, and a steep learning curve. Endocytoscopy uses probe-based systems to obtain histology-equivalent images of the mucosa, following pretreatment with mucolytic agents and staining with dyes such as methylene blue and crystal violet.[20] It has not been tested in dysplasia surveillance to date.

Conclusion

Dysplasia screening has seen a paradigm shift from the historical practice of random serial biopsies to lesion detection and targeted resection, where possible, using optical technologies, with HDE and CE, and using a risk-stratification approach currently supported by international guidelines. Current gaps in knowledge include competency training and procedural cost but also the true and long-term impact of dysplasia detection with modern techniques relating to IBD-CRC detection and survival. Meanwhile, newer optical techniques and noninvasive methods for dysplasia detection may have further and positive impact on dysplasia screening and its purported aims.

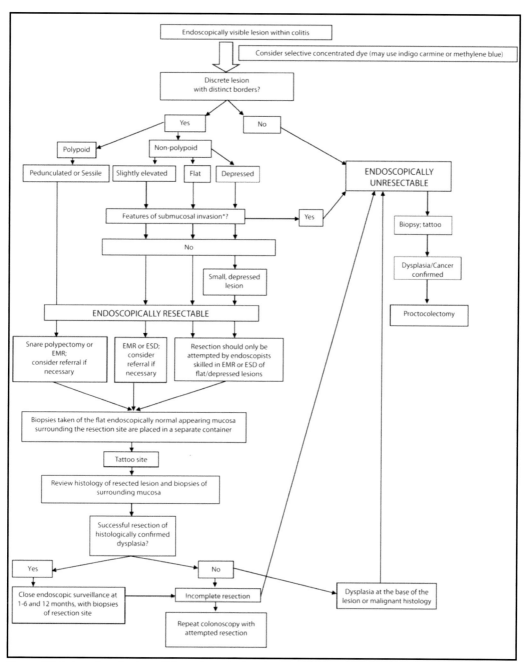

Figure 37-4. American Society of Gastrointestinal endoscopy algorithm for management of lesions detected at surveillance colonoscopy. (Reproduced with permission from American Society for Gastrointestinal Endoscopy Standards of Practice Committee, Shergill AK, Lightdale JR, et al. The role of endoscopy in inflammatory bowel disease. *Gastrointest Endosc*. 2015;81[5]:1101-1121.e1-13.)

References

1. American Society for Gastrointestinal Endoscopy Standards of Practice Committee, Shergill AK, Lightdale JR, et al. The role of endoscopy in inflammatory bowel disease. *Gastrointest Endosc.* 2015;81(5):1101-1121.e1-13.
2. Laine L, Kaltenbach T, Barkun A, et al. SCENIC international consensus statement on surveillance and management of dysplasia in inflammatory bowel disease. *Gastrointest Endosc.* 2015;81(3):489-501.e26.
3. Eaden JA, Abrams KR, Mayberry JF. The risk of colorectal cancer in ulcerative colitis: a meta-analysis. *Gut.* 2001;48(4):526-535.
4. Choi CH, Rutter MD, Askari A, et al. Forty-year analysis of colonoscopic surveillance program for neoplasia in ulcerative colitis: an updated overview. *Am J Gastroenterol.* 2015;110(7):1022-1034.
5. Castano-Milla C, Chaparro M, Gisbert JP. Systematic review with meta-analysis: the declining risk of colorectal cancer in ulcerative colitis. *Aliment Pharmacol Ther.* 2014;39(7):645-659.
6. Limdi JK, Farraye FA. An update on surveillance in ulcerative colitis. *Curr Gastroenterol Rep.* 2018;20(2):7.
7. Farraye FA, Odze RD, Eaden J, Itzkowitz SH. AGA technical review on the diagnosis and management of colorectal neoplasia in inflammatory bowel disease. *Gastroenterology.* 2010;138(2):746-774, 74.e1-4; quiz e12-3.
8. Rutter MD, Saunders BP, Wilkinson KH, Kamm MA, Williams CB, Forbes A. Most dysplasia in ulcerative colitis is visible at colonoscopy. *Gastrointest Endosc.* 2004;60(3):334-339.
9. Ananthakrishnan AN, Cagan A, Cai T, et al. Colonoscopy is associated with a reduced risk for colon cancer and mortality in patients with inflammatory bowel diseases. *Clin Gastroenterol Hepatol.* 2015;13(2):322-329.e1.
10. Annese V, Daperno M, Rutter MD, et al. European evidence based consensus for endoscopy in inflammatory bowel disease. *J Crohns Colitis.* 2013;7(12):982-1018.
11. Rutter MD, Riddell RH. Colorectal dysplasia in inflammatory bowel disease: a clinicopathologic perspective. *Clin Gastroenterol Hepatol.* 2014;12(3):359-367.
12. Konijeti GG, Shrime MG, Ananthakrishnan AN, Chan AT. Cost-effectiveness analysis of chromoendoscopy for colorectal cancer surveillance in patients with ulcerative colitis. *Gastrointest Endosc.* 2014;79(3):455-465.
13. Iannone A, Ruospo M, Palmer SC, et al. Systematic review with network meta-analysis: endoscopic techniques for dysplasia surveillance in inflammatory bowel disease. *Aliment Pharmacol Ther.* 2019;50(8):858-871.
14. Imperatore N, Castiglione F, Testa A, et al. Augmented endoscopy for surveillance of colonic inflammatory bowel disease: systematic review with network meta-analysis. *J Crohns Colitis.* 2019;13(6):714-724.
15. Marion JF, Waye JD, Israel Y, et al. Chromoendoscopy is more effective than standard colonoscopy in detecting dysplasia during long-term surveillance of patients with colitis. *Clin Gastroenterol Hepatol.* 2016;14(5):713-719.
16. Deepak P, Hanson GJ, Fletcher JG, et al. Incremental diagnostic yield of chromoendoscopy and outcomes in inflammatory bowel disease patients with a history of colorectal dysplasia on white-light endoscopy. *Gastrointest Endosc.* 2016;83(5):1005-1012.
17. Mooiweer E, van der Meulen-de Jong AE, Ponsioen CY, et al. Chromoendoscopy for surveillance in inflammatory bowel disease does not increase neoplasia detection compared with conventional colonoscopy with random biopsies: results from a large retrospective study. *Am J Gastroenterol.* 2015;110(7):1014-1021.
18. Carballal S, Maisterra S, Lopez-Serrano A, et al. Real-life chromoendoscopy for neoplasia detection and characterization in long-standing IBD. *Gut.* 2018;67(1):70-78.
19. Soetikno R, Sanduleanu S, Kaltenbach T. An atlas of the nonpolypoid colorectal neoplasms in inflammatory bowel disease. *Gastrointest Endosc Clin N Am.* 2014;24(3):483-520.
20. Subramanian V, Ragunath K. Advanced endoscopic imaging: a review of commercially available technologies. *Clin Gastroenterol Hepatol.* 2014;12(3):368-376.e1.

SECTION VI

SURGICAL TREATMENT

38
QUESTION

WHAT IS THE APPROPRIATE EVALUATION OF THE PREOPERATIVE PATIENT WITH IBD? (MALNUTRITION, STEROIDS, SMOKING)

Amy L. Lightner, MD

Prior to the advent of biologics with infliximab in 1998, corticosteroids were the cornerstone of medical management. Today, there is an increasing number of pharmaceutical immunosuppressives that are being used to treat medically refractory inflammatory bowel disease (IBD)—corticosteroids, immunomodulators (6-mercaptopurine, azathioprine, methotrexate), and biologics (infliximab, adalimumab, certolizumab pegol, vedolizumab, ustekinumab). Despite the increased armamentarium, many patients will succumb to primary and secondary loss of response, and up to 60% of patients with Crohn's disease (CD)[1] and 30% with ulcerative colitis (UC)[2] will still require a major abdominal operation during their lifetime.

By the time patients present for surgery, they are often quite ill and suffer from a chronic disease with poor nutrition, anemia, opioid dependency, and chronic immunosuppression. When taken to the operating room for an intestinal resection, up to 8% of patients with CD will suffer from intra-abdominal sepsis,[3] and up to 5% to 25%[4] of patients with UC will suffer from pelvic sepsis, the leading cause of ileal pouch–anal anastomosis (IPAA) failure. Several modifiable risk factors for intra-abdominal sepsis following ileocecal resection and pelvic sepsis following IPAA have been identified, including increased body mass index, anemia, poor nutritional status, and immunosuppression. It is therefore important to focus on modifiable areas of preoperative optimization to ensure the best possible postoperative outcomes in our patients with IBD. Key preoperative considerations include thoughtful perioperative management of immunosuppressive therapy, careful assessment of nutritional status, and strategies for smoking cessation, especially in patients with CD.

Rubin DT, Friedman S, Farraye FA, eds. *Curbside Consultation in IBD:*
49 Clinical Questions, Third Edition (pp 253-256).
© 2022 Taylor & Francis Group.

Immunosuppressive Therapy

At the time of surgery, 30% to 40% of patients with moderate to severe CD are steroid dependent. The literature has consistently reported that patients exposed to corticosteroids preoperatively have significantly increased rates of superficial surgical site infections, deep space infections, and anastomotic leaks.[5] Unfortunately, many patients are unable to wean off steroids prior to surgery due to the severity of their symptoms. Given that some reports have shown an increased risk of postoperative complications at doses > 20 mg to > 40 mg, it may be worth weaning corticosteroids preoperatively to less than 20 mg daily, when able.

Immunomodulators (6-mercaptopurine, methotrexate, azathioprine) are utilized as a glucocorticoid-sparing agent for the maintenance of remission or in conjunction with biologic therapy to decrease secondary loss of response due to antibody formation. Fortunately, evidence from both large retrospective reviews and systematic reviews suggest that the perioperative use of immunomodulators does not increase adverse postoperative outcomes.[6]

In contrast, the literature regarding the association of biologics with increased postoperative morbidity remains controversial and limited by retrospective study design, heterogeneous patient populations, inconsistent primary endpoints, and variability in the time from biologic exposure to surgery. In CD, numerous retrospective series and 3 prospective studies have reported no significant increase in postoperative complications in the setting of anti–tumor necrosis factor (TNF) therapy, while several other retrospective and prospective studies have reported a significant increase in the rate of postoperative infectious complications and intra-abdominal septic complications in patients exposed to anti-TNF therapy. In UC, while also controversial, there are large single-center series that report anti-TNF therapy increases the rate of peri-pouch sepsis postoperatively,[7] thereby increasing long-term pouch failure rates. For patients exposed to vedolizumab, the literature remains similarly controversial. While both single-center and multicenter studies report increased risk of postoperative infectious complications,[8] others have not found the same increased risk.[9] In patients exposed to vedolizumab undergoing IPAA, one study reported no increased risk of peri-pouch sepsis related to vedolizumab,[10] while another group found a significantly increased risk of superficial surgical site infection and clinically increased rate of peri-pouch sepsis compared to patients exposed to anti-TNF (31% vs 6%).[11] Both studies were limited by a small number of patients exposed to vedolizumab within 12 weeks of IPAA.

To date, only one study has evaluated the association of preoperative exposure to ustekinumab and postoperative complications. There were no differences in the number of 30-day postoperative complications among the 44 ustekinumab-treated patients vs 169 anti-TNF treated patients across 6 IBD referral centers, suggesting ustekinumab may be safe in the perioperative period.[12]

Nutritional Optimization

Patients with UC and CD are at particularly high risk of malnutrition, with rates ranging from 25% to 69%.[13] In surgical patients, this rate is even higher at 85%. Markers of malnutrition include weight loss > 10% of body weight within 6 months, a body mass index < 18.5 kg/m, and serum albumin levels less < 3.0 g/dL. Postoperative complications are known to be increased in the setting of poor nutritional status, making preoperative nutritional optimization vital for improvement of postoperative outcomes. Exclusive enteral feeding not only induces mucosal healing but significantly decreases the rate of intra-abdominal septic complications.[14] In fact, only 4 weeks of exclusive enteral feeding prior to surgery in patients with CD has shown to reduce both infectious and noninfectious postoperative complications and significantly improve nutritional and inflammatory status. Evidence for parenteral nutrition remains more controversial, with some studies reporting decreased postoperative complications but others reporting an increased rate of line sepsis.

Smoking Cessation

Smoking increases severity, frequency of flares, need for hospitalization, and ultimate need for surgical intervention in patients with CD. In addition, smoking is associated with increased risk for postoperative morbidity and, more specifically, is an important predictor of anastomotic leakage. Smoking cessation, at least 4 weeks prior to surgery, can effectively reduce the adverse postoperative risks associated with smoking.[15]

Preoperative Management Strategy Based on Aforementioned Evidence

1. *Corticosteroids:* Make all attempts to wean off corticosteroids prior to surgical intervention for CD. If unable to wean off completely, make all attempts to wean to a dose less than 20 mg prior to surgical intervention. For patients undergoing IPAA, consider a 3-stage or modified 2-stage IPAA where colectomy is performed at the first stage, allowing pouch construction at a date when patients have been weaned off all corticosteroids. There is no need to wean corticosteroids prior to subtotal colectomy as a first of 3 stages for IPAA.

2. *Immunomodulators:* The elimination half-life of 6-mercaptopurine and azathioprine is approximately 1 hour. Thus, patients can be counseled to hold immunomodulators on the day of surgery and resume them on postoperative day 1.

3. *Preoperative management of biologics:*
   a. If an elective CD surgical patient is on a Q8-week biologic dosing regimen, attempt to give the last dose of biologic 4 weeks prior to surgery and the postoperative dose (if continuing for prophylaxis or concurrent disease outside the resection margins) 4 weeks after surgery to maintain a consistent dosing regimen.
   b. If an elective CD surgical patient is on dual or triple immunosuppression, have the patient meet with stoma therapy. Combination immunosuppression is associated with a significantly increased rate of postoperative anastomotic leak, so appropriately counsel the patient that intestinal diversion may be the safest approach.
   c. For patients with UC undergoing IPAA:
      i. There is no need to delay the initial subtotal colectomy in the setting of corticosteroids, immunomodulators, maintenance biologic therapy, or induction therapy.
      ii. All patients on corticosteroids and/or biologic therapy are treated with a 3-stage approach or modified 2-stage approach, where proctectomy and construction of the pouch is performed at least 12 weeks from the prior colectomy. This minimizes the risk of pelvic sepsis, the leading cause of pouch failure.

4. *Nutrition:* Enteral nutritional support is preferred to parenteral due to decreased risk of infection, decreased cost, and improved gastrointestinal growth and function given its physiologic nature as compared to parenteral support.
   a. Consider delaying elective surgery until albumin is > 3.0 g/dL. Utilize enteral nutrition when able.
   b. If enteral nutrition cannot be tolerated, consider 2 to 4 weeks of parenteral nutrition prior to elective surgical intervention.
   c. If a prolonged ileus or nothing per os is anticipated postoperatively (eg, extensive adhesiolysis, proximal small bowel disease, extensive strictureplasty), consider initiation of parenteral nutrition 2 to 4 weeks prior to surgery with the intent of continuing postoperatively, until adequate oral intake has been achieved.

5. *Smoking:* Interventions to promote smoking cessation, including individual counseling, should be initiated at least 2 months prior to surgical intervention.

   a. Consider delaying elective surgery until smoking cessation has been achieved at least 4 weeks prior to surgery.

Conclusion

There is currently an expanding repertoire of immunosuppressive medications and escalating disease severity at the time of surgery. Thus, careful attention to the preoperative optimization in the perioperative management of immunosuppressive therapies, nutritional status, and smoking cessation is desperately needed. Weaning corticosteroids, initiating enteral feeds, and smoking abstinence for at least 4 weeks prior to surgery can all improve postoperative outcomes for patients with IBD. Future evidence-based algorithms for optimal perioperative management may be useful for both gastroenterologists and surgeons treating patients with IBD.

References

1. Peyrin-Biroulet L, Loftus EV Jr, Colombel JF, Sandborn WJ. The natural history of adult Crohn's disease in population-based cohorts. *Am J Gastroenterol.* 2010;105(2):289-297.

2. Feuerstein JD, Cheifetz AS. Ulcerative colitis: epidemiology, diagnosis, and management. *Mayo Clin Proc.* 2014;89(11):1553-1563.

3. Brouquet A, Maggiori L, Zerbib P, et al. Anti-TNF therapy is associated with an increased risk of postoperative morbidity after surgery for ileocolonic Crohn disease: results of a prospective nationwide cohort. *Ann Surg.* 2018;267(2):221-228.

4. Fazio VW, Kiran RP, Remzi FH, et al. Ileal pouch anal anastomosis: analysis of outcome and quality of life in 3707 patients. *Ann Surg.* 2013;257(4):679-685.

5. Subramanian V, Saxena S, Kang JY, Pollok RC. Preoperative steroid use and risk of postoperative complications in patients with inflammatory bowel disease undergoing abdominal surgery. *Am J Gastroenterol.* 2008;103(9): 2373-2381.

6. Colombel JF, Loftus EV Jr, Tremaine WJ, et al. Early postoperative complications are not increased in patients with Crohn's disease treated perioperatively with infliximab or immunosuppressive therapy. *Am J Gastroenterol.* 2004;99(5):878-883.

7. Mor IJ, Vogel JD, da Luz Moreira A, Shen B, Hammel J, Remzi FH. Infliximab in ulcerative colitis is associated with an increased risk of postoperative complications after restorative proctocolectomy. *Dis Colon Rectum.* 2008;51(8):1202-1207; discussion 1207-1210.

8. Lightner AL, Mathis KL, Tse CS, et al. Postoperative outcomes in vedolizumab-treated patients undergoing major abdominal operations for inflammatory bowel disease: retrospective multicenter cohort study. *Inflamm Bowel Dis.* 2018;24(4):871-876.

9. Yamada A, Komaki Y, Patel N, et al. Risk of postoperative complications among inflammatory bowel disease patients treated preoperatively with vedolizumab. *Am J Gastroenterol.* 2017;112(9):1423-1429.

10. Ferrante M, de Buck van Overstraeten A, Schils N, et al. Perioperative use of vedolizumab is not associated with postoperative infectious complications in patients with ulcerative colitis undergoing colectomy. *J Crohns Colitis.* 2017;11(11):1353-1361.

11. Lightner AL, McKenna NP, Moncrief S, Pemberton JH, Raffals LE, Mathis KL. Surgical outcomes in vedolizumab-treated patients with ulcerative colitis. *Inflamm Bowel Dis.* 2017;23(12):2197-2201.

12. Lightner AL, McKenna NP, Tse CS, et al. Postoperative outcomes in ustekinumab-treated patients undergoing abdominal operations for Crohn's disease. *J Crohns Colitis.* 2017;12(4):402-407.

13. Mijac DD, Jankovic GL, Jorga J, Krstic MN. Nutritional status in patients with active inflammatory bowel disease: prevalence of malnutrition and methods for routine nutritional assessment. *Eur J Intern Med.* 2010;21(4):315-319.

14. Li Y, Zuo L, Zhu W, et al. Role of exclusive enteral nutrition in the preoperative optimization of patients with Crohn's disease following immunosuppressive therapy. *Medicine (Baltimore).* 2015;94(5):e478.

15. Kulaylat AS, Kulaylat AN, Schaefer EW, et al. Association of preoperative anti-tumor necrosis factor therapy with adverse postoperative outcomes in patients undergoing abdominal surgery for ulcerative colitis. *JAMA Surg.* 2017;152(8):e171538.

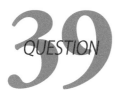

MY PATIENT WITH CROHN'S DISEASE HAS AN ILEAL ABSCESS. WHAT IS THE APPROPRIATE MANAGEMENT AND TIMING OF MEDICAL AND SURGICAL THERAPIES?

Victor G. Chedid, MD, MSc and Sunanda V. Kane, MD, MSPH

Crohn's disease (CD) is characterized by transmural inflammation of the bowel wall and may involve the gastrointestinal tract from mouth to anus. Approximately 80% of patients with CD have small bowel involvement, typically distal ileum, and around 50% of patients with CD have ileocolitis (inflammation involving the ileum and colon). Consequently, the disease is often complicated by fistula formation, bowel perforations, and abscesses. Intra-abdominal or pelvic abscesses develop in 10% to 28% of patients with CD. This may be the presenting feature of the disease or may develop during the course of the illness, either spontaneously or as a complication of surgery. In most cases, the abscess remains localized, resulting in localized peritonitis, abdominal pain, and fevers. In rare cases, the abscess may perforate, leading to diffuse peritonitis. The combination of an intra-abdominal abscess with active CD poses a clinical dilemma for the treating physician, who must weigh the benefits of using immunosuppressive therapies for inflammatory bowel disease (IBD) against the risks of immunosuppression in the presence of serious abdominal infection. Traditionally, intra-abdominal abscesses in CD were managed with early surgery that often involved external drainage procedures, bowel resection, and the creation of diverting ostomies in acutely ill patients. Today, intra-abdominal abscesses are frequently treated initially with antibiotics and percutaneous drainage, with surgical resection of diseased bowel performed later, if necessary, as an elective, 1-stage procedure. Additionally, in some tertiary centers, endoscopic nonsurgical management of ileal abscesses is performed either as an alternative to surgery or a bridge to surgery.

Rubin DT, Friedman S, Farraye FA, eds. *Curbside Consultation in IBD:*
49 Clinical Questions, Third Edition (pp 257-261).
© 2022 Taylor & Francis Group.

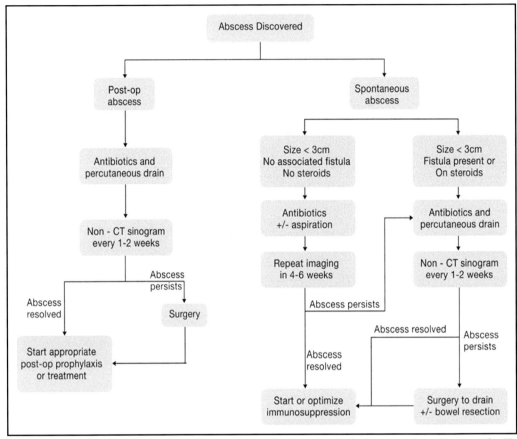

Figure 39-1. A suggested algorithm for managing intra-abdominal abscesses in patients with CD. (Adapted from Feagins LA, Holubar SD, Kane SV, Spechler SJ. Current strategies in the management of intra-abdominal abscesses in Crohn's disease. *Clin Gastroenterol Hepatol.* 2011;9[10]:842-850.)

Initial Management

The optimal initial management of intra-abdominal abscesses in patients with CD involves an integrated, multidisciplinary team that includes gastroenterologists, colorectal surgeons, radiologists, and possibly infectious disease specialists (Figure 39-1).[1] Once the diagnosis of an abscess is made, antimicrobial therapy should be initiated promptly, using agents effective against enteric gram-negative aerobic and facultative bacilli, enteric gram-positive streptococci, and obligate anaerobic bacilli. The duration of antibiotic treatment depends on the efficacy of the chosen drainage procedure. For an adequately drained abscess, antibiotics should be continued for at least 3 to 7 days. If the abscess is not effectively drained or if adequate clinical improvement is not seen within 3 to 5 days, a longer course of antibiotics is required, and reimaging should be performed to ensure that no undrained fluid collections remain.

Percutaneous Drainage

Over the past several decades, percutaneous drainage (aspiration and insertion of a drainage catheter) for CD-related abscesses has emerged as a first-line treatment option or as a bridge to surgery in acutely ill or malnourished patients in preparation for future elective surgery. A survey of the Nationwide Inpatient Sample showed a significant increase in the use of percutaneous surgery since 1998 compared to surgery.[2] Case series and retrospective studies of patients with both spontaneous and postoperative CD-related abscesses have shown that percutaneous drainage can be performed successfully in 74% to 100% of cases, although up to 20% require more than one percutaneous drainage procedure. Furthermore, initial treatment by percutaneous drainage may avoid surgery in some cases. For patients with postoperative abscesses in particular, available studies suggest that reoperation can be avoided with percutaneous drainage in 67% to 100% of cases. In cases where surgery is performed after percutaneous abscess drainage (typically for spontaneous abscesses), the surgeon is often able to perform a primary bowel anastomosis and avoid bowel diversion via ostomy construction, which is often required in primary surgical drainage procedures. With successful percutaneous drainage, defervescence and clinical improvement typically occur within 24 to 48 hours, and catheter output often decreases within 1 week. Additionally, early intervention for abscess drainage is associated with shorter hospital stay.

Several factors play into the success of percutaneous drainage of an abscess, including the nature of the abscess (spontaneous vs postoperative), abscess size, and whether the abscess is associated with a fistula. The effect of abscess size on the success rate of percutaneous drainage has not been evaluated specifically in any study. Nevertheless, it has been suggested that abscesses larger than 3 cm in diameter are amenable to, and will not resolve without drainage, whereas abscesses 3 cm or smaller are likely to respond to antibiotics alone or in combination with percutaneous aspiration (without an in-dwelling catheter). Furthermore, an abscess larger than 6 cm on imaging can be a predictor of the patient ultimately requiring bowel resection. The presence of a fistula should be suspected when an in-dwelling catheter in an abscess yields a persistently high drainage output. For abscesses with in-dwelling catheters that persistently drain more than 50 mL of fluid per day, some authorities recommend a fistulogram or contrast-enhanced magnetic resonance imaging or computed tomography to seek an enteric fistula, even if a prior study had been negative.

Unfortunately, there are no randomized controlled trials comparing percutaneous and surgical drainage of CD-related abscesses. Gutierrez et al performed a retrospective study comparing the outcomes of 37 patients who underwent percutaneous drainage as initial treatment for these abscesses with the outcomes of 29 patients who had surgery as initial treatment.[3] The investigators found that the time to resolution did not differ significantly between the 2 treatment groups (25 days vs 21.5 days, surgery vs percutaneous drainage, respectively, $P = .08$). After 1 year of follow-up, approximately one-third of patients treated with percutaneous drainage eventually had surgery. Nguyen et al performed a similar retrospective study with 55 patients who underwent percutaneous drainage as initial management and 40 patients who underwent surgery as their initial management.[4] They found similar rates of abscess occurrence and complications between patients treated with medical (percutaneous) vs surgical treatment. They also found that a history of perianal disease and active ileal disease (endoscopic or radiologic evidence) were associated with increased risk of abscess recurrence. In a recent meta-analysis comparing outcomes of percutaneous drainage alone vs primary surgery for CD-related intra-abdominal spontaneous abscesses, there was a significantly higher risk of abscess recurrence following percutaneous drainage, with 30% of these patients avoiding subsequent surgery.[5] There was no significant difference between approaches in post-procedural complication rate, ultimate permanent stoma requirement, or length of hospital stay.

For patients with spontaneous abscesses, once the acute suppurative issues have been addressed, endoscopic assessment of the bowel should be considered to help guide the next steps in patient management. Few data are available to guide the decision regarding the optimal timing for performing colonoscopy after treating an abscess; it is generally our practice to wait 4 to 6 weeks. The colonoscopy allows for the precise localization of the diseased bowel segments (in the colon and distal small bowel) and for the assessment of bowel disease severity; this information is important for planning surgery and for determining whether medical therapy for the IBD requires alteration.

Surgical Drainage

Surgical drainage of intra-abdominal abscesses due to CD involves exploration of the abdomen and pelvis, evacuation of all abscess contents, irrigation and debridement of the abscess cavity, and, typically, en bloc bowel resection with or without external suction drainage. It is important to recognize that while surgery may treat the acute septic complication of CD it usually does not cure CD because recurrence after bowel resection is the rule rather than the exception. At 1 year after the surgical resection of diseased bowel for patients with CD, endoscopic evidence of disease recurrence can be found at the anastomosis in 73% to 93% of cases, and clinical recurrence is seen in 20% to 30%. In addition, bowel resection for CD can be complicated by anastomotic septic complications and new fistula formation. Today, surgical drainage of intra-abdominal abscesses is typically reserved for cases that are not amenable to or have failed percutaneous drainage, or for those that have failed to resolve with maximal medical therapy. Furthermore, early operative intervention after percutaneous drainage (within 7 days) in perforating CD may be associated with a high incidence of diversions and readmissions compared to elective surgery.[6]

Adjuvant Immunosuppressive Use

SPONTANEOUS ABSCESSES

The use of immunosuppressive therapy (steroids, immunomodulators, and biologics) during the treatment of CD-related abscesses has not been well studied, and few evidence-based data are available to guide therapy. However, if immunosuppressive agents are going to be continued in the setting of intra-abdominal or pelvic sepsis, then it seems prudent to prescribe concomitant antibiotics and continue antibiotic therapy until the septic source has been eradicated.

After abscess drainage, patients with spontaneous abscesses should be considered for immunosuppressive therapy. No studies have specifically studied which agents are best in these situations or how long to wait after abscess drainage before starting these agents. In a post hoc analysis of the ACCENT II (A Crohn's Disease Clinical Trial Evaluating Infliximab in a New Long-Term Treatment Regimen in Patients With Fistulizing Crohn's Disease) study, patients who had an intra-abdominal abscess were mandated to have had abscess drainage at least 3 weeks prior to study entry. Of the 15 patients with 22 abdominal draining fistulas who were treated with infliximab, none developed abscesses during the study period. Moreover, in their retrospective analysis of medical vs surgical treatment, Nguyen et al found that treatment with an anti–tumor necrosis factor (monotherapy or in combination with an immunomodulator) after abscess resolution was protective against abscess recurrence.[3]

POSTOPERATIVE ABSCESSES

Recommendations for starting immunosuppressive therapy for patients with postoperative abscesses differ from those for patients with spontaneous abscesses. For patients with spontaneous abscesses, immunosuppressive therapy is started as soon as possible after percutaneous drainage based on the assumption that these abscesses arose from diseased bowel, and diseased bowel requires treatment to enable abscess healing and to prevent abscess recurrence. In contrast, post-operative abscesses result from complications of surgery, and that surgery often includes resection of the diseased bowel. In this setting, immediate immunosuppression is not required to prevent diseased bowel from interfering with abscess healing, and early immunosuppression might impair abscess healing and predispose patients to septic complications. Therefore, immunosuppressive therapy is generally withheld from patients with postoperative abscesses until those abscesses have healed. After abscess healing, immunosuppression can be started as indicated to prevent future flares of IBD.

References

1. Feagins LA, Holubar SD, Kane SV, Spechler SJ. Current strategies in the management of intra-abdominal abscesses in Crohn's disease. *Clin Gastroenterol Hepatol*. 2011;9(10):842-850.
2. Ananthakrishnan AN, McGinley EL. Treatment of intra-abdominal abscesses in Crohn's disease: anationwide analysis of patterns and outcomes of care. *Dig Dis Sci*. 2013;58(7):2013-2018.
3. Gutierrez A, Lee H, Sands BE. Outcome of surgical versus percutaneous drainage of abdominal and pelvic abscesses in Crohn's disease. *Am J Gastroenterol*. 2006;101(10):2283-2289.
4. Nguyen DL, Sandborn WJ, Loftus EV Jr, et al. Similar outcomes of surgical and medical treatment of intra-abdominal abscesses in patients with Crohn's disease. *Clin Gastroenterol Hepatol*. 2012;10(4):400-404.
5. Clancy C, Boland T, Deasy J, et al. A meta-analysis of percutaneous drainage versus surgery as the initial treatment of Crohn's disease-related intra-abdominal abscess. *J Crohns Colitis*. 2016;10(2):202-208.
6. Sangster W, Berg AS, Choi CS, et al. Outcomes of early ileocolectomy after percutaneous drainage for perforated ileocolic Crohn's disease. *Am J Surgery*. 2016;212(4):728-734.
7. Perl D, Waljee AK, Bishu S, et al. Imaging features associated with failure of nonoperative management of intraabdominal abscesses in Crohn disease. *Inflamm Bowel Dis*. 2019;25(12):1939-1944.
8. Graham E, Rao K, Cinti S. Medical versus interventional treatment of intra-abdominal abscess in patients with Crohn disease. *Infect Dis (Auckl)*. 2017;10:1179916117701736.
9. Mao R, Chen YJ, Chen BL. Intra-cavitary contrast-enhanced ultrasound: anovel radiation-free method for detecting abscess-associated penetrating disease in Crohn's disease. *J Crohns Colitis*. 2019;13(5):593-599.

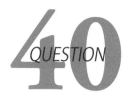

What Is the Updated Approach to Monitoring and Prevention in a Patient With Crohn's Disease After an Ileocecectomy and Primary Anastomosis?

Ashwin N. Ananthakrishnan, MD, MPH

There are an estimated 1 million individuals with Crohn's disease (CD) in the United States and millions more worldwide. Nearly half of patients with CD will require at least 1 intestinal surgery in their lifetime.[1] The most common operation in such patients is an ileocecal resection with primary anastomosis between the neo-terminal ileum and ascending colon. Even after removal of all macroscopically diseased segments, nearly 70% to 90% of patients will have endoscopic or histologic evidence of recurrence within 1 year following their first surgery (endoscopic recurrence).[2] The recurrence is frequently in the neo-terminal ileum, at or just proximal to the ileocolonic anastomosis. About half of the patients will have recurrence of symptoms associated with CD (clinical recurrence). One-third of patients who undergo resection may eventually require a second resection surgery (surgical recurrence) within 10 years. Following are the 5 steps I use in the management of CD postoperatively.

Step 1: Risk Stratification

My first step in managing patients postoperatively is to understand the patients' risk factors for recurrence. There are many studies that have attempted to define which clinical features are associated with clinical, endoscopic, or surgical recurrence (Table 40-1).[3] One of the most consistently defined risk factors is smoking. Continued smoking after the resection increases the risk of clinical recurrence by 50% and the risk of endoscopic and surgical recurrence 2-fold. In addition, surgery for penetrating CD is associated with higher likelihood of recurrence than for long-standing fibrostenotic disease. Other risk factors that have been associated with recurrence

Rubin DT, Friedman S, Farraye FA, eds. *Curbside Consultation in IBD:*
49 Clinical Questions, Third Edition (pp 263-267).
© 2022 Taylor & Francis Group.

Table 40-1

Definite and Possible Risk Factors for Postoperative Crohn's Disease Recurrence

Definite Risk Factors

Smoking

Surgery for penetrating disease

Possible Risk Factors

Male gender

Presence of granulomas

Prior intestinal resection

Longer resection segment length

Short duration of disease

Type of anastomosis

Histologic involvement at the margins

Genetic, microbiome, and serologic features

---

in some but not other studies include male gender, shorter duration of disease, longer resection length, anastomotic technique, histologic involvement at the resected margins, and presence of granulomas. Certain genetic (eg, NOD2) and microbiome features (depletion of *Faecalibacterium prausnitzii*) have been linked to recurrence in some small studies but not replicated in others and are not yet clinically useful.

Step 2: Assessment of Postoperative Recurrence

The second step in the management of postoperative CD is to actively assess for occurrence of endoscopic and clinical recurrence. The presence of symptoms of abdominal pain or diarrhea postoperatively correlate poorly with objective evidence of inflammation in the postoperative setting. Therefore, monitoring for recurrence based on symptoms alone is not sufficient. The most widely used and accepted method for assessing postoperative recurrence is colonoscopy. Postoperative recurrence is endoscopically quantified using the Rutgeerts score (Table 40-2).[2] This ranges from i0 (normal) to i4 disease (diffuse inflammation with large ulcers, nodules, and/or narrowing). A Rutgeerts score of i2 to i4 is considered significant endoscopic recurrence. The severity of endoscopic recurrence correlates with future risk of clinical recurrence. Patients with endoscopic scores of i0 or i1 have low clinical recurrence of rates of 0% to 10% at 3 years. In contrast, patients with i2, i3, and i4 recurrence can be expected to have clinical recurrence rates of 15%, 40%, and 90%, respectively. Emerging data from the POCER (Postoperative Crohn's Endoscopic Recurrence) study suggest that fecal calprotectin levels postoperatively correlate with Rutgeerts endoscopic score and can be used as a noninvasive marker for surveying for recurrence.[4] Levels of fecal calprotectin greater than 100 µg/g indicated endoscopic recurrence

Table 40-2
Rutgeerts Classification for Postoperative Recurrence

Rutgeerts score	*Description*
i0	Normal
i1	Fewer than 5 aphthous ulcers
i2	> 5 aphthous lesions Normal intervening mucosa Lesions confined to anastomosis
i3	Diffuse aphthous ileitis
i4	Diffuse inflammation with large ulcers, nodularity, and narrowing

with 89% sensitivity and 58% specificity, and a negative predictive value of 91%. Computed tomography, magnetic resonance imaging, and video capsule endoscopy can also be used but are less frequently employed.

Step 3: Defining the Optimal Postoperative Medical Regimen

There have been several clinical trials examining the efficacy of different therapeutic strategies in preventing clinical or endoscopic recurrence of CD. Probiotics and aminosalicylates are not effective for preventing recurrence postoperatively and should not be used.[5] Nitroimidazole antibiotics (metronidazole, ornidazole) have been shown to be effective for preventing endoscopic and clinical recurrence. In a small clinical trial of 80 patients, those randomized to ornidazole had lower rates of clinical recurrence (8% vs 38%) and endoscopic recurrence (54% vs 79%) compared to placebo. However, nearly one-third of patients did not tolerate this antibiotic class. Four randomized controlled trials examined the efficacy of azathioprine in preventing postoperative recurrence and suggest a modest benefit in reduction of clinical and severe endoscopic recurrence. An initial proof-of-concept clinical trial, followed by a multicenter randomized controlled trial, demonstrated infliximab to be very effective in preventing endoscopic and clinical recurrence following ileocecal resection.[6] In the PREVENT (Prospective, Multicenter, Randomized, Double-Blind, Placebo-Controlled Trial Comparing REMICADE [infliximab] and Placebo in the Prevention of Recurrence in Crohn's Disease Patients Undergoing Surgical Resection Who Are at an Increased Risk of Recurrence) trial of patients with CD at high risk of recurrence, a smaller proportion of patients treated with infliximab had endoscopic recurrence at week 76 compared to those treated with placebo (31% vs 60%).[6] The benefit was greatest in people beginning infliximab soon after the resection, with only a more modest benefit observed if infliximab was initiated following development of the recurrence.[7] Randomized trials and open-label studies have similarly demonstrated adalimumab to be effective in preventing recurrence with a similar magnitude of benefit.[5,8] We do not yet have high-quality data on the efficacy of vedolizumab or ustekinumab to prevent recurrence.

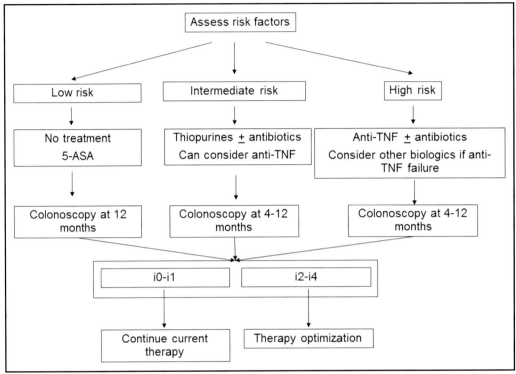

Figure 40-1. Strategy for postoperative management of CD.

Step 4: Determining the Timing of Initiation of Postoperative Therapy

The timing on initiation of postoperative therapy depends on the patient's prior history and risk factors for recurrence (Figure 40-1). Patients without any risk factors, such as those who undergo resection for long-standing isolated fibrostenotic disease, can be monitored postoperatively for recurrence with a colonoscopy 6 to 12 months after resection. If there is evidence of endoscopic recurrence, I then initiate therapy. I place patients who have 2 or more risk factors or have biologic prior to the resection on biologic therapy 2 to 4 weeks after the initial surgery to prevent recurrence. If patients had been on an agent for only a short while (< 3 months) before the surgery, then the resection may not be a primary failure of therapy and the same treatment can be continued. On the other hand, patients with secondary loss of response after an adequate trial should be switched to an alternate therapy. In very high-risk patients, I add on metronidazole for the first 3 months for additional benefit if the patient tolerates it.

Step 5: Assess Response and Optimize Therapy

It is important to objectively assess for efficacy of postoperative therapy and optimize the regimen. Typically, I do this with either fecal inflammatory markers such as calprotectin or a colonoscopy 6 to 12 months after initiating therapy. Patients with clinical and/or endoscopic evidence of failure of the initial postoperative regimen have their therapy optimized based on the clinical scenario.

Conclusion

The key principles in managing postoperative CD are initiation of therapy for postoperative prevention (depending on risk factors) and active surveillance for endoscopic and clinical recurrence. The discussion about postoperative treatment should begin preoperatively, as therapy is most effective when initiated within 2 to 4 weeks of the surgery. While anti–tumor necrosis factor agents have the most robust data supporting efficacy, weaker evidence supports a benefit to antibiotics and immunomodulators in the right clinical setting. Objectively evaluating therapy efficacy and optimizing accordingly is important to ensure best patient outcomes.

References

1. Cosnes J, Gower-Rousseau C, Seksik P, Cortot A. Epidemiology and natural history of inflammatory bowel diseases. *Gastroenterology.* 2011;140(6):1785-1794.
2. Rutgeerts P, Geboes K, Vantrappen G, Kerremans R, Coenegrachts JL, Coremans G. Natural history of recurrent Crohn's disease at the ileocolonic anastomosis after curative surgery. *Gut.* 1984;25(6):665-672.
3. Yamamoto T. Factors affecting recurrence after surgery for Crohn's disease. *World J Gastroenterol.* 2005;11(26):3971-3979.
4. Wright EK, Kamm MA, De Cruz P, et al. Measurement of fecal calprotectin improves monitoring and detection of recurrence of Crohn's disease after surgery. *Gastroenterology.* 2015;148(5):938-947.e931.
5. Regueiro M, Velayos F, Greer JB, et al. American Gastroenterological Association Institute technical review on the management of Crohn's disease after surgical resection. *Gastroenterology.* 2017;152(1):277-295.e273.
6. Regueiro M, Feagan BG, Zou B, et al. Infliximab reduces endoscopic, but not clinical, recurrence of Crohn's disease after ileocolonic resection. *Gastroenterology.* 2016;150(7):1568-1578.
7. Regueiro M, Kip KE, Baidoo L, Swoger JM, Schraut W. Postoperative therapy with infliximab prevents long-term Crohn's disease recurrence. *Clin Gastroenterol Hepatol.* 2014;12(9):1494-1502.e1491.
8. De Cruz P, Kamm MA, Hamilton AL, et al. Crohn's disease management after intestinal resection: a randomized trial. *Lancet.* 2015;385(9976):1406-1417.

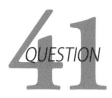

How Does Perioperative Immune Suppression Affect Surgical Outcomes in IBD?

Shintaro Akiyama, MD, PhD; Akihiro Yamada, MD, PhD; and
Atsushi Sakuraba, MD, PhD

Despite optimal medical management, up to 30% of patients with ulcerative colitis (UC) and 75% of patients with Crohn's disease (CD) will need surgery for refractory disease or its complications during the disease course.[1] Studies have demonstrated that patients with UC and CD carry a high risk of postoperative complications, including infection, with incidence ranging from 20% to 30%.[2] Hence, it is essential that gastroenterologists and surgeons understand the surgical values and risk factors affecting surgical outcomes in patients with inflammatory bowel disease (IBD).

Current and emerging therapies for IBD, including various biologics, mainly target the immune cells and inflammatory cytokines. They can induce and maintain remission in a substantial proportion of patients, which may result in a decreased need for surgery. However, due to the systemic immunosuppressive properties, some of these medications have characteristic side effects such as infections. The use of immunosuppressive and biologic drugs has been increasing; therefore, understanding the influence of these medications on surgical outcomes, including infectious complications, is important.

Corticosteroids are often administered to induce remission in acute episodes of IBD. A number of studies have assessed the risk of postoperative complications with corticosteroids in patients with IBD.[3] A meta-analysis reviewed a total of 7 observational studies and showed an increased risk of overall postoperative complications (OR 1.41, 95% CI, 1.07 to 1.87) among patients with IBD on corticosteroids. Furthermore, this meta-analysis demonstrated an increased risk of postoperative infectious complications (OR 1.68, 95% CI, 1.24 to 2.28) with the use of corticosteroids.[4] Another meta-analysis demonstrated that preoperative corticosteroid use in patients with CD may be a risk factor for postoperative intra-abdominal septic complications, including anastomotic leakage, intra-abdominal abscess, or enterocutaneous fistula (OR 1.99, 95% CI, 1.54 to 2.57).[5]

Rubin DT, Friedman S, Farraye FA, eds. *Curbside Consultation in IBD:*
49 Clinical Questions, Third Edition (pp 269-272).

Hence, it is important to acknowledge that corticosteroid use is a risk factor for postoperative complications, including infections, and dose reduction of corticosteroids should be considered before surgery, especially before elective surgeries, to improve surgical outcomes.

Thiopurines are immunomodulatory medications used to maintain remission in steroid-dependent patients with IBD or to prevent the development of antidrug antibodies in those receiving anti–tumor necrosis factor-α (TNF-α) agents.[6] The use of thiopurines is known as an independent risk factor for opportunistic infections in patients with IBD.[7] Most single-center studies revealed no increased risk of postoperative complications in patients with IBD treated with thiopurines alone or in combination with corticosteroids or anti-TNF-α agents.[8] A meta-analysis assessed the risk factors of intra-abdominal septic complications after surgery in patients with CD and showed no association with immunomodulator use (OR 1.07, 95% CI, 0.66 to 1.73).[5] Although further studies are needed to demonstrate the effect of combination therapies of thiopurines and corticosteroids or anti-TNF-α agents on surgical outcome in patients with IBD, thiopurine monotherapy does not appear to increase the risk of postoperative complications in patients with IBD.

Anti-TNF-α agents have been increasingly used in patients with IBD and are known to carry a small risk of infections.[9] A recent study reported that up to 60% of patients with CD received anti-TNF-α agents before their first abdominal surgery, and whether their use in the perioperative period is associated with increased risk of complications is an important issue. A majority of single-institutional studies did not report increased risk of postoperative complications with the use of anti-TNF-α agents.[10] However, when results were pooled by a meta-analysis, preoperative anti-TNF-α agent use slightly increased the incidence of overall postoperative complications in patients with IBD (OR 1.28, 95% CI, 1.04 to 1.57) compared to patients without anti-TNF-α agents, and particularly infectious complications among patients with CD (OR 1.45, 95% CI, 1.03 to 2.05).[11] Meanwhile, the risk of postoperative complications was not increased in patients with UC receiving anti-TNF-α agents.[11] Several meta-analyses have been conducted to elucidate the influence of anti-TNF-α agents on complications after surgery in patients with CD, but their results were inconsistent.[12,13] Thus, a meta-analysis including more recently published articles was conducted and showed no statistically significant differences in the risk of postoperative complications (OR 1.17, 95% CI, 0.82 to 1.66) and infectious complications (OR 1.23, 95% CI, 0.87 to 1.74) between patients with CD treated with infliximab and those without.[14] Therefore, the perioperative use of anti-TNF-α agents in patients with IBD is considered safe, with no significant risk of complications after surgery.

Vedolizumab, a novel humanized immunoglobulin G1 monoclonal antibody against $\alpha_4\beta_7$ integrin, acts by suppressing intestinal inflammation through blocking of leukocyte trafficking to the digestive tract. However, leukocytes are also known to play an important role in wound healing, so the effect of vedolizumab on postoperative outcomes needs to be carefully evaluated. Several studies have been conducted to determine the risk of postoperative complications among patients with IBD who preoperatively received vedolizumab.[15,16] The Mayo study reported that the frequency of postoperative complications in patients with IBD preoperatively treated with vedolizumab was higher than that of patients receiving anti-TNF-α agents or no biologic therapy.[15] On the other hand, our retrospective cohort study compared the surgical outcome within 4 weeks of an operation between vedolizumab-exposed patients with IBD and those exposed to either anti-TNF-α agents or nonbiological therapy.[16] The propensity score matched analysis demonstrated that the risks of postoperative complications were not different among patients preoperatively receiving vedolizumab, anti-TNF-α agents or nonbiological therapy (UC, $P = .40$; CD, $P = .35$).[16] Furthermore, when propensity score matching was performed among those who underwent major or minor surgery, the rates of postoperative complications were similar among those 3 treatment groups as well.[16] Two meta-analyses did not find an increased risk of postoperative complications with preoperative vedolizumab exposure, although they mentioned that further large prospective cohort studies are essential to define the impact of preoperative vedolizumab on surgical outcomes.[17,18]

Other new biologics and small molecules targeting inflammatory cytokines or their signaling pathways have been used as the treatment of IBD, and investigations regarding their effects on surgical outcomes are still ongoing. Ustekinumab, which is a human immunoglobulin G1 kappa monoclonal antibody against the p40 subunit of interleukin (IL) 12/IL-23, has been recently approved for the treatment of CD. Lightner et al investigated the risk of postoperative complications in patients with CD treated with ustekinumab within 12 weeks of surgery and showed no increased risk for postoperative surgical site infections compared to those treated with anti-TNF-α agents.[19] A recent retrospective study in which ustekinumab-treated CD patients were matched to vedolizumab-treated patients based on their demographic characteristics revealed no significant difference in the rate of postoperative complications among the matched pairs.[20] Tofacitinib is an oral, small-molecule Janus kinase inhibitor that was recently approved for the treatment of UC. Due to the lack of data on real-world experiences, the influence of tofacitinib on surgical outcomes in patients with UC still remains unclear.

The influence of perioperative immunosuppression on surgical outcomes has been extensively studied in IBD. There is a growing body of evidence that indicates corticosteroids can increase the risk of postoperative complications. Additionally, recent studies have shown that anti-TNF-α agents, thiopurines, vedolizumab, and ustekinumab may not promote the risk of complications after surgery. A large proportion of patients with IBD who undergo surgery are preoperatively increasingly exposed to medications with immunosuppressive properties. With the introduction of medications with various mechanism of action, further studies are required to identify the risk of postoperative complications with each medication.

References

1. Langholz E, Munkholm P, Davidsen M, Binder V. Course of ulcerative colitis: analysis of changes in disease activity over years. *Gastroenterology*. 1994;107(1):3-11.
2. European Society of Coloproctology collaborating group. Risk factors for unfavorable postoperative outcome in patients with Crohn's disease undergoing right hemicolectomy or ileocecal resection: an international audit by ESCP and S-ECCO. *Colorectal Dis*. 2017. https://doi.org/10.1111/codi.13889
3. Ferrante M, D'Hoore A, Vermeire S, et al. Corticosteroids but not infliximab increase short-term postoperative infectious complications in patients with ulcerative colitis. *Inflamm Bowel Dis*. 2009;15(7):1062-1070.
4. Subramanian V, Saxena S, Kang JY, Pollok RC. Preoperative steroid use and risk of postoperative complications in patients with inflammatory bowel disease undergoing abdominal surgery. *Am J Gastroenterol*. 2008;103(9):2373-2381.
5. Huang W, Tang Y, Nong L, Sun Y. Risk factors for postoperative intra-abdominal septic complications after surgery in Crohn's disease: a meta-analysis of observational studies. *J Crohns Colitis*. 2015;9(3):293-301.
6. Nielsen OH, Vainer B, Rask-Madsen J. Review article: the treatment of inflammatory bowel disease with 6-mercaptopurine or azathioprine. *Aliment Pharmacol Ther*. 2001;15(11):1699-1708.
7. Naganuma M, Kunisaki R, Yoshimura N, Takeuchi Y, Watanabe M. A prospective analysis of the incidence of and risk factors for opportunistic infections in patients with inflammatory bowel disease. *J Gastroenterol*. 2013;48(5):595-600.
8. Colombel JF, Loftus EV Jr, Tremaine WJ, et al. Early postoperative complications are not increased in patients with Crohn's disease treated perioperatively with infliximab or immunosuppressive therapy. *Am J Gastroenterol*. 2004;99(5):878-883.
9. Shah ED, Farida JP, Siegel CA, Chong K, Melmed GY. Risk for overall infection with anti-TNF and anti-integrin agents used in IBD: a systematic review and meta-analysis. *Inflamm Bowel Dis*. 2017;23(4):570-577.
10. Kasparek MS, Bruckmeier A, Beigel F, et al. Infliximab does not affect postoperative complication rates in Crohn's patients undergoing abdominal surgery. *Inflamm Bowel Dis*. 2012;18(7):1207-1213.
11. Billioud V, Ford AC, Tedesco ED, Colombel JF, Roblin X, Peyrin-Biroulet L. Preoperative use of anti-TNF therapy and postoperative complications in inflammatory bowel diseases: a meta-analysis. *J Crohns Colitis*. 2013;7(11):853-867.
12. Kopylov U, Ben-Horin S, Zmora O, Eliakim R, Katz LH. Anti-tumor necrosis factor and postoperative complications in Crohn's disease: systematic review and meta-analysis. *Inflamm Bowel Dis*. 2012;18(12):2404-2413.

13. Rosenfeld G, Qian H, Bressler B. The risks of post-operative complications following pre-operative infliximab therapy for Crohn's disease in patients undergoing abdominal surgery: a systematic review and meta-analysis. *J Crohns Colitis*. 2013;7(11):868-877.

14. Xu Y, Yang L, An P, Zhou B, Liu G. Meta-analysis: the influence of preoperative infliximab use on postoperative complications of Crohn's disease. *Inflamm Bowel Dis*. 2019;25(2):261-269.

15. Lightner AL, Raffals LE, Mathis KL, et al. Postoperative outcomes in vedolizumab-treated patients undergoing abdominal operations for inflammatory bowel disease. *J Crohns Colitis*. 2017;11(2):185-190.

16. Yamada A, Komaki Y, Patel N, et al. Risk of postoperative complications among inflammatory bowel disease patients treated preoperatively with vedolizumab. *Am J Gastroenterol*. 2017;112(9):1423-1429.

17. Law CCY, Narula A, Lightner AL, McKenna NP, Colombel JF, Narula N. Systematic review and meta-analysis: pre-operative vedolizumab treatment and postoperative complications in patients with inflammatory bowel disease. *J Crohns Colitis*. 2018;12(5):538-545.

18. Yung DE, Horesh N, Lightner AL, et al. Systematic review and meta-analysis: vedolizumab and postoperative complications in inflammatory bowel disease. *Inflamm Bowel Dis*. 2018;24(11):2327-2338.

19. Lightner AL, McKenna NP, Tse CS, et al. Postoperative outcomes in ustekinumab-treated patients undergoing abdominal operations for Crohn's disease. *J Crohns Colitis*. 2018;12(4):402-407.

20. Novello M, Stocchi L, Holubar S, et al. Surgical outcomes of patients treated with ustekinumab vs. vedolizumab in inflammatory bowel disease: a matched case analysis. *Int J Colorectal Dis*. 2019;34(3):451-457.

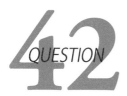

QUESTION 42

DOES THE TYPE OF SURGICAL ANASTOMOSIS (END-TO-END VERSUS SIDE-TO-SIDE) MAKE A DIFFERENCE IN LONG-TERM CROHN'S DISEASE OUTCOMES AND IN RECURRENCE?

Jana G. Hashash, MD, MSc; Andrew R. Watson, MD, MLitt; and David G. Binion, MD

Optimal short- and long-term management of patients with Crohn's disease (CD) requires coordination between medicine and surgery.[1,2] Surgeons play an essential role in the management of CD complications, which frequently include resection of strictures and/or fistulas in the small and large bowel with reanastomosis (ie, reconstruction of the bowel following resection). Surgeons are most focused on the immediate preoperative, intraoperative and short-term postoperative time period, with the goal of preventing surgical complications. Given that surgical complications are historically measured at the 30-day time point, longer-term outcomes following different procedures for CD have been less frequently explored. In contrast, gastroenterologists play a long-term role in the care of patients with CD. They are both the initial care givers, managing medical therapy for control of inflammation, and help manage patients in the early and late postoperative settings. This postoperative management frequently focuses on prevention of CD recurrence at the anastomotic site or in the neo-terminal ileum with the use of immunomodulator and/or biologic agents soon after reanastomosis, but will also address functional symptoms associated with long-term gastrointestinal injury/damage and the sequelae of resection.[2,3] It is readily appreciated that many patients with CD will experience diarrhea and abdominal pain after ileocecal resection, which may be due to a combination of factors, including loss of absorptive bowel length, bile acid malabsorption, and subsequent bile acid diarrhea, in addition to the recurrence of inflammation. There is new understanding that functional symptoms due to altered physiology related to the type of anastomotic reconstruction, specifically a side-to-side antiperistaltic anastomosis vs an end-to-end anastomosis, may also impact postoperative CD patient quality of life.[4] The operation, which is currently favored by surgeons with a stapled, side-to-side, antiperistaltic anastomosis, may in fact not yield the best long-term functional outcomes for patients with CD, leading to increased

Rubin DT, Friedman S, Farraye FA, eds. *Curbside Consultation in IBD: 49 Clinical Questions, Third Edition* (pp 273-283).
© 2022 Taylor & Francis Group.

abdominal pain and worse quality of life compared with an end-to-end anastomosis. Despite this need for coordinated care between gastroenterologists and surgeons, health care providers may function at cross purposes when balancing short- and long-term goals for the surgical and postoperative management of the patient with CD. In this chapter we review new understanding of the physiologic implications of choice of ileocecal anastomosis type on the long-term functional status and ultimately long-term quality of life in postoperative patients with CD.

Evolution of Surgery for Crohn's Disease: 1932 to the Present

Ileocecal resection is a hallmark feature of CD, dating back to the original 1932 description in *The Journal of the American Medical Association*, where 14 patients with terminal ileum strictures underwent resection and reanastomosis.[1] This historical perspective is still relevant today, as the majority of patients with CD, particularly those with ileocecal involvement, will require surgery during their lifetime. Surgery with resection of the diseased segment and reanastomosis is the most rapid approach to induce remission in patients with ileocecal CD. During much of the following 50 years, hand-sewn anastomoses, most commonly using an end-to-end or end-to-side configuration, were used to reconstruct the resected bowel. During this early period, there was no effective maintenance therapy for patients with CD, and the concept of postoperative prevention of recurrence with medical therapy had not yet been established. Therefore, postoperative management focused on relief of symptoms of diarrhea and alleviation of pain and cramping associated with bile acid malabsorption.

Over the past 6 decades, clinical advances in the care of patients with CD have included technical advances in surgery. Laparoscopic, minimally invasive approaches are now advocated as a superior strategy compared to the open laparotomy, with more rapid recovery, less postoperative pain, shorter postoperative ileus, as well as improved cosmetic results.[5,6] In addition to laparoscopy, advances in trauma surgery have led to the use of surgical stapling devices for the rapid creation of bowel anastomoses, which is technically less demanding compared with a hand-sewn anastomosis.

Commonly Used Ileocolonic Surgical Anastomoses

At least 50% patients with ileocolonic CD will undergo intestinal surgical resection at some point during their lifetime.[2,3] The most common surgery is an ileocecal resection. Surgeons have choices regarding reconstruction of the intestine following resection. Two of the most commonly utilized techniques are the side-to-side (Figures 42-1 and 42-2) and the end-to-end (Figure 42-3) ileocolonic anastomoses. Despite the differences in technique and anastomotic configuration, randomized, head-to-head comparative studies have not shown differences in the postoperative complication rates or recurrence rates between both anastomotic approaches assessed up to 1 year.[7-11] New long-term data, however, suggest that functional status will differ significantly between the different reconstructive approaches.[4] Restoring the bowel to a tube-like structure with an end-to-end (see Figure 42-3) anastomosis will improve postoperative quality of life and decrease the need for health care utilization in the 2 years following surgery compared with individuals who have undergone an antiperistaltic, side-to-side anastomosis (Table 42-1).[4]

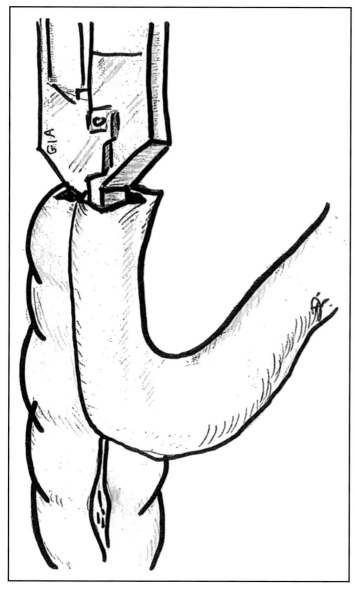

Figure 42-1. This image displays how the linear surgical stapler/cutting device is positioned along 2 intestinal lumens. After firing, the device will cut and staple simultaneously creating an anti-peristaltic side-to-side anastomosis. In this specific case, the staple is connecting a segment of normal small bowel (right) with normal colon (left).

SIDE-TO-SIDE ANASTOMOSIS

The side-to-side, antiperistaltic orientation compression anastomosis, with a linear surgical stapler/cutting device (Figure 42-4) was developed by Soviet trauma surgeons in the 1950s as a strategy to rapidly create a bowel anastomosis from 2 limbs of intestine.[12] The linear surgical stapler aligns 2 longitudinal intestinal segments in a side-to-side fashion (next to each other), most commonly in an antiperistaltic orientation (see Figure 42-1), deploying parallel rows of titanium staples, which are then separated with a cutting blade that slides between the staple lines to create a common channel. The anastomosis is then completed by firing a second staple line perpendicu-

Figure 42-2. A drawing showing the internal appearance (luminal side) of an antiperistaltic side-to-side anastomosis between colon (left) and small bowel (right). The parallel rows of titanium staples are transected by the cutting blade to create a common channel in the anastomotic reservoir. The anastomosis is completed by firing across perpendicularly.

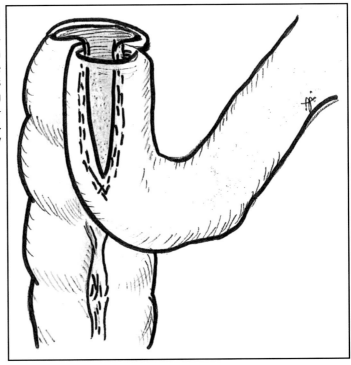

Figure 42-3. A drawing showing a hand sewn end-to-end anastomosis between colon and small bowel. The smaller lumen of the neoterminal ileum (left side) is transected at an angle to facilitate accommodating the size differential with the colonic lumen (right side).

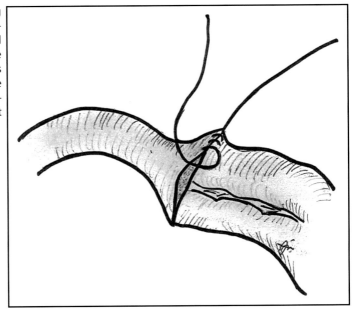

larly across the common channel to rapidly complete the bowel anastomosis. Closing the common channel can also employ 2 staple lines across the individual limbs of bowel. This device will rapidly divide bowel segments in a secure fashion and create an anastomosis between 2 segments of bowel. This approach has the advantage of speed, which is of paramount importance following traumatic injury. Also, the side-to-side anastomosis provides a ready solution for the reconstruction of 2 seg-

Table 42-1

Two-Year Outcomes of Crohn's Disease Patients Who Underwent Their First or Second Ileocecal Resection With an End-to-End Anastomosis Compared to a Side-to-Side Anastomosis

	ETEA (N = 68)	STSA (N = 60)	P Value (unadjusted)	Unadjusted Odds Ratio (95% CI)	Adjusted Odds Ratio (95% CI)
ED visit, N (%)	10 (14.7%)	20 (33.3%)	0.013	2.9 (1.2 to 6.8)	2.9 (1.2 to 6.9)
Hospitalization, N (%)	8 (11.8%)	18 (30%)	0.01	3.2 (1.3 to 8.1)	3.1 (1.2 to 7.8)
Abdominal CT scan, N (%)	9 (13.2%)	30 (50%)	< 0.001	6.6 (2.8 to 15.6)	6.5 (2.7 to 15.8)
Repeat resection surgery, N (%)	2 (2.9%)	4 (6.7%)	0.42	2.4 (0.4 to 13.4)	2.2 (0.4 to 12.6)
Endoscopic recurrence, N (%)	15/59 (25.4%)	22/56 (39.3%)	0.112	1.9 (0.9 to 4.2)	1.8 (0.8 to 4.2)
Mean SIBDQ ± SD	53.4 ± 10.04	47.9 ± 11.8	0.007	−5.2 (−9.1 to 1.4)	−5.1 (−8.7 to 1.5)
Median HBI (IQR)	3 (1.3, 5)	4 (1.5, 5)	0.15	0.9 (−0.3 to 2.2)	0.9 (−0.2 to 2.1)
Median CRP (mgI^{-1}, IQR)	0.33 (0.14, 0.69)	0.26 (0.1, 0.6)	0.53	0.08 (−0.2 to 0.4)	0.08 (−0.2 to 0.4)

CD = Crohn's disease; CI = confidence intervals; CRP = C-reactive protein; CT = computed tomography; ED = emergency department; ETEA = end-to-end anastomosis; HBI = Harvey-Bradshaw Index; IQR = interquartile range; SD = standard deviation; SIBDQ = Short Inflammatory Bowel Disease Questionnaire; STSA = side-to-side anastomosis.

Reproduced with permission from Gajendran M, Bauer AJ, Buchholz BM, et al. Ileocecal anastomosis type significantly influences long-term functional status, quality of life, and healthcare utilization in postoperative Crohn's disease patients independent of inflammation recurrence. *Am J Gastroenterol.* 2018;113(4):576-583.

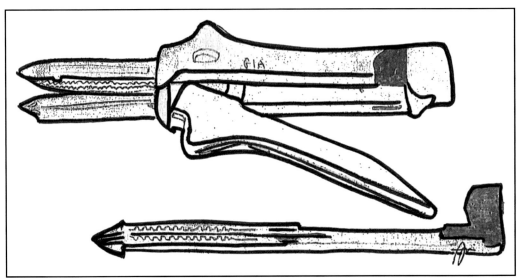

Figure 42-4. A drawing of a linear surgical stapling/cutting device which fires 2 rows of parallel titanium staples (used to connect the 2 bowel lumens) and a cutting blade in between the 2 rows of staples.

ments of bowel, which are of different caliber (ie, 1 larger tube and 1 smaller tube). The use of the titanium staples obviates the need for hand sewing multiple sutures and creates a simple and quick solution for joining 2 lumens of bowel of different caliber. For all of these reasons, the stapled side-to-side antiperistaltic anastomosis has emerged as the dominant type of reconstruction in CD, favored by surgeons due to the ease and speed of this technique.

Although the antiperistaltic side-to-side compression stapled anastomosis provides a rapid and elegant solution for creating a bowel anastomosis, the anatomic alterations can exert significant changes on intestinal postoperative physiology and function. The side-to-side, antiperistaltic anastomosis creates an aperistaltic reservoir, as the circular muscle layers, which propagate the muscular contractions of peristalsis, are transected in the common channel and the motility complex is abrogated by the antiperistaltic orientation of the bowel.

SIDE-TO-SIDE ANASTOMOSIS: POSTOPERATIVE ALTERATION IN BOWEL MOTILITY

The most commonly created ileocolonic anastomosis uses an antiperistaltic orientation of the 2 limbs of bowel in addition to transecting the circular muscle layers of the intestine in the common channel. Therefore, alterations in motility are an unavoidable side effect of this anastomotic approach.[4,13] This disruption in postoperative intestinal motility is not a deliberate objective of the side-to-side anastomosis, and there is a commonly held belief that the bowel adapts in the postoperative period to restore motor function.

In sharp distinction, purposefully disrupting motility with an antiperistaltic orientation of the bowel and transection of the circular muscle layers at the point of the common channel is a specific goal in the creation of a J pouch, ileoanal reconstruction following colectomy. The J pouch is not only an anatomic reservoir, but also deliberately disrupts migrating motor complexes and interdigestive motility during sleep to prevent nocturnal stooling, which will function more effectively as a "neo-colon." Physiologically, the antiperistaltic orientation of the bowel and the transection of the circular muscle layers are very successful in the J pouch, which will slow motility and ideally limit the number of bowel movements per day to 6 to 8 in patients who achieve optimal outcomes. However, the creation of an antiperistaltic fecal reservoir with this surgical approach is known to result in high concentrations of bacteria, which can trigger inflammation, commonly known as *pouchitis*. Patients with inflammatory bowel disease who suffer from pouchitis will typically require courses of antibiotics for treatment. J pouch ileoanal reconstruction is not routinely offered to patients with CD who have undergone colectomy, as they may experience more severe inflammation, with pouch complications including stenosis and fistula formation, resulting in pouch failure and a need for excision in up to 50% of individuals. What has not been fully explored is whether the inadvertent disruption of motility and the creation of a fecal reservoir at the ileocolonic antiperistaltic side-to-side anastomosis will create similar challenges with high bacterial concentrations, leading to increased long-term risk of inflammation at the anastomotic site. Additional unanswered challenges concern the effect of multiple, sequential antiperistaltic side-to-side anastomoses in patients with CD with multiple segments of small bowel and how this can further impact motility.

END-TO-END ANASTOMOSIS

The end-to-end anastomosis reconstructs the intestine as an intact tube (see Figure 42-3) and most frequently necessitates a hand-sewn procedure. This anastomosis is technically more difficult, as the ability to fit together 2 limbs of intestine with different calibers can be demanding, testing the skill of the surgeon. The technical challenge of the end-to-end anastomosis includes taking a longer intraoperative period, as the surgeon must fashion the 2 lumens of anastomotic segments to match a potential size differential. Either interrupted or noninterrupted sutures are used to create the connection. The potential advantage of the end-to-end anastomosis is the restoration of the bowel anatomy into an intact tube, which can restore intestinal physiology as this anastomosis facilitates downstream propagation of motility complexes more readily.[4,13] The end-to-end anastomosis avoids cutting across the circular muscle layers and avoids creation of an antiperistaltic reservoir, which is mandatory with the side-to-side anastomotic configuration. This physiologic advantage of the end-to-end anastomosis over the side-to-side anastomosis has been characterized in animal models of surgical research performed in dogs as well as rats. The restoration of motility in the end-to-end anastomosis will presumably help clear bacterial stasis, which may also help with long-term success in preventing CD recurrence at the anastomotic site.

Effect of Anastomosis Type on Quality of Life, Functional Status, and Health Care Utilization

In addition to concerns regarding fecal stasis at the side-to-side anastomosis leading to increased bacterial concentrations, there are additional consequences of this anatomic alteration, which may contribute to abdominal pain, as the sensory nerves in the intestine remain intact after the anastomotic construction. Distention at the side-to-side anastomosis could lead to cramping and colicky types of pain as solid material is pushed across this fecal reservoir. These functional changes in patient status were addressed in a recent study conducted by our group, which compared not only the short-term differences but also the long-term clinical status of patients who underwent a side-to-side antiperistaltic ileocolonic anastomosis with those who underwent an end-to-end ileocolonic anastomosis.[4] The data were obtained from a prospective observational natural history registry. Results showed that over a 2-year postoperative period, patients with an end-to-end anastomosis had significantly fewer emergency department visits, hospitalizations, and abdominal computed tomography scans compared to patients with a side-to-side anastomosis

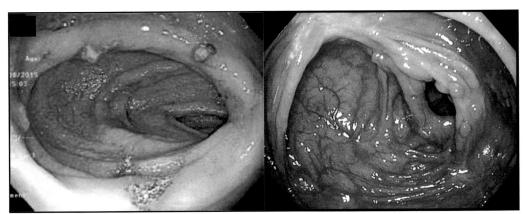

Figure 42-5. Examples of endoscopic appearance of a hand-sewn end-to-end anastomosis where in these specific photos, the colon is connected to the ileum in a continuous fashion to form a continuous tube.

(see Table 42-1).[4] This resulted in more than double the health care expenses in patients with the side-to-side anastomosis compared with an end-to-end anastomosis over the 2-year postoperative period. When evaluating inflammatory bowel disease–related quality of life in the 2-year postoperative period, patients with a side-to-side anastomosis had significantly worse quality of life compared to patients with an end-to-end anastomosis.[4] Additionally, there were no differences in the early postoperative complication rates between both groups.[4] Patients with a side-to-side anastomosis face many functional symptoms, presumably due to the antiperistaltic nature of the pouch created, which leads to stasis, fecalization, and subsequently symptoms of abdominal discomfort, pain, and distention.

ASSESSMENT OF POSTOPERATIVE DISEASE RECURRENCE: IMPACT OF ANASTOMOSIS TYPE

Concern that the type of surgical anastomosis could impact the rate of postoperative CD recurrence was the impetus for the prospective trial performed by McLeod and colleagues, where 170 patients undergoing ileocecal resection were randomized to have either a stapled side-to-side or an end-to-end anastomosis created.[14] The primary outcome variable was endoscopic recurrence at 1 year. This study demonstrated no difference in early surgical complications but a longer intraoperative time for the end-to-end anastomosis patients.

Rates of inflammation and disease recurrence were also assessed in the 2-year follow-up of ileocecectomy patients performed by our group.[4] Again, there was no difference in rates of inflammation (assessed by mean C-reactive protein levels), Rutgeerts endoscopic scores, and Harvey Bradshaw disease activity scores in patients with either side-to-side or end-to-end anastomosis at the 2-year point.[4] However, when these patients were followed beyond a 4-year postoperative period, the individuals with an end-to-end anastomosis demonstrated significantly better clinical status, as assessed by Rutgeerts scores.[15]

Endoscopic assessment of the anastomosis has emerged as a standard approach to guide medical treatment of early CD recurrence following surgery.[16] The end-to-end anastomosis is readily cannulated during routine colonoscopy (Figure 42-5), allowing for endoscopic assessment of the neo-terminal ileum, which is the highest risk anatomic segment for recurrence of CD inflammation.[17] The antiperistaltic side-to-side anastomosis poses technical challenges regarding endoscopic assessment (Figures 42-6 and 42-7).[17] There are limited data characterizing where in the side-to-side anastomosis recurrence will be most likely identified: in the neo-terminal ileum

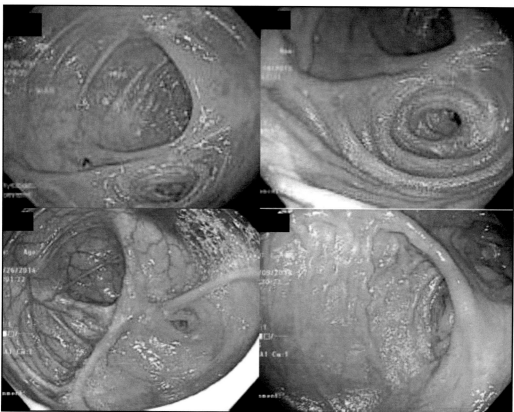

Figure 42-6. Examples of endoscopic appearance of side-to-side anastomoses. The view of the anastomotic reservoir demonstrates the stapled off limbs of colon on the top and the neoterminal ileum below. The inlet of the neoterminal ileum is not seen on these views, but is slightly upstream, opposite the visualized blind end.

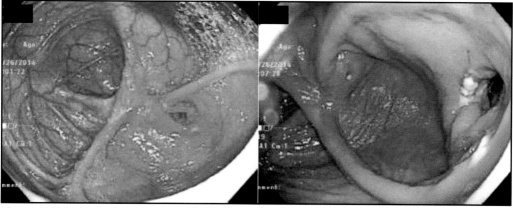

Figure 42-7. Endoscopic appearance of side-to-side anastomosis showing the stapled off limbs of colon on the top and the neoterminal ileum below (left image). The inlet of the neoterminal ileum (which appears ulcerated) is not seen on the image on the left, but seen on the image on the right, opposite to the visualized blind end.

along the staple line or at the proximal inlet. We assessed 82 postoperative patients with CD and found that endoscopic recurrence was most commonly seen at the anastomotic inlet (83% of recurrence) compared with 19% of the recurrence along the longitudinal staple line.[15] Therefore, it is essential that postoperative colonoscopic assessment of the side-to-side antiperistaltic anastomosis include a dedicated effort to assess the proximal inlet and not just the neo-terminal ileum along the staple line.

Conclusion

The majority of patients with CD with terminal ileum involvement will require surgery during their lifetime, and, until recently, there were no data informing which type of anastomotic reconstruction would offer the best chance for limiting long-term disease recurrence and improving long-term postoperative quality of life. Recent data from our center suggest that rebuilding the intestine as an intact "tube" with an end-to-end anastomosis will provide the best opportunity for an optimal functional outcome at 2 years, compared to an antiperistaltic side-to-side anastomosis, which creates a functional block to motility, leading to distention and pain at the anastomotic site in a subgroup of patients. Long-term follow-up data suggest that after 4 years the end-to-end anastomotic configuration exerts additional benefit with decreased endoscopic CD recurrence compared with the side-to-side anastomotic configuration. Finally, the ability of the gastroenterologist to perform endoscopic assessment of the anastomotic site is readily achieved with the end-to-end anastomosis. Side-to-side anastomosis will require a concerted effort to assess the neo-terminal ileum inlet, which is the site of the majority of recurrence. At the present time, the stapled side-to-side antiperistaltic anastomosis is the dominant procedure favored by surgeons for CD ileocecal reconstruction, but emerging data suggest that the more technically challenging end-to-end anastomosis may provide patients and gastroenterologists with a better chance for optimizing long-term health and quality of life.

References

1. Crohn BB, Ginzburg L, Oppenheimer GD. Regional ileitis: a pathologic and clinical entity. *JAMA*. 1932;99(16): 1323-1329.
2. Hashash JG, Regueiro M. A practical approach to preventing postoperative recurrence in Crohn's disease. *Curr Gastroenterol Rep*. 2016;18(5):25.
3. Hashash JG, Regueiro MD. The evolving management of postoperative Crohn's disease. *Expert Rev Gastroenterol Hepatol*. 2012;6(5):637-648. https://doi.org/10.1586/egh.12.45
4. Gajendran M, Bauer AJ, Buchholz BM, et al. Ileocecal anastomosis type significantly influences long-term functional status, quality of life, and healthcare utilization in postoperative Crohn's disease patients independent of inflammation recurrence. *Am J Gastroenterol*. 2018;113(4):576-583.
5. Beddy D, Dozois EJ, Pemberton JH. Perioperative complications in inflammatory bowel disease. *Inflamm Bowel Dis*. 2011;17(7):1610-1619.
6. Ananthakrishnan AN, McGinley EL, Saeian K, Binion DG. Laparoscopic resection for inflammatory bowel disease: outcomes from a nationwide sample. *J Gastrointest Surg*. 2010;14(1):58-65.
7. Strong S, Steele SR, Boutrous M, et al. Clinical practice guideline for the surgical management of Crohn's disease. *Dis Colon Rectum*. 2015;58(11):1021-1036.
8. Choy PY, Bissett IP, Docherty JG, Parry BR, Merrie A, Fitzgerald A. Stapled versus handsewn methods for ileocolic anastomoses. *Cochrane Database Syst Rev*. 2011;(9):CD004320.
9. He X, Chen Z, Huang J, et al. Stapled side-to-side anastomosis might be better than handsewn end-to-end anastomosis in ileocolic resection for Crohn's disease: a meta-analysis. *Digest Dis Sci*. 2014; 59(7):1544-1551.
10. Simillis C, Purkayastha S, Yamamoto T, Strong SA, Darzi AW, Tekkis PP. A meta-analysis comparing conventional end-to-end anastomosis vs. other anastomotic configurations after resection in Crohn's disease. *Dis Colon Rectum*. 2007;50(10):1674-1687.

11. Guo Z, Li Y, Zhu W, Gong J, Li N, Li J. Comparing outcomes between side-to-side anastomosis and other anastomotic configurations after intestinal resection for patients with Crohn's disease: a meta-analysis. *World J Surg.* 2013;37(4):893-901.

12. Steichen FM, Ravitch MM. History of mechanical devices and instruments for suturing. *Curr Probl Surg.* 1982;19(1): 1-52.

13. Arnold JH, Alevizatos CA, Cox SE, Richards WO. Propagation of small bowel migrating motor complex activity fronts varies with anastomosis type. *J Surgical Research.* 1991;51(6):506-511.

14. McLeod RS, Wolff BG, Ross S, Parkes R, McKenzie M. Investigators of the CT. Recurrence of Crohn's disease after ileocolic resection is not affected by anastomotic type: results of a multicenter, randomized, controlled trial. *Dis Colon Rectum.* 2009;52(5):919-927.

15. Ertem F, Watson AR, Ramos Rivers C, et al. Endoscopic patterns and location of post-operative recurrence in Crohn's disease patients with side to side anastomosis following ileocecal resection. *Gastroenterology.* 2019;156(6):S-850-S-851.

16. Hommes DW, van Deventer SJ. Endoscopy in inflammatory bowel diseases. *Gastroenterology.* 2004;126(6): 1561-1573.

17. Hashash JG, Binion DG. Endoscopic evaluation and management of the postoperative Crohn's disease patient. *Gastrointest Endosc Clin N Am.* 2016;26(4):679-692.

SECTION VII

HEALTH MAINTENANCE

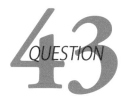

WHAT IS THE MOST SUCCESSFUL STRATEGY TO PROMOTE SMOKING CESSATION IN PATIENTS WITH CROHN'S DISEASE?

Michael Buie, BHSc and Gilaad G. Kaplan, MD, MPH

Tobacco use is the leading cause of preventable chronic disease and death in developed countries worldwide. A meta-analysis has shown a consistent association between smoking and the diagnosis of Crohn's disease (CD).[1] Furthermore, individuals who continue to smoke after diagnosis worsen their prognosis. Smoking is associated with relapsing flares and CD-related hospitalizations.[2] Smokers with CD are more likely to be prescribed immunosuppressants, corticosteroids, and biological agents.[2] Patients with CD who smoke are at greater susceptibility for requiring intestinal resections, particularly if they smoked throughout their adult life and were diagnosed after the age of 40 years.[3] Patients with CD who smoke postoperatively also have a greater likelihood of recurrence after ileocecal resection.[2]

The positive benefits of smoking cessation for those with CD are measurable. For example, one study demonstrated that the risk of a flare was comparable between patients who quit smoking and nonsmokers.[4] Also, the Tabacrohn study group showed that patients with CD who quit smoking have similar outcomes to nonsmokers, whereas patients who continue smoking have high rates of relapse.[5] A cost-utility analysis demonstrated that a smoking cessation program for persons with CD saved the US health care system $60 million over a 5-year period.[6] Thus, for both the sustainability of health care systems and the well-being of afflicted individuals, it is critical that clinicians educate patients on and promote the importance of smoking cessation.

So, what is the most successful strategy to promote smoking cessation in patients with CD? The foundation of smoking cessation is awareness, education, counseling, pharmacology, and behavioral interventions.

Rubin DT, Friedman S, Farraye FA, eds. *Curbside Consultation in IBD:*
49 Clinical Questions, Third Edition (pp 287-292).
© 2022 Taylor & Francis Group.

Education and Awareness

Effective smoking cessation strategies require appropriate education of patients and clinicians. Advising smoking abstinence to patients with CD is important because those who are aware of the risks smoking has on their disease course may find it easier to quit. The majority of patients with CD are not aware that smoking is particularly harmful for their disease prognosis, and patients with CD who actively smoke are the least aware.[7] Moreover, half of the patients with CD who smoke are in a precontemplative state such that they lack the intention and motivation to quit.[8]

Educating patients is crucial to promoting healthy behaviors. In a 2003 study, only 6.9% of patients were informed of the impact smoking has on CD by their gastroenterologist. After patients are informed, the intent of quitting smoking is greater, compared to those who are uninformed (78.6% vs 47.8%).[9] These findings further emphasize the importance of informing patients of the adverse effects smoking has on the disease course of their CD. Educating patients on the harmful effect of smoking on their CD is paramount, but providing effective strategies to quit smoking is challenging. In a 2018 study, 94% of gastroenterologists felt comfortable discussing the benefits of smoking cessation, yet only 56% of gastroenterologists felt comfortable discussing smoking cessation strategies with patients.[10] Educating patients on the harm of smoking without providing smoking cessation strategies is often not successful: The majority of smokers with CD will not quit smoking with educational materials alone.[7] The combination of education and counseling for smoking cessation strategies is necessary to realize further reductions in the prevalence of smoking.

Counseling

While there are multiple smoking cessation frameworks used worldwide, such as the ABCs or the five A's of smoking cessation, they commonly encompass similar components.[11] Unfortunately, smoking cessation frameworks are designed for application to the general population, and there is limited literature applying this framework to those with CD.

The National Comprehensive Cancer Network (NCCN) guidelines for smoking cessation recommend that clinicians first determine a patient's smoking status when beginning a smoking cessation program. Table 43-1 provides questions clinicians can ask to assess the risk of smoking relapse as well as nicotine dependency.[12] However, clinicians must be conscious that patients underestimate self-reported active smoking rates. Next, clinicians should determine a patient's nicotine dependency, which predicts the difficulty for smokers to achieve smoking abstinence. The Fagerström Nicotine Dependence Test is a common, standardized tool used to rate nicotine dependence from 1 to 10 (Table 43-2).[13] Smoking status assessment should be updated and recorded at regular intervals, noting changes in smoking status and attempts to quit; by doing so, clinicians will have a personalized smoking assessment for future follow-ups.[12]

Motivational interviewing (MI) is a counseling strategy to engage individuals in smoking cessation. MI aims to express empathy by highlighting inconsistencies between a patient's values (eg, living a healthy lifestyle) and the harms associated with smoking. Furthermore, clinician advice can be tailored to bridge the gap between inconsistent values and respecting the patient's autonomy regarding smoking cessation. Clinicians must expect resistance to advice and respond with empathy and positive reinforcement.

The US Preventative Services Task Force recommends use of the five R's as a framework for MI: *relevance*, *risks*, *rewards*, *roadblocks*, and *repetition*.[14] Effective MI is relevant to patients with CD as it identifies personalized risks and rewards; identifies a patient's potential roadblocks to quit; and has repetition by incorporating MI into follow-up visits. A patient's risk of relapse is

Table 43-1

National Comprehensive Cancer Network Assessment of a Patient's Smoking Status by Determining Risk of Relapse and Nicotine Dependence

1. Has the patient ever smoked before?
2. Is the patient currently a smoker?
3. Has the patient smoked in the past 30 days?
4. Does the patient smoke everyday, some days, or not at all?
5. If or what other types of tobacco products are used?
6. For former smokers, when was the last time a patient smoked? And for current smokers, what cessation aids have been used?

Adapted from Shields PG, Herbst RS, Arenberg D, et al. Smoking cessation, Version 1.2016, NCCN clinical practice guidelines in oncology. *J Nat Comp Cancer Net.* 2016;14(11):1430-1468.

highest among those with cravings, anxiety, stress, or depression, who are living or working with smokers, and/or who abuse alcohol or drugs.[12] These factors put patients at risk for recidivism, and clinicians should discuss the risk of relapse and provide guidance and support to promote continued smoking cessation attempts.

Pharmacological Therapies

Pharmacotherapies are effective medications that facilitate smoking cessation by addressing nicotine withdrawal symptoms. Immediate initiation of pharmacotherapy is recommended. One study found that cancer patients have similar quit rates whether they undertake abrupt or gradual smoking cessation; however, because smoking is so deleterious to disease progression in CD, abrupt smoking cessation is recommended where possible. The US Food and Drug Administration has approved several pharmacotherapy interventions: nicotine replacement therapy (NRT), varenicline, and bupropion. NRTs are available as long- (nicotine patch) and short-acting (lozenge, nicotine gum) over-the-counter pharmacotherapies. NRTs administer nicotine without smoking and aim to reduce withdrawal symptoms and the motivation to smoke. A Cochrane network meta-analysis published in 2013 supports combination NRT therapy over single forms of NRT alone.[15]

Varenicline is a prescription non-nicotinic partial agonist of the $\alpha_4\beta_2$ subtype of the nicotinic acetylcholine receptor that works by mimicking the effects of nicotine. It is the most effective single pharmacotherapy option for smoking cessation and typically prescribed for 12 weeks. The Cochrane network meta-analysis reports that varenicline increases the odds of smoking cessation almost 3-fold when compared to placebo.[15] The safety of varenicline has been extensively studied. A systematic review and meta-analysis of 39 randomized controlled smoking cessation trials identified no evidence to suggest that varenicline increases risk of suicide or suicide attempts, suicidal ideation, depression, or death.[16]

Bupropion, initially an antidepressant, is an effective pharmacotherapy for smoking cessation. Bupropion acts as a norepinephrine and dopamine reuptake inhibitor. Its safety has been studied, and recent systematic reviews report that it is rarely associated with serious neuropsychiatric

Table 43-2
Fagerström Test for Nicotine Dependence

Question	Points
1. How soon after you wake up do you smoke your first cigarette? • After 60 minutes • 31 to 60 minutes • 6 to 30 minutes • Within 5 minutes	0 1 2 3
2. Do you find it difficult to refrain from smoking in places where it is forbidden? • Yes • No	1 0
3. Which cigarette would you hate most to give up? • The first one in the morning • Any other	1 0
4. How many cigarettes per day do you smoke? • 10 or less • 11 to 20 • 21 to 30 • 31 or more	0 1 2 3
5. Do you smoke more frequently during the first hours after waking than during the rest of the day? • Yes • No	1 0
6. Do you smoke even if you are so ill that you are in bed most of the day? • Yes • No	1 0
Total points	

Scoring: 7 to 10 = high dependence; 4 to 6 points = moderately dependent; less than 4 points = minimally dependent.

Adapted with permission from Heatherton TF, Kozlowski LT, Frecker RC, Fagerström KO. The Fagerström Test for Nicotine Dependence: a revision of the Fagerström Tolerance Questionnaire. *Br J Addict*. 1991;86(9):1119-1127.

adverse events, including in those with existing mental illness.[15] Meta-analyses show that vareni-cline is more effective than bupropion, leading the NCCN panel to recommend combination NRT and varenicline as primary therapy options, and bupropion as a second-line therapy.[12]

Behavioral Therapies and Alternate Approaches

Behavioral therapies work by enhancing a patient's motivation to quit smoking and are effec-tive in combination with pharmacotherapies.[12] The foundation of behavioral therapies is counsel-ing with MI, providing social support, and supporting problem solving. For example, patients at risk for relapse often respond to behavioral therapy that targets habitual factors or social cues in their environment that promote relapse. Behavioral therapies build coping skills (eg, relaxation techniques) to address stressful scenarios that often serve as barriers to quitting.[11] Clinicians can integrate short (< 20 minutes in 1 clinical visit) and comprehensive (> 20 minutes in multiple follow-up visits) behavioral therapy sessions, though smoking cessation rates are optimized via comprehensive programs.[17] For example, patients should receive at least 4 in-person counseling sessions within 12 weeks.[12] Behavioral therapy interventions lasting more than 6 months have demonstrated additional benefits toward smoking cessation.[17]

Literature shows that combination pharmacotherapy and behavioral therapy are most effective—when acceptable and feasible for an individual patient.[11] Behavioral therapies can take place in person (one-on-one or in a group session), remotely by telephone, or via self-help web-based interventions. Self-help materials may be available in print form or through mobile applica-tions. Clinicians should consider a patient's preferences, as well as the availability of resources, before choosing an appropriate behavioral therapy delivery method. For example, a study on the preferences of smoking cessation information among Canadian cancer patients reported that most preferred support were print materials (45%), advice on a telephone (39%), dialogue directly with a clinician (29%), website-based information (15%), and support groups (11%).[18]

The most effective smoking cessation strategy combines pharmacotherapy and behavior therapy.[17] When compared to pharmacotherapy alone, the addition of behavioral interventions (eg, in-person counseling, telephone advice, and self-help materials) increases cessation rates.[14] As patients progress through pharmacotherapy, behavioral therapy should intensify and may be accompanied with referrals to psychologists.[12] Patients with anxiety or depression may need refer-ral to a psychiatrists. If patients are still unable to quit, they should be referred to smoking cessa-tion clinics if available or quit lines (eg, US National Quitline: 1-800-QUIT-NOW), which can provide behavioral therapy when in-person counseling is limited.[12]

Alternative smoking cessation treatments, more specifically electronic nicotine delivery sys-tems (ENDS), such as e-cigarettes, have recently become a popular phenomenon. ENDS are not approved by the US Food and Drug Association for smoking cessation, though e-cigarette usage for over 6 months has been associated with smoking cessation.[19] Although e-cigarettes could be an effective strategy, a recent study found that the need for previous surgical resection was higher in cigarette smokers (44.2%) and e-cigarette users (35.7%) vs nonsmokers (26.8%).[20] Thus, e-cigarettes may adversely affect the disease course of CD similar to smoking. The literature for ENDS, such as e-cigarettes, is sparse, particularly in patients with CD. Therefore, clinicians should not recommend the use of ENDS or other alternative cessation strategies until further evidence accumulates.

Conclusion

Cigarette smoking is associated with disease exacerbations in patients with CD. Given the adverse effect of smoking on CD, gastroenterologists should collaborate with primary care providers to integrate smoking cessation into their clinics. Successful smoking cessation starts with awareness and education of the harm associated with smoking on the prognosis of CD. Clinicians trained in MI can use counseling strategies to enhance the likelihood that their patients will quit smoking. Evidence-based pharmacotherapies in conjunction with behavioral therapies are often required to maximize smoking cessation success. Additionally, when appropriate, clinicians should refer patients to psychologists and psychiatrists to break the cycle of addiction. Implementing comprehensive multipronged smoking cessation strategies is the foundation for abstinence of smoking in persons with CD, which in turn can significantly improve disease course and outcomes.

References

1. Mahid SS, Minor KS, Soto RE, Hornung CA, Galandiuk S. Smoking and inflammatory bowel disease: a meta-analysis. *Mayo Clin Proc*. 2006;81(11):1462-1471.
2. Lakatos PL, Szamosi T, Lakatos L. Smoking in inflammatory bowel diseases: good, bad or ugly? *World J Gastroenterol*. 2007;13(46):6134-6139.
3. Frolkis AD, de Bruyn J, Jette N, et al. The association of smoking and surgery in inflammatory bowel disease is modified by age at diagnosis. *Clin Transl Gastroenterol*. 2016;7(4):e165-e165.
4. Cosnes J, Carbonnel F, Carrat F, Beaugerie L, Cattan S, Gendre J. Effects of current and former cigarette smoking on the clinical course of Crohn's disease. *Aliment Pharmacol Therap*. 1999;13(11):1403-1411.
5. Nunes T, Etchevers MJ, García-Sánchez V, et al. Impact of smoking cessation on the clinical course of Crohn's disease under current therapeutic algorithms: a multicenter prospective study. *Am J Gastroenterol*. 2016;111(3):411-419.
6. Coward S, Heitman SJ, Clement F, et al. Funding a smoking cessation program for Crohn's disease: an economic evaluation. *Am J Gastroenterol*. 2015;110(3):368-377.
7. Ducharme-Bénard S, Côté-Daigneault J, Lemoyne M, et al. Patients with inflammatory bowel disease are unaware of the impact of smoking on their disease. *J Clin Gastroenterol*. 2016;50(6):490-497.
8. Leung Y, Kaplan GG, Rioux KP, et al. Assessment of variables associated with smoking cessation in Crohn's disease. *Dig Dis Sci*. 2012;57(4):1026-1032.
9. Ryan WR, Ley C, Allan RN, Keighley MRB. Patients with Crohn's disease are unaware of the risks that smoking has on their disease. *J Gastrointest Surg*. 2003;7(5):706-711.
10. Nulsen B, Sands BE, Shah BJ, Ungaro RC. Practices, attitudes, and knowledge about Crohn's disease and smoking cessation among gastroenterologists. *Eur J Gastroenterol Hepatol*. 2018;30(2):155-160.
11. Siu AL, U.S. Preventive Services Task Force. Behavioral and pharmacotherapy interventions for tobacco smoking cessation in adults, including pregnant women: U.S. Preventive Services Task Force recommendation statement. *Ann Intern Med*. 2015;163(8):622-634.
12. Shields PG, Herbst RS, Arenberg D, et al. Smoking cessation, Version 1.2016, NCCN clinical practice guidelines in oncology. *J Nat Comp Cancer Net*. 2016;14(11):1430-1468.
13. Heatherton TF, Kozlowski LT, Frecker RC, Fagerström KO. The Fagerström test for nicotine dependence: a revision of the Fagerström Tolerance Questionnaire. *British J Addiction*. 1991;86(9):1119-1127.
14. Patnode CD, Henderson JT, Thompson JH, Senger CA, Fortmann SP, Whitlock EP. Behavioral counseling and pharmacotherapy interventions for tobacco cessation in adults, including pregnant women. *Evidence Syntheses, No. 134*. Agency for Healthcare Research and Quality (US); 2015.
15. Cahill K, Stevens S, Perera R, Lancaster T. Pharmacological interventions for smoking cessation: an overview and network meta-analysis. *Cochrane Database System Rev*. 2013;(5):CD009329.
16. Thomas KH, Martin RM, Knipe DW, Higgins JPT, Gunnell D. Risk of neuropsychiatric adverse events associated with varenicline: systematic review and meta-analysis. *BMJ*. 2015;350:h1109.
17. Stead LF, Koilpillai P, Lancaster T. Additional behavioral support as an adjunct to pharmacotherapy for smoking cessation. *Cochrane Database System Rev*. 2015;(10):CD009670.
18. Sampson L, Papadakos J, Milne V, et al. Preferences for the provision of smoking cessation education among cancer patients. *J Cancer Ed*. 2018;33(1):7-11.
19. Rahman MA, Hann N, Wilson A, Mnatzaganian G, Worrall-Carter L. E-cigarettes and smoking cessation: evidence from a systematic review and meta-analysis. *PLOS ONE*. 2015;10(3):e0122544.
20. K. Loonat, R. Sagar CS. P716 Current smoking trends in British IBD patients in the age of e-cigarettes. *BMJ Open Gastroenterol*. 2019;21;6(1):e000309.

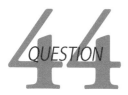

QUESTION

WHICH VACCINES SHOULD PATIENTS WITH IBD RECEIVE?

Freddy Caldera, DO, MS, and Francis A. Farraye, MD, MSc

Treatment of inflammatory bowel disease (IBD) has evolved with anti–tumor necrosis factor (TNF) inhibitors, interleukin (IL) 12/IL-23 antibodies, anti-integrin antibodies, and novel small molecules that have enhanced the overall quality of life for many patients with IBD. These agents have increased the rates of clinical remission and mucosal healing and reduced the need for surgery, but in some cases they are also associated with an increased risk for serious and opportunistic infections.[1] Many of these infections may be preventable with routine vaccination.[2] Serious infections can develop in patients with IBD, and those on combination therapy (anti-TNF therapy and an immunomodulator) have the highest annual incidence of infection, affecting 1 in 45 patients.[3] Patients with IBD historically have lower rates of vaccination than the general population due to lack of knowledge, concerns about vaccine safety, and lack of clarity as to which provider (primary care provider or gastroenterologist) is responsible for recommending and providing age-appropriate vaccines. Clinical practice guidelines for vaccination of the immunosuppressed host recommend that specialists share responsibility for ensuring their patients receive appropriate vaccines.[4] Therefore, gastroenterologists should be aware of necessary vaccines for their patients with IBD and play an active role in ensuring that their patients receive immunizations either by providing the vaccinations in the office or by outlining clear recommendations for the patient and primary care provider.

Rubin DT, Friedman S, Farraye FA, eds. *Curbside Consultation in IBD: 49 Clinical Questions, Third Edition* (pp 293-298).
© 2022 Taylor & Francis Group.

Inactive Vaccines

The optimal time to obtain immunization history to provide appropriate vaccines is at first diagnosis of IBD or during transfer of care. All patients with IBD, regardless of whether they are immunosuppressed, should follow the immunization schedule for inactive vaccines outlined by the Advisory Committee on Immunization Practice (ACIP; Table 44-1).[5] Whenever possible, vaccines should be given prior to starting immunosuppressive therapy. Patients with IBD on aminosalicylates or thiopurines can mount a normal vaccine response, but the response may be blunted in those on anti-TNF agents, especially those on combination therapy with thiopurines.[2,6] Whether newer immunosuppressive agents added to the IBD treatment armamentarium (vedolizumab, ustekinumab, or tofacitinib) will also induce a lower vaccine response is unknown. Vedolizumab targets $\alpha_4\beta_7$ integrin and selectively inhibits the migration of memory T cells into the gastrointestinal mucosa.[7,8] This gut selectivity may not affect vaccine response in patients with IBD to parenteral vaccines such as hepatitis B. There is a paucity of studies evaluating if the vaccine response can be improved by providing booster or higher doses of certain vaccines. Immunosuppressed patients with IBD might benefit from a different immunization schedule based on their immunosuppressive regimen. Thus, studies evaluating if the immune response can be improved are needed.

Live Vaccines

In general, the administration of live vaccines is contraindicated in immunosuppressed patients due to concern it poses a risk of infection by the vaccine strain. Disseminated varicella infections have been reported in immunosuppressed patients receiving a live varicella zoster virus vaccine.[9] The current live vaccines available for adults with IBD can be divided into 3 groups: (1) travel vaccines intended for those undergoing international travel; (2) adult vaccine (attenuated herpes zoster [HZ] and intranasal influenza); and (3) pediatric vaccines normally administered to children prior to entering school. Several live vaccines are used for international travel, including anthrax, oral polio, smallpox, Bacillus Calmette-Guérin, oral typhoid, and yellow fever vaccines, and are therefore contraindicated in the immunosuppressed patient. Consultation with an infectious disease/travel medicine expert should be considered for patients to determine the advisability of travel or to provide alternate methods of prevention.

The live attenuated HZ vaccines and intranasal influenza vaccines are 2 vaccines available for adults. The live influenza vaccine is intended for nonpregnant individuals age 2 to 49 years of age and contraindicated in anyone on immunosuppressive agents. Live attenuated and recombinant vaccines to prevent HZ are currently available. The live attenuated HZ vaccine (ZVL) is relatively contraindicated in patients on anti-TNF therapy but could be given to patients with IBD on standard doses of methotrexate (< 0.4 mg/kg per week), azathioprine (< 3.0 mg/kg per week), or 6-mercaptopurine (< 1.5 mg/kg per day). The recombinant HZ vaccine (RZV) is provided as an intramuscular injection as 2 doses over 6 months and is indicated for all immunocompetent adults 50 years and older. The RZV should be the preferred vaccine for patients with IBD since it is more efficacious in preventing HZ, safe to provide to immunosuppressed patients, and is preferred over ZVL. The ZVL vaccine is no longer available in the United States as of July 2020. Ensuring patients with IBD are vaccinated is of utmost importance since they are at increased risk for HZ compared to the general population and since immunosuppression is an independent risk factor.[10]

Table 44-1

Vaccines for Adult Patients With IBD

Vaccine	IBD Patients on Non-Immunosuppressing Regimens	IBD Patients on Immunosuppressing Regimens	Comments
Seasonal inactivated influenza	Annually	Annually	Do not use live attenuated influenza vaccine in immunocompromised patients
Measles-mumps-rubella (MMR)	If indicated, 2 doses 4 to 8 weeks apart	Contraindicated	
Varicella	If indicated, 2 doses 4 to 8 weeks apart	Contraindicated	
Herpes zoster (recombinant inactive, RZV)	Two-dose series separated by 2 to 6 months for age ≥ 50	Two-dose series separated by 2 to 6 months for age ≥ 50	Preferred vaccine by ACIP and safe to administer to those immunosuppressed
Hepatitis A	If indicated, 2 doses at least 6 months apart	If indicated, 2 doses at least 6 months apart	
Hepatitis B	If indicated, 3 doses on 0-, 1-, 6-month schedule	If indicated, 3 doses on 0-, 1-, 6-month schedule	Consider checking HBsAb 4 to 8 weeks after completing series
Hepatitis B recombinant vaccine[11]	If indicated, 2 doses at 0 and 1 month	If indicated, 2 doses 0 and 1 month	Consider checking HBsAb 4 to 8 weeks after completing series
Human papillomavirus (HPV)	Three doses, 0-, 1- to 2-, and 6-month schedule for age ≤ 26 years	Three doses, 0-, 1- to 2-, and 6-month schedule	Recent FDA approval to age 45, awaiting ACIP recommendations

(continued)

Table 44-1 (continued)

Vaccines for Adult Patients With IBD

Vaccine	IBD Patients on Non-Immunosuppressing Regimens	IBD Patients on Immunosuppressing Regimens	Comments
Meningococcal vaccines (ACYW) or serogroup B	If indicated, use recommended regimen for adult immunization	If indicated, use recommended regimen for adult immunization	
Pneumococcal conjugate vaccine (PCV13)	If < 65 years old, not recommended If age ≥ 65 years, use as part of PCV13-PPSV23 regimen	Single dose followed by PPSV23 in 1 year	Consider administering to those anticipating immunosuppressing therapy
Pneumococcal polysaccharide vaccine (PPSV23)	If age ≥ 65 years, use as part of PCV13-PPSV23 regimen	Dose 1 year after PCV13; Repeat if 5 years and single dose for age ≥ 65 years	Consider administering to those anticipating immunosuppressing therapy
Tetanus-diphtheria-acellular pertussis (Td/Tdap)	If no prior vaccination, 3 doses on 0-, 1-, 6- to 12-month schedule with 1 dose of Tdap included If previously immunized, single dose of Tdap, then Td every 10 years	If no prior vaccination, 3 doses on 0-, 1-, 6- to 12-month schedule with 1 dose of Tdap included If previously immunized, single dose of Tdap, then Td every 10 years	

ACIP = Advisory Committee on Immunization Practices; anti-HB = antibody to hepatitis B surface antigen; IBD = inflammatory bowel disease.

Table 44-2

Acceptable Presumptive Evidence of Immunity to Varicella, Measles, and Rubella

Evidence of immunity to measles and rubella includes any of the following:	Evidence of immunity to varicella includes any of the following:
1. Documentation of 2 doses of measles vaccination	1. Documentation of age-appropriate vaccination with 2-dose varicella vaccine series
2. Documentation of 1 dose of a live rubella vaccination	2. Laboratory evidence of immunity*
3. Laboratory confirmation of disease	3. Birth in the United States before 1980**
4. Birth before 1957	4. Diagnosis or verification of a history of varicella disease by a health care provider
	5. Diagnosis or verification of a history of herpes zoster by a health care provider

*Commercial assays can be used to assess disease-induced immunity, but they lack sensitivity to always detect vaccine induced immunity (ie, they might yield false-negative results).

**Should not be used for individuals who are immunosuppressed, pregnant, or health care workers.

Assessing Immunity to Live Pediatric Vaccines

The live pediatric vaccines are varicella and measles, mumps, and rubella (MMR), which are both administered as a 2-dose series. The majority of patients will have received the vaccines prior to their diagnosis since the second dose of these vaccines is typically administered at ages 4 to 6 years.[12,13] Preventive care guidelines recommend assessing immunity to these viruses due to recent measles outbreaks and the potential risk of life-threatening complications from disseminated varicella in immunosuppressed patients with IBD. The ACIP states that appropriate immunization history is acceptable evidence for immunity for MMR and varicella. They recommend against serologic screening in persons with presumptive immunity by these criteria (Table 44-2) due to a potential false negative serologic test.[13] Patients with IBD who have received the MMR vaccines series have similar antibody concentrations to MMR compared the healthy controls.[14] Therefore, gastroenterologists should follow the ACIP recommendations and rely on immunization history to determine immunity to MMR and varicella in immunosuppressed patients with IBD.

Conclusion

In conclusion, providing vaccines and obtaining an immunization history is essential health care maintenance for patients with IBD. Gastroenterologists should be familiar with which vaccines are required and how to determine immunity to pediatric live vaccines. In addition, they should share responsibility with primary care providers in ensuring their patients are up-to-date and receive appropriate vaccines.

References

1. Lichtenstein GR, Loftus EV, Isaacs KL, Regueiro MD, Gerson LE, Sands BE. ACG clinical guideline: management of Crohn's disease in adults. *Am J Gastroenterol*. 2018;113(4):481-517.
2. Farraye FA, Melmed GY, Lichtenstein GR, Kane SV. ACG clinical guideline: preventive care in inflammatory bowel disease. *Am J Gastroenterol*. 2017;112(2):241-258.
3. Kirchgesner J, Lemaitre M, Carrat F, Zueriek M, Carbonnel F, Dray-Spira R. Risk of serious and opportunistic infections associated with treatment of inflammatory bowel diseases. *Gastroenterology*. 2018;155(2):337-346.e310.
4. Rubin LG, Levin MJ, Ljungman P, et al. 2013 IDSA clinical practice guideline for vaccination of the immunocompromised host. *Clin Infect Dis*. 2014;58(3):e44-e100.
5. Kim DK, Riley LE, Hunter P, et al. Recommended immunization schedule for adults aged 19 years or older, United States, 2018. *Ann Intern Med*. 2018;168:210-220.
6. Dotan I, Werner L, Vigodman S, et al. Normal response to vaccines in inflammatory bowel disease patients treated with thiopurines. *Inflamm Bowel Dis*. 2012;18(2):261-268.
7. Feagan BG, Rutgeerts P, Sands BE, et al. Vedolizumab as induction and maintenance therapy for ulcerative colitis. *New Eng J Med*. 2013;369:699-710.
8. Wyant T, Fedyk E, Abhyankar B. An overview of the mechanism of action of the monoclonal antibody vedolizumab. *J Crohns Colitis*. 2016;10(12):1437-1444.
9. Alexander KE, Tong PL, Macartney K, Beresford R, Sheppeard V, Gupta M. Live zoster vaccination in an immunocompromised patient leading to death secondary to disseminated varicella zoster virus infection. *Vaccine*. 2018;36(27):3890-3893.
10. Khan N, Patel D, Trivedi C, et al. Overall and comparative risk of herpes zoster with pharmacotherapy for inflammatory bowel diseases: a nationwide cohort study. *Clin Gastroenterol Hepatol*. 2018;16(12):1919-1927.e1913
11. Schilliem S, Harris A, Link-Gelles R. Recommendations of the Advisory Committee on Immunization Practices for use of a hepatitis B vaccine with a novel adjuvant. *Morb Mortal Wkly Rep*. 2018;67(15):455-458.
12. Marin M GD, Chaves SS, Schmid S, Seward JF, Advisory Committee on Immunization Practices, Centers for Disease Control and Prevention (CDC). Prevention of varicella: recommendations of the Advisory Committee on Immunization Practices (ACIP). *MMWR Recomm Rep*. 2007;56(RR-4):1-40.
13. McLean HQ, Fiebelkorn AP, Temte JL, Wallace GS, Centers for Disease Control and Prevention. Prevention of measles, rubella, congenital rubella syndrome, and mumps, 2013: summary recommendations of the Advisory Committee on Immunization Practices (ACIP). *Morb Mortal Wkly Rep*. 2013;62(RR-04):1-33.
14. Caldera F, Misch EA, Saha S, et al. Immunosuppression does not affect antibody concentrations to measles, mumps, and rubella in patients with inflammatory bowel disease. *Dig Dis Sci*. 2018;64(1):189-195.

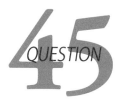

How Can Gastroenterologists Address IBD-Related Health Maintenance in Clinical Practice?

Erica R. Cohen, MD and Gil Y. Melmed, MD, MS

Patients with inflammatory bowel disease (IBD) receive fewer preventive services than general medical patients[1] despite a higher risk of complications from preventable diseases. Gastroenterologists are uniquely positioned to address health maintenance and should work closely with primary care providers (PCPs) to ensure appropriate services are rendered. Although many health maintenance measures typically fall within the purview of PCPs, gastroenterologists prescribing biologic medications should be aware of related health maintenance issues and be able to effectively communicate recommendations to patients and PCPs.[2] Since the added time to address these issues can be cumbersome, providers need effective, practical, and efficient strategies to incorporate these discussions into their clinical workflow.

Depression

Depression and anxiety are common disorders affecting individuals with IBD. The risk of major depressive disorder is nearly 2 times greater than the general population.[3] Depression is associated with decreased medication compliance and worse disease-specific outcomes in patients with IBD.[4] Patients treated for depression use fewer health care services compared to those who went untreated.[5] This makes screening for depression a critical component of the holistic approach to patient care in IBD. Several valid instruments exist for screening, including the Patient Health Questionnaire (PHQ) 2, and 9, the Beck Depression Inventory, among others.

The PHQ-2 is a brief, 2-item question set easily incorporated into the clinical workflow (Table 45-1). Administration may occur at either check-in or during the patient visit itself. The

Rubin DT, Friedman S, Farraye FA, eds. *Curbside Consultation in IBD:*
49 Clinical Questions, Third Edition (pp 299-305).
© 2022 Taylor & Francis Group.

Table 45-1
Patient Health Questionnaire-2 Depression Screen

Over the Last 2 Weeks, How Often Have You Been Bothered by the Following Problems?	Not at All (0 points)	Several Days (1 point)	More Than Half the Days (2 points)	Nearly Every Day (3 points)
Little interest or pleasure in doing things				
Feeling down, depressed, or hopeless				

PHQ-2 score ranges from 0 to 6, where a score of 3 represents a cut-off point for positive depression screen (83% and 90% sensitivity and specificity, respectively).[6] The questionnaire can be administered by nonlicensed clinic staff. The ability to do so, without the need for a social worker or mental health provider, makes for operationally efficient incorporation into the clinic. Nevertheless, a positive depression screen should prompt further discussion during the visit with subsequent referral to a trained mental health provider. Future clinical visits should assess the patient's mental health progress and incorporate that diagnosis into the overall IBD treatment plan.

Tobacco Cessation

All patients with IBD should undergo smoking cessation counseling, particularly those with Crohn's disease (CD). Tobacco use in CD is associated with more severe presentation, more frequent flares, higher rates of surgery, and increased utilization of immunosuppressive therapy compared to nonsmokers.[7,8] Encouragingly, when smokers with CD quit using tobacco, the risk of flares, need for steroids, and the need for immunosuppressive therapy returns to a similar risk level as their nonsmoking counterparts.[9]

The negative effects of smoking do appear dose dependent, so while gastroenterologists should counsel patients to completely abstain from tobacco, even a partial decrease in daily use is beneficial. In a controlled trial, the primary predictors of successful smoking cessation were the physician, previous intestinal surgery, high socioeconomic status, and females taking oral contraceptives.[10] All participants in this study were offered a smoking cessation program. This highlights the need for physicians to provide smoking cessation materials and offer coordination and assistance to help facilitate utilization of these services.

Skin Cancer Screening

Patients with IBD treated with immunosuppressive therapy are at an increased risk of developing nonmelanoma skin cancers (NMSC). The increased risk is associated with persistent use of thiopurines and, to a lesser extent, anti–tumor necrosis factor (TNF) agents, which may be associated with a slightly increased risk of melanoma. Combination thiopurine plus anti-TNF therapy conferred a cumulative risk of NMSC.[11] Although the risk of NMSC is thought to be lower with vedolizumab and ustekinumab, current clinical guidelines do not differentiate NMSC screening recommendations by the type of agent.

While there are no randomized controlled trials defining the optimal preventive approach, current recommendations maintain that patients on immunosuppressive therapy should have annual skin examinations and wear full-spectrum sunscreen with protective clothing.[12] A 12-study meta-analysis cited in the American College of Gastroenterology guidelines found that IBD alone was associated with a 37% increased risk of melanoma (RR 0.37; 95% CI, 1.10 to 1.70) compared to the general population.[13] The risk of melanoma was higher in studies performed prior to the biologic era (8 studies before 1998). It is thus recommended that patients with IBD should undergo screening for melanoma independent of immunosuppressive therapy use. Referral for and the facilitation of skin cancer screening, like behavioral health screening, can be built into the clinic staff's task list to optimize efficiency while providing well-rounded care.

Cervical Cancer Screening

Persistent infection with certain strains of human papillomavirus (HPV) is associated with the development of cervical cancer. It is unknown if simply having IBD can increase one's risk for cervical malignancy, but many concomitant risk factors exist such as immunosuppressive therapy.[14] There is an approximately 6-time higher incidence of abnormal pap smears in women with IBD vs age-, race-, and parity-matched controls, particularly after immunosuppressant exposure.[15] Furthermore, women with IBD with abnormal tests were more likely to harbor high-risk HPV serotypes 16 and 18. This suggests an important benefit to HPV screening and vaccination before initiating immunosuppressive therapy. The American College of Obstetricians and Gynecologists recommends annual screening after starting immunosuppressive agents.[16] The HPV vaccine should be offered to all women (and men) between the ages of 9 to 26 but does not replace annual cervical dysplasia screening. In the event a woman on immunosuppressive therapy is diagnosed with HPV in the presence of cervical dysplasia, discontinuing immunosuppression should be discussed on a case-by-case basis in conjunction with the treating gynecologist.

Osteoporosis Screening

Patients with IBD are at higher risk of impaired bone mineral density and skeletal fractures.[17] The pathophysiology of IBD-related osteoporosis is not completely understood; however, certain risk factors have been identified and are listed in Table 45-2.[18] There is insufficient evidence to suggest that chronic intestinal inflammation in and of itself represents an independent predictor of bone mineral loss in IBD. Screening for impaired bone density is recommended in the non-IBD general population for patients over age 60, have low body mass index, are postmenopausal, use tobacco, or have prolonged steroid use for at least 3 months. Those with ulcerative colitis and any of the risk factors for abnormal bone mineral density should undergo osteoporosis screening, even if they have already had ileal pouch surgery with anal anastomosis.[18]

Current guidelines recommend that patients with IBD with any of the risk factors should undergo a dual-energy X-ray absorptiometry (DEXA) scan at the time of diagnosis.[12] If the bone density is normal, preventative strategies should be employed, including calcium and vitamin D supplementation, weight-bearing exercise, limited corticosteroid use, and smoking cessation.[19] For those diagnosed with osteopenia, similar recommendations should be discussed and a repeat DEXA is recommended in 24 months. If a patient with IBD has osteoporosis or sustains an aty-

Table 45-2

Cancer Screening and Osteoporosis

	Risk Factors	Initial Visit Counseling	Follow-Up		
Melanoma	IBD Family history Intense sun exposure	Annual skin surveillance Broad spectrum sunscreen Protective clothing	Consider adjusting medication regimen if malignancy found (avoid exposure to anti-TNF if melanoma; avoid exposure to thiopurine if NMSC)		
Non-Melanoma Skin Cancer	Immunomodulator or biologic Family history Intense sun exposure				
Cervical Cancer	Immunomodulator or biologic HPV	Annual gynecologic examination HPV vaccination			
Bone Mineral Density	Smoking Chronic inflammation Malnutrition Vitamin D deficiency Recurrent steroid use Postmenopausal women Men 50 years of age or older History of low trauma fractures	Vitamin D (OH) 25 levels Baseline DEXA scan Calcium supplementation Preventive weight bearing exercise	**Low 25, (OH)D** Give supplementation Reassess levels periodically	**Osteopenia** Counsel DEXA 2 years	**Osteoporosis** Consider referral DEXA 2 years

pical fracture, screening for secondary causes (hypogonadism, vitamin D deficiency, celiac) should be considered. Bisphosphonates and other pharmacologic treatment options should be considered, with appropriate DEXA scan follow-up.

Vaccinations

Patients with IBD are at increased risk for vaccine-preventable infections. (Please see Question 44 for a full discussion on the background and rationale for vaccination recommendations.) Practices may incorporate checklists,[20] patient handouts, and utilization of nonphysician office staff to improve vaccine recommendation awareness and education. Studies have demonstrated improvement in influenza vaccination rates in IBD clinics using simple patient education materials or short surveys prior to seeing their provider and offering vaccination by nurses.[21,22]

Conclusion

Addressing general health maintenance in patients with IBD improves overall well-being and prevents untoward consequences of both the disease itself and the medications used to treat it. Despite increased recognition of the importance of health maintenance, the additional tasks associated with addressing health maintenance issues may be neglected in a busy clinical practice. However, including health maintenance into the practice of IBD need not overly burden the clinician.

Some practical options to effectively implement health maintenance into practice include (1) administering web-based or electronic surveys prior to the clinical visit either at home or in the waiting room to screen for depression, smoking status, and vaccine history; (2) creating a template in the electronic medical record that includes hard-stop placeholders to address depression screening, smoking status, bone health, and vaccinations; and (3) health maintenance screening by the ancillary clinic staff upon initial patient intake. Incorporating a short checklist into the medical record template note can facilitate quick review of the recommended health maintenance prior to completing the patient visit (Table 45-3).[20] Embedding IBD-specific health maintenance into the clinical visit—prior to, during, and after the time spent seeing the clinician—optimizes the likelihood of effective, proactive care.

Table 45-3
Potential Clinical Checklist

Cancer Prevention	Date Completed	Next Due
Cervical Cancer (annual Pap smear when immunocompromised)		
Skin Cancer (annual skin surveillance, sunscreen, protective clothing)		
Colon Cancer (see Question 37) (every 1 to 2 years after 8 to 10 years of disease; if ulcerative colitis beyond the rectum or Crohn's in at least one-third of colon)		
Bone Mineral Density	*Date Completed*	*Next Due*
Vitamin D 25 (OH) Level (periodic testing)		
Bone Density Assessment With DEXA (see Risk Factors in Table 45-2)		
Calcium, Vitamin D, and Weight-Bearing Exercises (recommend with each course of steroids or if impaired, low vitamin D levels or abnormal DEXA)		
Other	*Date Completed*	*Next Due*
Tobacco Cessation Counseling (at every clinic visit)		
Depression Screening (at every clinic visit)		

References

1. Selby L, Kane S, Wilson J, et al. Receipt of preventive health services by IBD patients is significantly lower than by primary care patients. *Inflamm Bowel Dis*. 2008;14(2):253-238.
2. Melmed GY. Immunizations and IBD: whose responsibility is it? If I'm the prescribing doctor, shouldn't it be mine? *Inflamm Bowel Dis*. 2012;18(1):41-42.
3. Walker JR, Ediger JP, Graff LA, et al. The Manitoba IBD cohort study: a population-based study of the prevalence of lifetime and 12-month anxiety and mood disorders. *Am J Gastroenterol*. 2008;103(8):1989-1097.
4. Nigro G, Angelini G, Grosso SB, Sategna-Guidetti C. Psychiatric predictors of noncompliance in inflammatory bowel disease: psychiatry and compliance. *J Clin Gastroenterol*. 2001;32(1):66-68.
5. Deter HC, Keller W, von Wietersheim J, et al. Psychological treatment may reduce the need for healthcare in patients with Crohn's disease. *Inflamm Bowel Dis*. 2007;13(6):745-752.

6. Nimalasuriya K, Compton MT, Guillory VJ, Prevention Practice Committee of the American College of Preventative Medicine. Screening adults for depression in primary care: a position statement of the American College of Preventive Medicine. *J Fam Pract*. 2009;58(10):535-538.

7. Nunes T, Etchevers MJ, Domenech E, et al. Smoking does influence disease behavior and impacts the need for therapy in Crohn's disease in the biologic era.*Aliment Pharmacol Ther*. 2013;38(7):752-760.

8. Nunes T, Etchevers MJ, Merino O, et al. Does smoking influence Crohn's disease in the biologic era? The TABACROHN study. *Inflamm Bowel Dis*. 2013;19(1):23-29.

9. Ryan WR, Allan RN, Yamamoto T, Keighley MRB. Crohn's disease patients who quit smoking have a reduced risk of reoperation for recurrence. *Am J Surg*. 2004;187(2):219-225.

10. Cosnes J, Beaugerie L, Carbonnel F, et al. Smoking cessation and the course of Crohn's disease: an intervention study. *Gastroenterology*. 2001;120:1093-1099.

11. Peyrin-Biroulet L, Khosrotehrani K, Carrat F, et al. Increased risk for nonmelanoma skin cancers in patients who receive thiopurines for inflammatory bowel disease. *Gastroenterology*. 2011;141(5):162128.e1-28.e5.

12. Farraye FA, Melmed GY, Lichtenstein GR, Kane SV. ACG clinical guideline: Preventive care in inflammatory bowel disease. *Am J Gastroenterol*. 2017;112(2):241-258.

13. Singh S, Nagpal SJ, Murad MH, et al. Inflammatory bowel disease is associated with an increased risk of melanoma: a systematic review and meta-analysis. *Clin Gastroenterol Hepatol*. 2014;12(2):210-218.

14. Rungoe C, Simonsen J, Riis L, Frisch M, Langholz E, Jess T. Inflammatory bowel disease and cervical neoplasia: a population-based nationwide cohort study. *Clin Gastroenterol Hepatol*. 2015;13(4):693-700.e1.

15. Kane S, Khatibi B, Reddy D. Higher incidence of abnormal Pap smears in women with inflammatory bowel disease. *Am J Gastroenterol*. 2008;103(3):631-636.

16. Practice bulletin no. 157: cervical cancer screening and prevention. *Obstet Gynecol*. 2016;127:e1-e20.

17. Bernstein CN, Leslie WD, Lebo MS. AGA technical review on osteoporosis in gastrointestinal diseases. *Gastroenterology*. 2003;124(3):795-841.

18. Shen B, Remzi FH, Oikonomou IK, et al. Risk factors for low bone mass in patients with ulcerative colitis following ileal pouch-anal anastomosis. *Am J Gastroenterol*. 2009;104(3):639-646.

19. Raisz LG. Clinical practice. Screening for osteoporosis. *N Engl J Med*. 2005;353(2):164-171.

20. IBD Checklist for Monitoring & Prevention. Cornerstones Health. Updated February 9, 2020. Accessed June 18, 2021. https://www.cornerstoneshealth.org/wp-content/uploads/2020/08/NEW-IBD-Checklist-for-Monitoring-Prevention-526a.pdf

21. Parker S, Chambers White L, Spangler C, et al. A quality improvement project significantly increased the vaccination rate for immunosuppressed patients with IBD. *Inflamm Bowel Dis*. 2013;19(9):1809-1814.

22. Reich JS, Miller HL, Wasan SK, et al. Influenza and pneumococcal vaccination rates in patients with inflammatory bowel disease. *Gastroenterol Hepatol*. 2015;11(6):396-401.

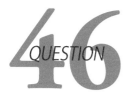

How Should We Screen Our Patients With IBD for Depression and Anxiety?

Alyse Bedell, PhD and Laurie Keefer, PhD

Inflammatory bowel diseases (IBD) are associated with a significant degree of psychosocial burden, including anxiety, depression,[1] and reduced quality of life.[2] The clinical repercussions of untreated depression and anxiety are far-reaching, including increased hospitalization, testing, and therapies[3]; lower response to treatment; and higher rates of relapse,[4] though it should be noted that these may be both a cause and a consequence of psychological distress.[5,6] As such, the American College of Gastroenterology clinical guidelines for both ulcerative colitis[7] (UC) and Crohn's disease[8] (CD) recommend that patients with IBD be routinely screened for anxiety and depression and provided with appropriate resources for treatment.

Depression, Anxiety, and Other Symptoms and Diagnoses of Clinical Interest in IBD

DEPRESSION AND ANXIETY

Major depressive disorder (MDD), which is the most common form of depression, is characterized by sadness and/or loss of interest or pleasure in usual activities with other cognitive or physiological symptoms (eg, insomnia, impaired concentration, worthlessness). In 2017, 17.3 million adults in the United States had at least one major depressive episode, representing 7.1% of all US adults.[9] Generalized anxiety disorder (GAD), the most common of the anxiety disorders, affects 6.8 million adults, or 3.1% of the US population.[10] GAD is characterized by persistent and

Rubin DT, Friedman S, Farraye FA, eds. *Curbside Consultation in IBD:*
49 Clinical Questions, Third Edition (pp 307-312).
© 2022 Taylor & Francis Group.

excessive worry in a number of different domains, as well as other symptoms of anxiety such as restlessness, muscle tension, and irritability.[11] The prevalence of anxiety (20.5%) and depression (15.2%) among patients with IBD is greater than that of the general population[12] and is more prevalent among patients with active inflammation than those in remission.[13]

ADJUSTMENT DISORDER

In cases of acute and/or mild psychological distress, an adjustment disorder may be a more appropriate diagnostic label than MDD or GAD. According to the Fifth Edition of the *Diagnostic and Statistical Manual of Mental Disorders* (DSM-5), an adjustment disorder consists of emotional or behavioral symptoms (eg, depression, anxiety, behavioral problems) within 3 months of a stressful event that are not better explained by another mental health diagnosis.[11] An adjustment disorder should be considered when symptom onset is associated with a change in disease status, such as an initial diagnosis, flare, or change in treatment, and the patient does not meet criteria for MDD, GAD, or another mood or anxiety disorder.

GASTROINTESTINAL-SPECIFIC ANXIETY

While not a psychiatric diagnosis in its own right, gastrointestinal-specific anxiety is a common cognitive-affective phenomenon among gastrointestinal patients that refers to cognitions, emotions, and behaviors resulting from fear and anxiety about gastrointestinal sensations and symptoms rather than general life stressors.[14] In IBD, this can lead to amplification of pain and avoidance behavior and isolation and is thought to be driven by alterations in the activity of the gut-brain axis.[15,16]

Assessment

SELF-REPORT SCREENING TOOLS

The use of validated, self-reporting screening tools can help facilitate a quick assessment of psychological distress. While cut-off scores provide an easy reference for symptom severity, consistent use of these tools during clinic visits also allows a provider to draw comparisons in their patients across time. For depression, we recommend use of the Patient Health Questionnaire-9[17] (PHQ-9; Table 46-1), which has the highest validity in IBD.[18] Often, item 9 will be removed (suicidal ideation) to avoid liability. The Patient-Reported Outcomes Measurement Information System Anxiety Short Form v1.0 8a[19] (PROMIS Anxiety; Table 46-2) similarly has the strongest support for assessing anxiety in this population.[18]

CLINICAL INTERVIEW

A clinical interview, which may also include a review and discussion of the patient's measured questionnaire data, is an integral component of screening for depression and anxiety in IBD. Questions assessing psychological distress should be asked in every visit, not just when depression or anxiety is suspected. By making these questions a routine aspect of the clinic visit, patients are less likely to feel that they are being singled out and more likely to respond openly and honestly. Open-ended questions such as, "How are you coping with all of this?" or "What areas of your life are being impacted by your illness?" take an unassuming tone, allowing for a variety of responses. For patients who appear embarrassed or ashamed to admit to psychological distress, normalizing

Table 46-1
Patient Health Questionnaire-9

Over the Last 2 Weeks, How Often Have You Been Bothered by Any of the Following Problems?	Not at All	Several Days	More Than Half the Days	Nearly Every Day
1. Little interest or pleasure in doing things	0	1	2	3
2. Feeling down, depressed, or hopeless	0	1	2	3
3. Trouble falling or staying asleep, or sleeping too much	0	1	2	3
4. Feeling tired or having little energy	0	1	2	3
5. Poor appetite or overeating	0	1	2	3
6. Feeling bad about yourself—or that you are a failure or have let yourself or your family down	0	1	2	3
7. Trouble concentrating, such as reading the newspaper or watching television	0	1	2	3
8. Moving or speaking so slowly that other people could have noticed? Or the opposite—being so fidgety or restless that you have been moving around a lot more than usual	0	1	2	3
9. Thoughts that you would be better off dead or of hurting yourself in some way	0	1	2	3

questions such as, "Many people with IBD struggle sometimes with depression and anxiety, or feel they need more support with coping; have you been experiencing anything like this recently?" can be a more helpful approach.

Providing Resources

EDUCATION ON THE RELATIONSHIP BETWEEN STRESS, ANXIETY, DEPRESSION, AND IBD

Education should be provided about the relationship between stress, anxiety, depression, and IBD, either before or after screening and regardless of whether a patient endorses psychological distress in that visit. Box 46-1 gives an example script.

Table 46-2
PROMIS Anxiety

Please Respond to Each Question or Statement by Marking One Box per Row. **In the Past 7 Days . . .**	Never	Rarely	Sometimes	Often	Always
I felt fearful.					
I found it hard to focus on anything other than my anxiety.					
My worries overwhelmed me.					
I felt uneasy.					
I felt nervous.					
I felt like I needed help for my anxiety.					
I felt anxious.					
I felt tense.					

Box 46-1
Education on the Relationship Between Stress, Anxiety, Depression, and IBD

"The brain and the body are integrally connected. If you were to put your hand on a hot stove, the injury would be to your hand—no argument there, right? But in order for you to actually *feel* the sensation of pain, your body needs your brain to interpret the signals coming from the nerve endings in your hand, and then send the message back down to the hand to be experienced as pain. So pain, and really any physical sensations, are based in the brain. In a similar way, your brain and gut are communicating all the time about your digestion, your hunger, your stress level, and all kinds of things. When you feel stressed, whether it is about your gastrointestinal symptoms or other things in your life, this causes very real changes to your body that change the way your gastrointestinal tract functions and this can make your symptoms worse, whether or not you are having a disease flare. If you experience more symptoms, this causes *additional* stress, creating a vicious cycle."

Box 46-2
Providing Referrals

"Given how important it is to your IBD treatment and your overall quality of life to address your stress/anxiety/depression/fears about your illness, I would like you to meet with a colleague of mine, a psychologist/social worker for an evaluation. This person has experience working with patients with IBD and can help us have a clearer picture of other factors that might be contributing to how you're feeling so that we can make a plan to address them. How does that sound to you?"

REFERRALS

After providing education on the relationship between psychological distress and IBD, you should provide your patient with a referral for evaluation with a mental health provider for psychotherapy and/or medication. The manner in which a gastroenterologist presents a referral can make a significant impact on whether a patient chooses to schedule an appointment with a mental provider and their degree of openness, so developing a solid elevator pitch is a good investment of your time. Box 46-2 gives an example script.

TYPES OF TREATMENT

A direct referral for general mental health psychotherapy and/or psychiatric medication management is appropriate for patients who appear to have severe and/or long-standing depression or anxiety that is not closely tied to their IBD. For patients experiencing psychological distress that is closely tied to their IBD, or that appears to be a more acute presentation, an ideal referral would be to a psychologist or other mental health provider with specific training in brain-gut psychotherapies. If a gastrointestinal psychologist is part of your integrated service, they are an excellent resource and can provide a more thorough psychological assessment and treatment recommendations. In cases where a gastrointestinal psychologist is not available, a good option is to establish a relationship with a psychologist or other mental health provider who specializes in working with patients with medical conditions.

Regardless of which referral pathway your patient takes, be sure to check in with your patient on their treatment progress and connect with their mental health provider, if possible. Establishing this connection can ease a patient's concerns that they are being dumped onto another provider and instead demonstrates use of an integrated approach to their care.

Conclusion

Depression, anxiety, and other symptoms associated with psychological distress are common among patients with IBD and have been traditionally underdiagnosed.[13] Depression and anxiety are associated with multiple negative clinical outcomes, which in turn contributes to worsened depression and anxiety, creating a vicious cycle. Patients with IBD are likely to have frequent contact with their gastroenterologists, and in some cases more than with any other health provider. As such, gastroenterologists are well-positioned to provide screening for depression and anxiety and to provide resources, as appropriate.

References

1. Mikocka-Walus A, Knowles SR, Keefer L, Graff L. Controversies revisited: a systematic review of the comorbidity of depression and anxiety with inflammatory bowel diseases. *Inflamm Bowel Dis.* 2016;22(3):752-762.
2. Knowles SR, Graff LA, Wilding H, Hewitt C, Keefer L, Mikocka-Walus A. Quality of life in inflammatory bowel disease: a systematic review and meta-analyse—part I. *Inflamm Bowel Dis.* 2018;24(4):742-751.
3. Navabi S, Gorrepati VS, Yadav S, et al. Influences and impact of anxiety and depression in the setting of inflammatory bowel disease. *Inflamm Bowel Dis.* 2018;24(11):2303-2308.
4. Graff LA, Walker JR, Bernstein CN. Depression and anxiety in inflammatory bowel disease: a review of comorbidity and management. *Inflamm Bowel Dis.* 2009;15(7):1105-1118.
5. Keefer L, Kane SV. Considering the bidirectional pathways between depression and IBD: recommendations for comprehensive IBD Care. *Gastroenterol Hepatol.* 2017;13(3):164-169.
6. Bitton A, Dobkin PL, Edwardes MD, et al. Predicting relapse in Crohn's disease: a biopsychosocial model. *Gut.* 2008;57(10):1386-1392.
7. Rubin DT, Ananthakrishnan AN, Siegel CA, Sauer BG, Long MD. ACG clinical guideline: ulcerative colitis in adults. *Am J Gastroenterol.* 2019;114(3):384-413.
8. Lichtenstein GR, Loftus EV, Isaacs KL, Regueiro MD, Gerson LB, Sands BE. ACG clinical guideline: management of Crohn's disease in adults. *Am J Gastroenterol.* 2018;113(4):481-517.
9. National Institute of Mental Health. Major depression. https://www.nimh.nih.gov/health/statistics/major-depression.shtml#part_155029. Accessed June 9, 2020.
10. Anxiety and Depression Association of America. Generalized anxiety disorder (GAD). https://adaa.org/understanding-anxiety/generalized-anxiety-disorder-gad. Accessed June 9, 2020.
11. American Psychiatric Association. *Diagnostic and statistical manual of mental disorders.* 5th ed. 2013.
12. Neuendorf R, Harding A, Stello N, Hanes D, Wahbeh H. Depression and anxiety in patients with inflammatory bowel disease: a systematic review. *J Psychosom Res.* 2016;87:70-80.
13. Bennebroek Evertsz' F, Thijssens NAM, Stokkers PCF, et al. Do inflammatory bowel disease patients with anxiety and depressive symptoms receive the care they need? *J Crohns Colitis.* 2012;6(1):68-76.
14. Labus JS, Bolus R, Chang L, et al. The Visceral Sensitivity Index: development and validation of a gastrointestinal symptom-specific anxiety scale. *Aliment Pharmacol Ther.* 2004;20(1):89-97.
15. Gracie DJ, Hamlin PJ, Ford AC. The influence of the brain-gut axis in inflammatory bowel disease and possible implications for treatment. *Lancet Gastroenterol Hepatol.* 2019;4(8):632-642.
16. Labanski A, Langhorst J, Engler H, Elsenbruch S. Stress and the brain-gut axis in functional and chronic-inflammatory gastrointestinal diseases: a transdisciplinary challenge. *Psychoneuroendocrinology.* 2020;111:104501.
17. Kroenke K, Spitzer RL, Williams JB. The PHQ-9: validity of a brief depression severity measure. *J Gen Intern Med.* 2001;16(9):606-613.
18. Bernstein CN, Zhang L, Lix LM, et al. The validity and reliability of screening measures for depression and anxiety disorders in inflammatory bowel disease. *Inflamm Bowel Dis.* 2018;24(9):1867-1875.
19. Pilkonis PA, Choi SW, Reise SP, et al. Item banks for measuring emotional distress from the Patient-Reported Outcomes Measurement Information System (PROMIS): depression, anxiety, and anger. *Assessment.* 2011;18(3):263-283.

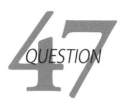

WHAT IS THE ROLE OF DIET IN THE TREATMENT OF IBD AND HOW DO I DISCUSS THIS WITH MY PATIENTS?

James D. Lewis, MD, MSCE and Tamar Pfeffer Gik, RD, MSc

The primary goal of the gastrointestinal tract is to digest and absorb nutrients. Nutritional care for patients with inflammatory bowel disease (IBD) can have 2 principle goals: correct nutritional deficiencies and serve as a primary or complementary therapy.

Nutritional Screening

It is important that all patients with IBD undergo nutritional screening to assess for malnutrition. This can be facilitated by employing a validated tool to detect the patients who are at risk for malnutrition. To date, the best studied tool among patients with IBD is the Malnutrition Universal Screening Tool ('MUST')[1] (Figure 47-1). Patients who are identified as at risk for malnutrition may benefit from formal evaluation by a registered dietitian or related health care professional. When discussing the need for nutritional support during a flare, one can emphasize that the purpose is to aid patients during a time when eating is difficult yet the nutritional needs remain substantial. One can also emphasize that weight loss due to active inflammation is not a favorable outcome and may be associated with a poor prognosis.

When Should You Recommend Nil Per Os?

Nil per os (NPO) is a common recommendation for patients admitted to the hospital with exacerbation of IBD, but should be only used in one of the following situations[2,3]:

Rubin DT, Friedman S, Farraye FA, eds. *Curbside Consultation in IBD: 49 Clinical Questions, Third Edition* (pp 313-320).
© 2022 Taylor & Francis Group.

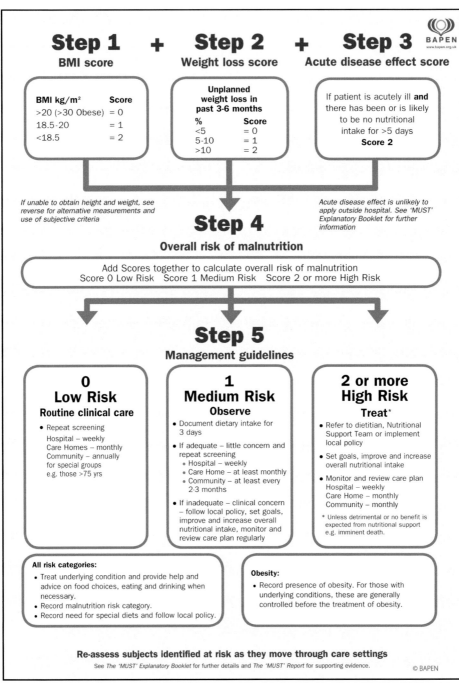

Figure 47-1. The Malnutrition Universal Screening Tool ('MUST'), developed by the Malnutrition Advisory Group of the British Association for Parenteral and Enteral Nutrition, is a screening tool aimed to detect malnutrition and risk for malnutrition. It includes an assessment of current body mass index (BMI), weight loss, and prospect of nutritional intake. The sum of these subscores indicates the risk for malnutrition: low risk (0), medium risk (1), or high risk (≥ 2). The algorithm goes on to advise how to manage the patient. (The 'Malnutrition Universal Screening Tool' ('MUST') is reproduced here with the kind permission of BAPEN [British Association for Parenteral and Enteral Nutrition]. For further information on 'MUST' see www.bapen.org.uk Copyright © BAPEN 2012.)

1. Patients are being prepared for endoscopy, surgery, or imaging study.
2. Enteral feed is contraindicated; the risks exceed the benefits such as in the setting of bowel obstruction, toxic megacolon, intractable nausea, and vomiting.

When Should One Consider Using Oral Nutritional Supplements in IBD?

Oral nutritional supplements (ONS) are liquid formulas that can be used as meal replacements and supply patients with macronutrients (carbohydrates, protein, and lipids) as well as balanced micronutrients (vitamins and trace elements). The ONS may be a polymeric, elemental, or semi-elemental formula.

During periods of active disease, patients may find it difficult to eat an adequate diet and as a first-line defense should meet with a registered dietitian to improve oral intake. If the patient continues to lose weight and their nutritional status is compromised, ONS may be used—the exact amount should be calculated based on a measure of nutritional intake and assessment of the deficit.

When ONS are required, polymeric formulas are more palatable and should generally be attempted first as most patients can digest nutrients in the proximal small bowel and therefore do not need an elemental formula. In patients with extensive small bowel disease or severe proximal small bowel disease who cannot tolerate polymeric feeds, semi-elemental or elemental feeds can be considered. In patients with diabetes mellitus, the glucose levels should be monitored, and if possible, ONS designed specifically for patients with diabetes should be used.

An increased frequency of bowel movements may be an initial side effect of ONS. However, most patients will adapt within 1 week. Because the increase in bowel frequency may be due to high osmolarity of the ONS, patients should be advised to drink the ONS slowly and/or dilute the ONS with water. If the increased bowel movement persists, less osmotic formulas or elemental/semi-elemental formulas can be tried.

When Should Tube Feeding Be Used?

To ensure adequate nutrient supply in case the oral intake is not possible (low appetite, difficulty swallowing, anorexia, etc) a nasogastric feeding tube may be used. The enteral route is always preferred to the parenteral route when it is possible; even in cases of reduced absorption, the enteral route should be chosen with some parenteral support.[4] Even small amounts of enteral nutrition are believed to help sustain the integrity of the gut mucosa, which is a major barrier to infection from the microbes that reside in the gut.

When Should Parenteral Nutrition Be Used?

Parenteral nutrition is not the first choice in patients with IBD in need of nutritional support and should not be used as a means of bowel rest for remission induction purposes.[4] Parenteral nutrition is indicated in a minority of patients, such as those who are not able to obtain sufficient nutrients via an enteral route (ie, either orally or via tube feeds) in the setting of a high output fistula and in severely malnourished patients in urgent need of a surgical intervention.[3,4]

What Should We Be Doing for Our Patients Who Are Surgical Candidates?

The nutritional status of patients undergoing surgery should be optimized. The European Society for Parenteral and Enteral Nutrition's (ESPEN) general surgical guidelines recommend that patients who cannot obtain more than 50% of their nutritional needs 7 days before the surgery with oral intake should begin nutritional support with ONS and tube feeds if needed.[3,4] Parenteral nutrition is associated with higher infection rate; therefore, the enteral route should be preferred for infection prevention.[3]

Parenteral nutrition in the preoperative setting should be used in one of the following scenarios:

1. In case that regular oral intake, ONS, and TF support provide less that 50% of the nutritional need for more than 7 days, parenteral nutrition should be administered while still using the enteral route.
2. The gastrointestinal tract is compromised: intestinal obstruction, ileus, severe shock, intestinal ischemia, high output fistula, severe intestinal hemorrhage.

After surgery patients should gradually return to a full and diverse diet and should reintroduce all food groups, beginning with a soft texture and returning to a full and healthy diet. Returning to a regular diet may occasionally be difficult for patients as they are accustomed to functional side effects from food items. If necessary, counseling by a registered dietitian can facilitate resumption of a regular diet.

Exclusive Enteral Nutrition

Exclusive enteral nutrition (EEN) has been primarily used as a primary therapy in pediatric Crohn's disease (CD). EEN is a dietary regimen in which the patient with active CD consumes a diet restricted to only ONS. Approximately 80% of children who adhere to this regimen will achieve a clinical remission, and EEN is considered comparably effective to corticosteroids when used in children.[5] A small study (n = 34) has also demonstrated a 58% early endoscopic response rate.[6] This led to the positioning of EEN as a recommended first-line therapy in pediatric IBD in the 2014 ECCO-ESPGHAN joint guidelines.[7,8] The main obstacle in implementing EEN in adult care is the low adherence rate, but in selected adult patients with CD who are in need of a remission agent and the use of steroids or other immunomodulation is contraindicated, this may be a feasible option. When you discuss EEN with the patient, you can emphasis that EEN is typically employed for only 6 to 8 weeks and that that within 10 to 14 days patients will sense clinical improvement.

In the setting of perioperative nutrition for elective surgery, a course of EEN in preparation for surgery has been shown to reduce surgical complications as well as prepare the patient nutritionally for surgery regardless of perioperative nutritional status.[9] The potential benefits of using EEN prior to surgery include less corticosteroid use prior to surgery (ie, a means to avoid or lower the dose) and nutritional repletion, both of which are believed to result in improved postoperative outcomes.

There is no evidence to support the use of EEN in patients with ulcerative colitis.

Should Patients With IBD Adhere to a Specific Diet?

Patients with IBD are often advised to avoid high-fiber foods, but there is scarce evidence on the effectiveness of low-fiber diet. A head-to-head study in patients with non-stricturing CD compared a low-residue to a normal diet found that adherence to a low-fiber diet did not improve outcomes; therefore, we should not overly restrict our patients.[10] Furthermore, low-fiber diets are known to decrease microbial diversity, which may play a role in perpetuating bowel inflammation. As such, most people with IBD should be advised to eat a healthy diverse diet, including high-fiber foods.[4,11] However, patients with severe fibrostenotic disease who have recurrent obstructive symptoms should avoid high-fiber foods. Patients with strictures that do not suffer from obstructive symptoms may eat fruits and vegetables in moderation and in adjusted texture (eg, vegetable soup, pureed fruits, and vegetables or fruit shakes). All must be consumed in moderation and should have formal nutritional counseling.[4]

When discussing the importance of fruits and vegetables in the patient's diet, you should explain that these are chronic diseases and patients must live a healthy life just like people without IBD. A healthy diet and physical activity can be beneficial in preventing metabolic disease such as diabetes and fatty liver.

Many diets are popular in patients with IBD and are highly publicized on the internet. To date, none of these diets have been shown to be the best IBD diet. For patients with UC, we often recommend the avoidance of red and processed meats, although clinical trials proving the efficacy of this intervention are lacking. In a large randomized clinical trial of asymptomatic patients with CD who are members of the IBD Partners internet cohort, there was no difference in relapse rates among patients consuming high vs low levels of red and processed meat.[12] Nonetheless, there are likely other health benefits, and this is a sustainable dietary recommendation. For patients with CD or UC, the peer-reviewed literature contains mostly uncontrolled reports of success rates of the specific carbohydrate diet,[13] variations of the Paleolithic diet, personalized diets guided by immunoglobulin G levels,[14] and others. A small randomized controlled trial comparing the CD exclusion diet (CDED) to EEN in children with mild to moderate CD demonstrated that both were effective in remission induction but the CDED was better tolerated.[15] Secondary outcomes demonstrated higher remission rates once the EEN group had resumed their regular diet, with only 25% of calories coming from enteral nutrition formula. A common feature of all these diets is the avoidance of commercially prepared foods. Thus, a simple recommendation is to eat a diet based of homemade meals prepared from fresh ingredients (Figure 47-2).

What Are the Common Micronutrient Deficiencies?

There are multiple reasons for micronutrient deficiencies among patients with IBD, such as impaired absorption, decreased consumption, and increased losses in the lumen of the gut. Common micronutrient deficiencies should be monitored, and supplementation should be advised when deficiencies are found (Table 47-1). It is important to note that some tests for nutrient deficiencies are influenced by inflammation; as such, the evaluation should optimally be performed in a period of clinical remission.[4,16] The most common deficiencies are vitamin D, iron, and vitamin B_{12}. The latter is particularly common among patients who have undergone an ileal resection or have an ileal pouch–anal anastomosis. Such patients should be advised to monitor their B_{12} levels as they are at a greater risk for deficiency.

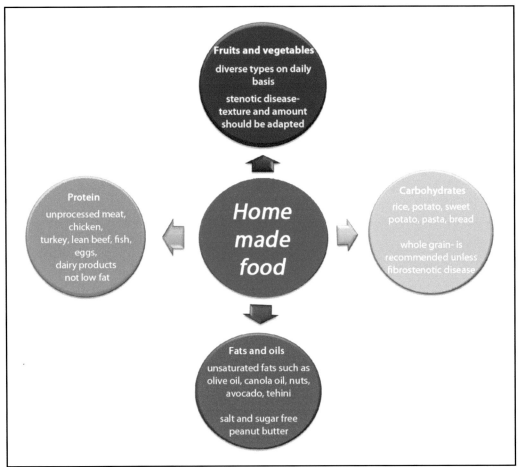

Figure 47-2. There is currently no single diet that can be recommended for patients with IBD. The current recommendation is to eat a well-balanced diet comprised of homemade food that includes all food groups.

Table 47-1

Micronutrient Monitoring and Recommended Repletion Strategy

Micronutrients	*Monitoring Frequency*	*Serum Biomarker*	*What Is Considered a Low Level*	*Repletion Management*
All Patients With IBD				
Vitamin D	Annually	25-OH vitamin D	Insufficiency: 20 to 30 ng/mL Deficiency: < 20 ng/mL	Oral 1400 IU/day High dose once weekly supplementation is also commonly employed
Folate	Annually	Folate	< 17 ng/mL	Oral 600 mcg–5 mg/day
Vitamin B_{12}	Annually	Vitamin B_{12}	< 300 pg/mL	Sublingual B12-1000 mcg Refractory cases IM injection
Iron	Every 6 months	Hb, ferritin, transferrin saturation	Hb ≤ 10 Ferritin < 30 Transferrin saturation < 20%	IV supplementation if unable to replete with oral iron supplement. Commonly used IV options include: Iron sucrose Ferric carboxymaltose Iron isomaltoside
Patients With SBS				
Micronutrients	*Monitoring Frequency*	*Serum Biomarker*	*What Is Considered a Low Level*	*Repletion Management*
Zinc	Annually	Zinc	< 70 µg/dL	Oral 20 to 40 mg/day
Magnesium	Annually	Magnesium	< 1.8 mg/dL	Oral ~200-400 mg/day may worsen diarrhea Intravenous supplementation can be used if needed
Copper	Annually	Free copper	< 10 µg/dL	Oral 1.5 to 3 mg/day
Vitamin B_{12}	Every 6 months	Vitamin B_{12}	< 300 pg/mL	Sublingual B12-1000 mcg Refractory cases intramuscular injection

References

1. Sandhu A, Mosli M, Yan B, et al. Self-screening for malnutrition risk in outpatient inflammatory bowel disease patients using the Malnutrition Universal Screening Tool (MUST). *J Parenter Enter Nutr.* 2014;40(4):507-510. https://doi.org/10.1177/0148607114566656
2. Gallinger ZR, Rumman A, Pivovarov K, Fortinsky KJ, Steinhart AH, Weizman AV. Frequency and variables associated with fasting orders in inpatients with ulcerative colitis: the Audit of Diet Orders—Ulcerative Colitis (ADORE-UC) Study. *Inflamm Bowel Dis.* 2017;23(10):1790-1795. https://doi.org/10.1097/MIB.0000000000001244
3. Weimann A, Braga M, Carli F, et al. ESPEN guideline: clinical nutrition in surgery. *Clin Nutr.* 2017;36(3):623-650. https://doi.org/10.1016/j.clnu.2017.02.013
4. Forbes A, Escher J, Hébuterne X, et al. ESPEN guideline: clinical nutrition in inflammatory bowel disease. *Clin Nutr.* 2017;36(2):321-347. https://doi.org/10.1016/j.clnu.2016.12.027
5. Buchanan E, Gaunt WW, Cardigan T, Garrick V, McGrogan P, Russell RK. The use of exclusive enteral nutrition for induction of remission in children with Crohn's disease demonstrates that disease phenotype does not influence clinical remission. *Aliment Pharmacol Ther.* 2009;30(5):501-507. https://doi.org/10.1111/j.1365-2036.2009.04067.x
6. Grover Z, Muir R, Lewindon P. Exclusive enteral nutrition induces early clinical, mucosal and transmural remission in paediatric Crohn's disease. *J Gastroenterol.* 2014;49(4):638-645. https://doi.org/10.1007/s00535-013-0815-0
7. Ruemmele FM, Veres G, Kolho KL, et al. Consensus guidelines of ECCO/ESPGHAN on the medical management of pediatric Crohn's disease. *J Crohns Colitis.* 2014;8(10):1179-1207.
8. Koletzko ÃÃS, Ridder L De, Escher JC, et al. Nutrition in pediatric inflammatory bowel disease: a position paper on behalf of the Porto Inflammatory Bowel Disease Group of the European Society of Pediatric. 2018;66(4):687-708. https://doi.org/10.1097/MPG.0000000000001896
9. Heerasing N, Thompson B, Hendy P, et al. Exclusive enteral nutrition provides an effective bridge to safer interval elective surgery for adults with Crohn's disease. *Aliment Pharmacol Ther.* 2017;45(5):660-669. https://doi.org/10.1111/apt.13934
10. Levenstein S, Prantera C, Luzi C, D'Ubaldi A. Low residue or normal diet in Crohn's disease: a prospective controlled study in Italian patients. *Gut.* 1985:26(10):989-993.
11. Lewis JD, Abreau MT. Diet as a trigger or therapy for inflammatory bowel diseases. *Gastroenterology.* 2018;152(2):398-414.e6. https://doi.org/10.1053/j.gastro.2016.10.019
12. Albenberg L, Brensinger CM, Wu Q, et al. A diet low in red and processed meat does not reduce rate of Crohn's disease flares. *Gastroenterology.* 2019;157(1):128-136.e5. https://doi.org/10.1053/j.gastro.2019.03.015
13. Obih C, Wahbeh G, Lee D, et al. Specific carbohydrate diet for pediatric inflammatory bowel disease in clinical practice within an academic IBD center. *Nutrition.* 2016;32(4):418-425. https://doi.org/10.1016/j.nut.2015.08.025
14. Gunasekeera V, Mendall MA, Chan D, Kumar D. Treatment of Crohn's disease with an IgG4-guided exclusion diet: a randomized controlled trial. *Dig Dis Sci.* 2016;61(4):1148-1157. https://doi.org/10.1007/s10620-015-3987-z
15. Levine A, Wine E, Assa A, et al. Crohn's disease exclusion diet plus partial enteral nutrition induces sustained remission in a randomized controlled trial. *Gastroenterology.* 2019;157(2):440-450.e8. https://doi.org/10.1053/j.gastro.2019.04.021
16. Halmos EP, Gibson PR. Dietary management of IBD-insights and advice. *Nat Rev Gastroenterol Hepatol.* 2015;12(3):133-146. https://doi.org/10.1038/nrgastro.2015.11

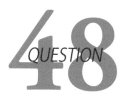

WHAT ADVICE SHOULD I GIVE THE PATIENT WITH IBD WHO IS TRAVELING?

Kay Greveson, BA, MSc and Shomron Ben-Horin, MD

Traveling away from the controlled environment of home can be somewhat overwhelming to a patient with inflammatory bowel disease (IBD), regardless if the purpose of travel is for work, studies, or leisure. Research has shown that having Crohn's disease or colitis does prevent people from traveling, including limitations on the amount of travel and the destination, mainly due to concerns about access to health care, the availability of medications, and concerns about sanitation in the travel destination.[1] However, research has shown that patients do not have adequate knowledge and are likely to travel without adequate insurance or without proper advice regarding immunizations.[2] Likewise, many gastroenterologists may not feel confident to provide comprehensive pre-travel consultations to their patients.[3] Planning ahead and ensuring patients are adequately advised and educated can make travel safer and enjoyable.

There are multiple aspects of travel to be considered: how to manage illness during travel, how to seek help if flaring during a trip, how to travel with medications and/or medical devices, considerations regarding immunization, and how to avoid and manage traveler's diarrhea. These points will be addressed in this chapter.

Advice Prior to Travel

THE PRE-TRAVEL CONSULTATION

Adequate consultations prior to travel are extremely important and should be done in conjunction with a travel clinic/travel health specialist wherever possible.[4] Patients should travel when

Rubin DT, Friedman S, Farraye FA, eds. *Curbside Consultation in IBD:*
49 Clinical Questions, Third Edition (pp 321-330).
© 2022 Taylor & Francis Group.

their disease is in remission and should be strongly discouraged from traveling when unwell. The travel destination, reason, and duration will impact the amount of planning and preparation required.

PATIENT PREPARATION

Advanced preparation is key to worry-free travels. Advise patients to do the following:

- Plan at least 6 to 8 weeks in advance if they plan to visit developing or tropical countries where they may need vaccinations or take special health precautions.
- When planning the trip patients should consider their itinerary and the availability of health care and medications in each destination.
- Have an emergency kit (placed in the carry-on baggage) that includes extra underwear, wet wipes, a plastic bag for soiled items, tissues, hand sanitizer, and deodorizing spray. This kit can also include special medications such as oral rehydration solutions, corticosteroids in case of a flare, antispasmodics, and antibiotics in case of traveler's diarrhea.
- Obtain a written summary in English of their medical history from the gastroenterology team to include allergies, past surgeries, past medical history, and current medication list.
- Obtain copies of all prescription medication that the patient is regularly receiving and those that will be taken on the trip.
- Have contact information (phone and email) of their IBD team and insurance company.
- Carry copies of all insurance cards and immunization records.
- In cases where patients have dietary restrictions, they can notify the travel company/airline ahead of time to allow them to accommodate certain diets. Common special dietary meals available include diabetic diets, gluten-free diets, and vegetarian diets. More complex needs may not be addressed. Airline websites typically provide this information, which can be researched ahead of time. A multilingual dietary card is also available to purchase via www.dietarycard.org.uk. This can help when visiting non–English-speaking countries.

TRAVEL INSURANCE

Research has shown that many patients fail to obtain adequate travel insurance.[2] This can be due to increased premiums or difficulty obtaining cover if they have other comorbidities or have had recent hospital admissions.

- Always declare all medical conditions as costs can be significant if medical advice is required.
- Advise patients to use an insurance broker/mediator and compare different premium as quotes can differ significantly between companies based on their individual risk assessment.
- Read the small print and know what is and is not covered, including any particular medical conditions or medical assistance.
- Know whether the travel insurance will cover repatriation home in case of emergency.
- Consider buying travel insurance that will cover costs if the trip needs to be cancelled in situations where the patient's health deteriorates or changes prior to the trip.

IMMUNIZATIONS

Immunizations may be essential for travel to developing countries. Ideally patients should be already be immunized against common diseases at diagnosis,[4] but this may not always be possible.

Table 48-1
Live Vaccines

Oral polio
Measles, mumps, and rubella (MMR)
Chickenpox/shingles (herpes zoster)
Yellow fever
Cholera (oral version also available as inactive)
Oral typhoid (injectable version is inactive)
Bacillus Calmette-Guérin (tuberculosis vaccination)
Flumist influenza vaccine (nasal spray only)
Rotavirus (used in infants only)
Adenovirus
Smallpox
Reproduced with permission from IBD Passport, www.ibdpassport.com.

The following should be considered:

- Find out immunizations required for the site of travel. The Centers for Disease Control and Prevention (CDC) has a relatively complete list of countries, immunization recommendations, and travel checklist online.[5]

- The patient should be advised to have a consultation at a travel medical clinic if there are vaccination concerns in the destination.
  - The immunosuppressed patient with IBD should not receive live vaccines (Table 48-1). However, if such vaccines are essential and travel plans cannot be altered, the following should be considered[4]:
    - Stop immunosuppression for 3 months before any live vaccine is given.
    - Once vaccinated, immunosuppressant medication can be restarted after 3 weeks.

- The risks of disease in certain areas of the world should be discussed and travel plans altered if the risk is high for exposure to pathogens for which the traveler cannot safely receive immunizations. The CDC has several references on their website that review advice on the needs of immunosuppressed travelers.[6] These may be helpful for the physician to review with the patient.

- Patients receiving immunosuppressant medications may have an attenuated response to certain vaccinations.

- Where a health professional advises that an individual should not be vaccinated on medical grounds, a medical letter of exemption should be provided, which should be taken into consideration by the port/border health authorities in the destination country.[7] The *International Certificate of Vaccination or Prophylaxis* is the official documentation used as proof of vaccination against a disease when a country entry requirement exists. An example exception letter with space for an official hospital stamp is available in the international certificate document.

Mode of Travel

Patients may travel for work or leisure, and the type of travel can be domestic or international using various modes of transport.

The patient should be advised to consider the following:

- Try and book advance seat selection wherever possible to reduce any anxiety regarding toilet access. An aisle seat close to the restrooms will make it easier to attend to bathroom needs during the flight or during train or bus journeys.
- The airline should be notified during booking of any special needs (eg, assistance getting on and off the plane, bathroom access, excess luggage due to medication and/or medical supplies). They will very often be able to help if patients need more time during security. The Transportation Security Administration (TSA) has information available for travelers with disabilities and medical conditions that cover many security questions.[8]
- Obtain a "toilet access card" from the local Crohn's and colitis patient organization that can help facilitate toilet access in transport centers. These are often on the back of the organization's members card, but patients may not necessarily have to join to obtain one.
- Stay hydrated during the flight with noncaffeinated beverages. If the traveler is prone to dehydration, commercial electrolyte solutions can be taken through security with a physician's prescription. If this is not possible, an oral rehydration solution can be made with bottled water using 1 L of water, 6 teaspoons of sugar, and one-half teaspoon of salt.[9]

DEEP VEIN THROMBOSIS

Long-haul flights (greater than 6 hours) are known to increase the risk of deep vein thrombosis, and therefore adequate advice and measures should be in place prior to the trip[10]:

- Walk around the cabin periodically to decrease the risk of blood clots, especially on long flights. Many patients with IBD may be prone to hypercoagulability, especially if there has been recent surgery or hospitalization.
- Other measures that might help include contracting the calf muscles while sitting (isometrics), avoiding crossing the legs, and staying hydrated.
- If a patient is at very high risk, such as those who have previously had a venous thrombosis, compression stockings and prophylaxis with low molecular-weight heparin may be considered.

TRAVEL AT HIGH ALTITUDE

Limited research has also been conducted into travel to high-altitude destinations (above 6500 ft/2000 m), such as mountain regions for skiing or hiking, and has demonstrated there is an increased risk of flare within 4 weeks of travel to areas of high altitude or long-haul air flights.[11] Patients planning trips such as these should be counseled on the possible risk of disease activity either during or after their trip.

Medications During Travel

Patients often are taking a variety of medications in different forms such as oral, liquid, enema, injectables, and temperature-sensitive medications. These can all pose problems when traveling, particularly for long distances or when going through customs or border security.[12]

The patient should be advised the following:

- Bring enough medication and supplies for the entire trip and extra in case of delay or lost medicines. Include any over-the-counter medications such as antidiarrheal medication and pain relievers.
- Many airlines and travel companies will give extra baggage allowance for patients needing to carry medications or medical appliances/equipment. Patients should contact the travel company at the time of booking to arrange.
- Always carry a good supply of medications in both hand and checked luggage in case items go missing.
- Carry a copy of all prescriptions and keep medications in original packaging where possible. If going to a foreign country, it would be helpful to know the names of the medications in that country's language. The Crohn's and Colitis Foundation of America has a partial list of medication names in other countries.[13]
- Try to adjust schedules of periodically administered medications so that, whenever possible, they will not be due during the travel period. For instance, patient may consult their gastroenterologist to explore administering an infusion of biologic up to 1 to 2 weeks earlier, if the scheduled date of infusion falls within a planned trip.
- If patients are carrying temperature-sensitive medications such as pre-filled syringes of biologics drugs (adalimumab, golimumab, certolizumab pegol) they should contact the airline in advance to ensure they can take them onboard the aircraft. Special wallets can be obtained online that keep medications cool for up to 8 hours.
- If medications need to be kept refrigerated, patients should contact the accommodation where they plan to stay to ensure there is a fridge in the room or that one can be arranged.
- Travel with injectable medications will require a physician letter explaining the diagnosis and need for the patient to carry medications with them.
- If patients are planning to travel though different time zones they should check with their physician/nurse practitioner to see if any changes in the timing of medications are required.

ENTERAL/PARENTERAL NUTRITION

Special consideration also needs to be given to those on enteral or parenteral nutrition. Travel is possible but again requires planning. The following aspects should be considered:

- Allow at least 6 weeks before departure date to plan the logistics of traveling with a feed. The home care company that delivers the feed can deliver to many overseas destinations. Exceptions to this are developing countries and those in war conflict or where delivery is not possible due to customs restrictions. Advise patients to contact the feed delivery company before they book their trip to ensure delivery is possible.
- Obtain a letter from the IBD/nutrition specialist outlining medical history, medication, and an explanation of why the patient requires enteral/parenteral nutrition. A sample clinician letter for patients traveling with intravenous or tube feeds can be found at the Oley Foundation website.[14]
- Ensure patients have a written plan from their specialist of what to do in an emergency.
- A complication management chart and travel advice pack that covers the symptoms and steps to take for common problems related to parenteral or tube feeding nutrition and an essential supply inventory list plus useful tips can be obtained from the Oley Foundation.[14]

LEGAL CONSIDERATIONS

Some prescription and over-the-counter medications patients use for things like pain relief, sleep aids, allergies, and even cold and flu remedies are illegal in some countries. The United Arab Emirates and Japan, for example, are among the most restrictive nations, but many ban or restrict importing narcotics, sedatives, amphetamines, and other common over-the-counter medications.[15] Special consideration should be given if patients are taking medication containing a controlled drug or drugs with an active ingredient that is banned in another country (eg, a typical 25 mg tablet of Tylenol (acetaminophen) exceeds the 10 mg maximum amount in a tablet patients can bring into Japan). Patients may get a fine or even be imprisoned if they travel with medicine that is illegal in another country.

- Patients should be aware of the active ingredients in all medications. Advise them to check with the embassy of the country they are traveling to see if the medications they will carry are restricted or prohibited.

- Carrying medication for personal use often does not pose significant problems, but travel for longer than 3 months with medications to last the duration of this time could be against the law in some countries.

- Advise patients that medications must be carried in their original packaging with an accompanying prescription and physician letter.

- In countries where a medication is allowed, but its amount is capped, reducing the dosage or switching to another available medication may be advised.

SPECIAL CONSIDERATIONS FOR PATIENTS RECEIVING BIOLOGICS

Patients' diseases are often at their best and in remission on biologics, and they should be encouraged to travel where possible. Advanced planning is essential for longer trips or to destinations outside America.

- Check with the manufacturer/pharmaceutical company in the case of biologic medications to make sure that the temperature requirements of the drug are adhered to. This may mean traveling with a cooler and ice packs and ensuring there is appropriate refrigeration along the way. Many medical-grade cool wallets are available online.

- If travel is in the United States, it may be possible to arrange collecting the biologic medicine at a pharmacy during the course of the trip.

- Advise patients who are in need for an infusion of biologics while abroad or who travel for long time and will need local dispensing of their drugs that once they arrive at the travel destination they will probably have to register with the local health care system or with a private medical insurance company, depending on local arrangements and the reason for the visit (eg, travel for business or an education visa may be covered by private medical insurance).

- The IBD team at the travel destination may have to apply for funding according to their local guidelines before treatment can commence. Most regular travel insurance policies will not cover treatment with biologics, even if the insurance policy covers preexisting illness such as Crohn's disease or ulcerative colitis.

- Use resources such as the IBD Passport website[16] to obtain the name and contact details of a gastroenterologist at the travel destination. The manufacturer of the biologic drug may also be able to help locate and contact a reputable gastroenterologist at the destination.

- Be aware that not all countries have access to the same medications. Some countries, for example, may use biosimilars, which would mean a switch for the patient. Some countries also do not have access to tofacitinib or vedolizumab. It is recommended to liaise with an IBD center in the patient's destination of travel to clarify these issues. This can be done either by personal connections or the IBD Passport network.

Obtaining Medical Advice When Traveling

SELF-MANAGEMENT PLAN

The unpredictable nature of IBD means that an alteration in symptoms may occur during travel. The physician/nurse practitioner should provide a personalized self-management plan to the patient in case of flares or a change in symptoms during travel. This should include alterations of medications and may include providing rescue medications to be used in an emergency, such as antibiotics or corticosteroids. Dietary recommendations can also be included. It is helpful to outline a plan in a document (paper or electronic) that is carried by the patient on their trip. Electronic resources and symptom trackers such as Oshi Health[17] may help patients self-manage their disease while traveling and give them more confidence. They may also provide a communication bridge from the patient to the hospital. As mentioned previously, IBD Passport[16] is also an excellent and well-evaluated online resource that provides a vast array of information to support and educate patients and health care professionals regarding travel with IBD. The website contains in-depth advice on many aspects covered in this chapter, such as the importance of and how to obtain travel insurance, vaccinations, and travel with medications.

CONTACTING THE HOME IBD TEAM

The health care provider should consider providing a means of email access to the traveler for emergencies or medical advice during the trip. Depending on the destination, phone contact with the provider may prove difficult due to time zone differences, the availability of the provider during periods when the patient is able to call, or access to international calls. Advising patients to obtain an international calling card, renting a cell phone, or changing their existing plan to allow international calls may also be helpful.

Email access may be the best way to communicate when away from home. Internet access is often widely available in airports and commercial establishments.

FINDING A DOCTOR WHEN TRAVELING

Obtaining medical advice when overseas is a common concern to patients who are traveling.[1,2] Hotels will often have a physician on call, which would be the first line of medical help. The International Association for Medical Assistance to Travelers maintains a list for its members of doctors in clinics in a large number of countries.[18] The US Department of State maintains a list of the websites of embassies, consulates, and diplomatic missions. On these sites, under the professional services category, there is a listing of physicians by specialty and whether they understand English.[19] In addition, the consulate may be able to help with family notification and helping the patient gain access to their home bank account for any needed funds. The traveler can register with the Department of State before leaving on the trip.

Traveler's Diarrhea

Travel to less-developed countries has the added risk of contracting a bacterial or viral infection that may lead to a diarrheal illness. There have been large-scale epidemics of norovirus reported on cruise ships. Fifty to 90% of patients traveling to nonindustrialized countries may be afflicted by diarrhea.[20]Advice regarding safe drinking and dietary changes may minimize the risk.

AVOIDING TRAVELER'S DIARRHEA

The patient should be advised the following:
- Avoid drinking water from questionable sources without boiling it. Bottled water may be safer and should be used both for drinking and brushing teeth. Avoid ice in drinks.
- Avoid swallowing water when showering, as well as swimming pool water, fresh water, and potentially contaminated ocean water.
- Stick with cooked vegetables, fish, and meats and avoid salads from buffet food as this may have been washed in tap water.
- Avoid dairy products unless they know that the conditions in which the product were prepared involves pasteurization and sterilization.
- Avoid food from food carts, street food, or food that may have been sitting out at room temperature for a long time. Prepared foods, such as salads, are often sources of bacterial contamination.
- Avoid fresh fruits unless they can be peeled at the time of ingestion.
- Prior to travel discuss with a physician whether prophylaxis of traveler's diarrhea with fluoroquinolones, azithromycin, or rifaximin should be considered. This can be carried in the emergency kit, along with instructions in a self-management plan regarding symptoms to be alert for and when to use the medications.

MANAGING TRAVELER'S DIARRHEA

If traveling to a destination where traveler's diarrhea may be common, it is important to provide patients with advice on how to manage this as part of a written or electronic self-management plan.

If traveler's diarrhea is suspected, patients should be advised of the following:
- Maintaining hydration is important. Drinking an oral rehydration solution as previously described may help maintain fluid and electrolyte balance. Soups provide both fluid and salt. Saltine crackers will also provide salt. This can be part of the traveler's emergency kit and brought from home.
- For mild diarrhea, antidiarrheal medication, such as bismuth subsalicylate and loperamide, can be used to control symptoms. For more severe diarrhea, these medications need to be combined with antibacterial therapy.
- For severe diarrhea, medical advice in the travel destination should be sought wherever possible. Antibiotic therapy should be in part directed by the typical enteric pathogens seen in the travel destination. Fluoroquinolones, rifaximin, and azithromycin have all been used for management of traveler's diarrhea. Regimens include 200 mg of rifaximin 3 times a day for 3 days, 750 mg of ciprofloxacin once a day for 1 to 3 days, 500 mg of levofloxacin once a day for 3 days, and 1 g of single-dose azithromycin.

- If a patient is going to a high-risk area, it is reasonable to give the patient a prescription for one of these regimens with guidance on when to start and when to seek medical attention in the case of diarrheal illness while traveling.

Overall, with careful planning, the patient with IBD can travel safely and enjoyably.

Travel With an Ostomy

Patients who had a surgery and stoma formation may be apprehensive about travel and how this may impact on stoma function, but there is no reason why they cannot continue to travel with advanced planning. It is important to liaise with the surgical and stoma care teams to reassure patients and provide the appropriate support and education. Many of the stoma supply companies will have information in local languages regarding travel with a stoma, but concerns that patients may have and ways to reassure them include the following:

- The stoma bag will behave the same during air travel as it does on the ground, but cabin pressure in aircraft can sometimes cause excess flatus (wind). If the stoma appliance has a filter, it will enable air to escape and hide any embarrassing odors.
- Advise patients to avoid food that may cause bloating and excess wind the day prior to travel.
- Before going through airport security, it is advisable to change the stoma appliance at the last minute to ensure it is empty. Security staff are duty bound to investigate any anomalies, but this will always be done in a discreet way. Advise patients to carry a stoma passport or travel certificate, as described earlier, to avoid awkward situations.[21]
- Patients who have had a colectomy and ileostomy will be more susceptible to dehydration due to the reduced ability to absorb fluid and electrolytes from the diet as effectively. Advise patients to be aware of the signs of dehydration and seek medical advice if they think they are becoming symptomatic.
- Advise patients to discuss their travel plans with their stoma nurse, as they may need additional products they would normally not need for activities such as swimming and for hot temperatures that cause perspiration, which means they will have to change their appliance more frequently.
- Due to increased security, carrying scissors in checked luggage is more difficult. Advise patients to precut all barriers at home. Alternatively, some stoma companies have a moldable system that does not need cutting to size.
- As with medication, pack stoma care supplies in both carry-on and checked luggage.
- Store stoma supplies in a cool place—do not leave ostomy products in hot places (eg, in the car) for long periods, since the heat may damage the baseplate adhesive.
- In the case that patients run out of supplies when abroad, advise them to take a note of the product name and code (usually found on the prescription) as well as the telephone number of their stoma supply company so that they can contact them.
- Stoma passport or travel certificates are available from most stoma companies or a stoma care nurse. These state the need for patients to carry stoma care supplies in case they are questioned at airport security/customs. In addition, it is helpful to take a copy of their prescription, which shows all the product codes and description.
- Similarly, for international travel, the stoma companies and ostomy associations[21] can provide stoma care and product information in different languages.

The Returning Traveler

Many travel-related infections will develop within 4 weeks of returning.[4] It is therefore important to be vigilant for new symptoms, especially those that do not fit with the patient's usual IBD symptoms. A history of foreign travel, stool, and parasite cultures should always be considered for patients with a recent history of foreign travel.

References

1. Soonawala D, van Eggermond AM, Fidder H, Visser LG. Pre-travel preparation and travel-related morbidity in patients with inflammatory bowel disease. *Inflamm Bowel Dis*. 2012;18(11):2079-2085.
2. Greveson, K, Shepherd T, Mulligan JP. Travel health and pre-travel preparation in the patient with inflammatory bowel disease. *Frontline Gastroenterology*. 2015;7(1):60-65.
3. Wasan SK, Coukos JA, Farraye FA. Vaccinating the inflammatory bowel disease patient: deficiencies in gastroenterologists knowledge. *Inflamm Bowel Dis*. 2011;17(12):2536-2560.
4. Rahier JF, Magro F, Abreu C, et al. Second European evidence-based consensus on the prevention, diagnosis and management of opportunistic infections in inflammatory bowel disease. *J Crohns Colitis*. 2014;8(6):443-468.
5. Destinations. Centers for Disease Control and Prevention. http://wwwnc.cdc.gov/travel/destinations/list. Accessed December 12, 2018.
6. Immunocompromised travelers. Centers for Disease Control and Prevention. https://wwwnc.cdc.gov/travel/yellowbook/2020/travelers-with-additional-considerations/immunocompromised-travelers. Accessed December 12, 2018.
7. Medical letter of exemption. Yellow Fever Zone. https://nathnacyfzone.org.uk/factsheet/6/medical-letter-of-exemption. Accessed September 25, 2019.
8. Travelers with disabilities and medical conditions. Transportation Safety Administration. https://www.tsa.gov/travel/special-procedures. Accessed December 12, 2018.
9. Oral rehydration solutions: made at home. Rehydration Project. http://rehydrate.org/solutions/homemade.htm. Accessed December 12, 2018.
10. Nguyen CG, Bernstein CN, Bitton A, et al. Consensus statements on the risk, prevention and treatment of venous thromboembolism in inflammatory bowel disease: Canadian Association of Gastroenterology. *Gastroenterology*. 2014;146(3):835-848.e6.
11. Vavrika S, Rogler G, Maetzler S, et al. High altitude journeys and flights are associated with an increased risk of flares in inflammatory bowel disease patients. *J Crohns Colitis*. 2014;8:191-199.
12. Travel with medication. Transport Security Administration. https://www.google.com/search?client=safari&rls=en&q=Travel+with+medication.+Transport+Security+Administration. https://www.tsa.gov/blog/2014/09/05/tsa-travel-tips-traveling-medication.&ie=UTF-8&oe=UTF-8. Accessed March 21, 2021.
13. International Names of Common IBD Medications. Crohn's & Colitis Foundation of America. http://www.ccfa.org/resources/traveling-with-ibd.html. Accessed December 12, 2018.
14. Oley Foundation. www.oley.org. Accessed December 12, 2018.
15. Department of Health. Travelling with controlled drugs. https://www.gov.uk/travelling-controlled-drugs. Accessed December 12, 2018.
16. IBD Passport. www.ibdpassport.com. Accessed December 12, 2018.
17. OSHI Health. https://www.oshihealth.com. Accessed December 12, 2018.
18. Doctors and clinics. International Association for Medical Assistance to Travellers. http://www.iamat.org/doctors_clinics.cfm. Accessed April 19, 2013.
19. US Department of State. http://www.usembassy.gov. Accessed April 19, 2013.
20. Kollaritsch H, Paulke-Korinek M, Wiedermann U. Traveler's diarrhea. *Infect Dis Clin North Am*. 2012;26(3):691-706.
21. United Ostomy Associations of America. https://www.ostomy.org/ostomy-travel-and-tsa-communication-card. Accessed December 12, 2018.

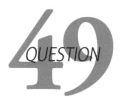

QUESTION 49

HOW SHOULD WE APPROACH THE DIAGNOSIS AND EVALUATION OF SEXUAL DYSFUNCTION IN PATIENTS WITH IBD?

Punyanganie S. de Silva, MBBS, MPH and Sonia Friedman, MD

Inflammatory bowel disease (IBD) often affects both men and women during their peak reproductive years,[1] and it is not uncommon for patients to develop complications and concerns regarding sexual function. Previous studies have shown that about 40% to 66% of women and up to 44% of men with IBD report sexual dysfunction.[2,3] In women, sexual dysfunction can occur at any of the 3 phases of sexual response, namely desire, arousal, and orgasm. In men, sexual dysfunction consists of erectile dysfunction, decreased libido, and abnormal ejaculation.

Patients with IBD can develop sexual dysfunction due to a variety of causes, which include active inflammation; surgical treatment in the abdominal, pelvic, or perianal regions; medication use, including corticosteroids, narcotics, and neuropsychiatric medications; hypogonadism; and depression. For many patients with IBD, their gastroenterologist remains their primary medical provider, so effective evaluation or screening for sexual dysfunction in both male and female patients is important. Although this is a sensitive and somewhat difficult conversation, patients with IBD have demonstrated willingness to engage and often welcome their provider's questions regarding their sexual function.[4]

Previously, one of the key limitations in assessing for sexual dysfunction was the lack of a validated, IBD-specific scoring system to evaluate sexual function. Existing tools such as the Female Sexual Function Index and the International Index of Erectile Function do not take into account problems that are unique to patients with IBD such as passing stool during intercourse, embarrassment due to setons or stomas, and/or severe perianal disease. In order to address this limitation, validated IBD-specific sexual dysfunction surveys for men and women have recently been introduced and are currently being used in research studies.[5,6] These surveys use a 10-point

Rubin DT, Friedman S, Farraye FA, eds. *Curbside Consultation in IBD:*
49 Clinical Questions, Third Edition (pp 331-336).
© 2022 Taylor & Francis Group.

Table 49-1
IBD-Male Sexual Dysfunction Scale

1. In the past year, how frequently has CD or UC affected your desire for sexual activity?
2. In the past year, has having CD or UC prevented you from having sex?
3. In the past year, has having CD or UC caused problems during sex?
4. In the past year, has having CD or UC caused you to feel guilty about intimacy or intercourse?
5. In the past year, to what extent has fatigue or lack of energy impacted your sex life?
6. In the past year, to what extent has abdominal or pelvic pain affected your sex life?
7. In the past year, how much has increased bowel movement frequency affected your sex life?
8. In the past year, how much has anal bleeding or discharge affected your satisfaction with your sex life?
9. In the past year, how much has anal pain, discomfort, or irritation affected your satisfaction with your sex life?
1. Are you ever afraid of participating in sexual activity due to your CD or UC?

CD = Crohn's disease; UC = ulcerative colitis.

---

scale for men (IBD-Male Sexual Dysfunction Scale) and 15-point scale for women (IBD-Female Sexual Dysfunction Scale) to identify features of sexual dysfunction (Tables 49-1 and 49-2).

In clinical practice, it is useful to initiate the conversation regarding sexual dysfunction by asking direct questions. This helps determine whether there is a possible problem with sexual function. Sometimes a broad question, "Do you experience any difficulties during sexual activity?" provides the patient with the necessary window to elaborate further. Other questions to consider asking are whether there are any problems during sexual activity due to either IBD activity (anal bleeding or discharge, pelvic or abdominal pain) or ostomy/fistulae/other perianal disease. The physician should also ask their patients whether they experience any mental distress or anxiety when undertaking sexual activity due to concerns related to IBD or effects of IBD treatment or surgery. Female patients should be asked whether they have dyspareunia or pelvic or abdominal pain during intercourse. Male patients should be asked if they have any erectile or ejaculatory concerns. Since fatigue and insomnia can also lead to sexual dysfunction, this should also be queried. Once a disorder has been identified, further determination should be made to establish whether this is a sexual interest/arousal disorder or orgasmic or genito-pelvic pain disorder (Figures 49-1 and 49-2).

When evaluating patients for sexual dysfunction, it is helpful to consider separating potential problems into different categories.[7] This should increase confidence in engaging patients in these sometimes difficult conversations. In this way, we can separate the problem into one or more specific categories and initiate appropriate treatments. Broadly, we can separate the problems to those related to IBD-specific inflammation or activity, IBD-related postsurgical complications or effects, medication use (including corticosteroids, neuropsychiatric medications, and opiates), hypogonadism, and mood disorders such as anxiety and depression.

Table 49-2
IBD-Female Sexual Dysfunction Scale

1. In the past year, do you feel that your CD or UC disease contributed to distress in your sex life?
2. In the past year, has your CD or UC disease prevented you from starting a sexual relationship?
3. In the past year, has your CD or UC disease delayed your starting a sexual relationship?
4. In the past year, did your CD or UC diagnosis prevent you from having sex?
5. In the past year, did your CD or UC diagnosis cause problems during sex?
6. In the past year, have you been conscious of your CD or UC during intercourse?
7. In the past year, did you have abdominal or pelvic pain during intercourse?
8. In the past year, did you have rectal/anal pain during intercourse?
9. In the past year, did you fear experiencing abdominal/pelvic pain during sexual activity?
10. In the past year, did you have a reduced desire or interest, or did you have trouble getting aroused during intercourse due to your CD or UC?
11. In the past year, did your CD or UC make you feel too tired to participate in sexual activities?
12. In the past year, how often did you feel that your CD or UC has negatively affected your sexual life?
13. In the past year, did you feel guilty about CD or UC and its effect on your partner?
14. In the past year, how much has anal bleeding or discharge affected your satisfaction with your sex life?
15. In the past year, how much has abdominal or pelvic pain affected your satisfaction with your sex life?

CD = Crohn's disease; UC = ulcerative colitis.

IBD-Specific Inflammation

Several studies have demonstrated that active disease can lead to discomfort during sexual activity, both mentally and physically. Therefore, it is important to consider asking follow-up questions pertaining to sexual activity when patients describe active IBD symptoms. Perianal complications such as abscesses or cutaneous fistulae, skin lesions such as fissures or skin tags, arthritic deformities, and abdominal and pelvic pain can all severely impair sexual function. In addition, the presence of active disease can lead to fatigue, which in turn can cause patients to experience difficulties, trepidation, lack of interest, and even fear of sexual activity. If a patient reports such IBD symptoms, the physician can then take this opportunity to inquire about any concerns they may have.

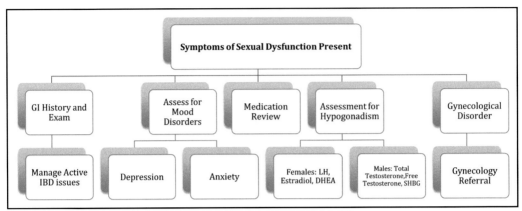

Figure 49-1. Causes of sexual dysfunction in men and women with IBD.

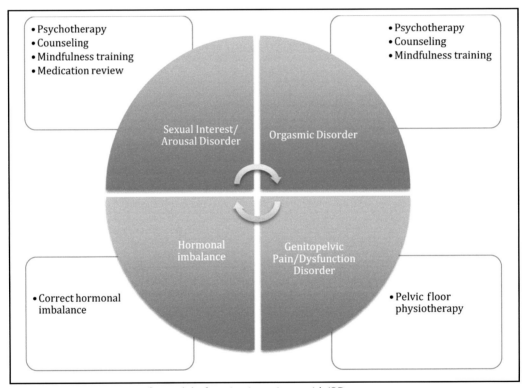

Figure 49-2. Management of sexual dysfunction in patients with IBD.

Postsurgical Complications

Certain IBD surgeries, such as ileoanal anastomosis (J pouch) surgery, have been associated with increased symptoms of dyspareunia, stool leakage, inability to attain orgasm, retrograde ejaculation, erectile dysfunction, reduced sexual satisfaction, and impaired body image.[8] Colostomies and ileostomies have also been linked to impaired body image and increased incidence of depression and anxiety, which in turn can lead to symptoms of sexual dysfunction. As health care providers, we should discuss with our patients the effect of surgery on sexual function during the preoperative evaluation. After surgery, health care providers should regularly screen patients for problems that interfere with sexual intercourse, such as perceptions of decreased attractiveness and dyspareunia in ileoanal J pouch and ostomy patients.

IBD Medications That Affect Sexual Function

Corticosteroids are frequently used in the management of IBD and are known to adversely affect sexual function. Actions such as avoiding long-term corticosteroid use, preventing steroid-induced diabetes, and referring appropriately to endocrinology are recommended if steroid-dependent patients report symptoms of sexual dysfunction. Opioids, antiepileptics, antipsychotics, antidepressants, anxiolytics, and psychoanaleptics have also been linked to symptoms of fatigue, low mood, insomnia, and erectile dysfunction in men[9] and sexual dysfunction in women. It is therefore imperative that health care providers review the effects of these medications on sexual function with symptomatic patients. This may then encourage the patient to, under specialist guidance, either reduce the dose of the culprit medication or seek a suitable alternative.

Hypogonadism

Hypogonadism is a major cause of sexual dysfunction among men. Prior studies have shown that up to 40% of men with IBD have hypogonadism. Testosterone replacement has been successfully used to treat erectile and arousal disorders, although the role of testosterone in sexual dysfunction in men with IBD remains unknown. If erectile/sexual dysfunction is suspected in a male patients with IBD, then it is recommended to screen for hypogonadism measuring total and free testosterone levels as well as sex hormone-binding globulin. In female patients, screening for hypogonadism can be undertaken by asking about amenorrhea, menstrual irregularities, hot flashes, and infertility. It is also helpful to check luteinizing hormone, estradiol, and dehydroepiandrosterone levels or refer appropriately to gynecology or endocrinology for testing.

Mood Disorders

As previously mentioned, depression is a major risk factor for decreased sexual function, and sexual dysfunction can also lead to depression.[5-7] Patients with IBD often suffer from mood disorders, so appropriate referral for counseling, psychotherapy, and possibly drug treatment can be helpful. Patients may sometimes find the prospect of seeking psychiatric support daunting, and a supportive environment in the IBD clinic, with an integrated team approach with trained professionals who are sensitive to the specific needs and concerns of patients with IBD, can be tremendously helpful.

Treatment Advice

Once sexual dysfunction is suspected and the potential cause/causes elicited, these should be systematically addressed. Before therapy for sexual dysfunction, address mood, self-image, stressors, and relationship issues (see Figures 49-1 and 49-2). If the patient's active IBD symptoms are the likely cause, then optimizing medical therapy would be the next step. In addition, the health care provider should refer their patient appropriately for further evaluation and treatment. Pelvic floor physical therapy has been shown to be an effective therapy for sexual dysfunction in patients with myofascial pelvic pain, survivors of gynecologic cancer, and those following prostatectomy and colectomies. Therefore, referral for myofascial release and pelvic floor strengthening exercises may be of benefit.

Conclusion

The symptoms, disease complications, and treatments for IBD can influence body image, intimacy, and sexual function. This in turn can significantly impair our patients' quality of life. Given the often high level of trust patients with IBD share with their IBD health care provider, they are willing and have been shown to be comfortable discussing these concerns. Therefore, it is important that we routinely ask about any symptoms of sexual dysfunction when evaluating patients in clinic and address them accordingly.

References

1. Moody G, Probert CSJ, Srinivastava EM, et al. Sexual dysfunction amongst women with Crohn's disease: a hidden problem. *Digestion*. 1992;52(3-4):179-183.
2. Marin L, Manosa M, Garcia-Planella E, et al. Sexual function and patients perceptions in inflammatory bowel disease: a case-control study. *J Gastroenterol*. 2013;48(6):713-720.
3. Timmer A, Bauer A, Kemptner D, Fürst A, Rogler G. Determinants of male sexual function in inflammatory bowel disease: a survey-based cross-sectional analysis in 280 men. *Inflamm Bowel Dis*. 2007;13(10):1236-1243.
4. Eluri S, Cross RK, Martin C, et al. Inflammatory bowel diseases can adversely impact domains of sexual function such as satisfaction with sex life. *Dig Dis Sci*. 2018;63(6):1572-1582.
5. O'Toole A, de Silva PS, Marc LG, et al. Sexual dysfunction in men with inflammatory bowel disease: a new ibd-specific scale. *Inflamm Bowel Dis*. 2018;24(2):310-316.
6. de Silva PS, O'Toole A, Marc LG, et al. Development of a sexual dysfunction scale for women with inflammatory bowel disease. *Inflamm Bowel Dis*. 2018;24(11):2350-2359.
7. Friedman S. Sexual dysfunction in inflammatory bowel disease: "don't ask, don't tell" doesn't work. *Inflamm Bowel Dis*. 2015;21(4):948-950.
8. Jedel S, Hood M, Keshavarzian A. Getting personal: a review of sexual functioning, body image, and their impact on quality of life in IBD patients. *Inflamm Bowel Dis*. 2015;21(4):923-938.
9. Friedman S, Magnussen B, O'Toole A, Fedder J, Larsen MD, Nørgård BM. Increased use of medications for erectile dysfunction in men with ulcerative colitis and Crohn's disease compared to men without inflammatory bowel disease: a nationwide cohort study. *Am J Gastroenterol*. 2018;113(9):1355-1362.

FINANCIAL DISCLOSURES

Dr. Bincy P. Abraham has no financial or proprietary interest in the materials presented herein.

Dr. Shintaro Akiyama has no financial or proprietary interest in the materials presented herein.

Dr. Jessica R. Allegretti is on the scientific advisory board for Finch Therapeutics, Artugen, and Servatus. She reports research support from Merck.

Dr. Ashwin N. Ananthakrishnan is on the scientific advisory boards for Abbvie and Gilead.

Dr. Jordan E. Axelrad has no financial or proprietary interest in the materials presented herein.

Dr. Filip J. Baert has no financial or proprietary interest in the materials presented herein.

Dr. Edward L. Barnes has no financial or proprietary interest in the materials presented herein.

Dr. Alyse Bedell has no financial or proprietary interest in the materials presented herein.

Dr. Shomron Ben-Horin has received consulting and advisory board fees and/or research support from AbbVie, MSD, Janssen, Takeda, BMS, Pfizer, Roche, Ferring, Galmed, and Celltrion

Dr. Madeline Bertha has no financial or proprietary interest in the materials presented herein.

Dr. David G. Binion has no financial or proprietary interest in the materials presented herein.

Dr. Diana Bolotin has no financial or proprietary interest in the materials presented herein.

Dr. Brian P. Bosworth has no financial or proprietary interest in the materials presented herein.

Michael Buie has no financial or proprietary interest in the materials presented herein.

Dr. Anthony Buisson has no financial or proprietary interest in the materials presented herein.

Dr. Freddy Caldera is a consultant for GSK and has received grant funding from Sanofi Pharmaceuticals.

Dr. Victor G. Chedid has no financial or proprietary interest in the materials presented herein.

Dr. Adam Cheifetz is a consultant for Abbvie, Janssen, Procise, Prometheus, Artugen, Bacainn, BMS, and Arena.

Dr. Britt Christensen has received consulting fees or research grants from Takeda, Janssen, Abbvie, Gilead, Novartis, Falk, Ferring, Pfizer, and Chiesi.

Dr. William T. Clarke has no financial or proprietary interest in the materials presented herein.

Dr. Jennie Clough has no financial or proprietary interest in the materials presented herein.

Dr. Erica R. Cohen has no financial or proprietary interest in the materials presented herein.

Dr. Jean-Frederic Colombel has no financial or proprietary interest in the materials presented herein.

Dr. Susan Connor has received honoraria for advisory board participation, speaker fees, educational support, and/or research support for Liverpool Hospital, South Western Sydney Local Health District Academic Unit or the IBD charity Crohn's Colitis Cure from Abbvie, Aspen, BMS, Celgene, Celltrion, Chiesi, Dr. Falk, Ferring, Fresenius Kabi, Gilead, Janssen, MSD, Novartis, Pfizer, and Takeda. She has received nonpharmacological research support from Agency for Clinical Innovation, Gastroenterological Society of Australia, Medical Research Future Fund, The Leona M. and Harry B. Helmsley Charitable Trust, and South Western Sydney Local Health District.

Dr. Ferdinando D'Amico has no financial or proprietary interest in the materials presented herein.

Dr. Silvio Danese has served as a speaker, consultant, and advisory board member for Schering-Plough, Abbvie, Actelion, Alphawasserman, AstraZeneca, Cellerix, Cosmo Pharmaceuticals, Ferring, Genentech, Grunenthal, Johnson and Johnson, Millenium Takeda, MSD, Nikkiso Europe GmbH, Novo Nordisk, Nycomed, Pfizer, Pharmacosmos, UCB Pharma, and Vifor.

Dr. Punyanganie S. de Silva has no financial or proprietary interest in the materials presented herein.

Dr. Jean A. Donet has no financial or proprietary interest in the materials presented herein.

Dr. Iris Dotan has no financial or proprietary interest in the materials presented herein.

Dr. David Drobne has no financial or proprietary interest in the materials presented herein.

Dr. Francis A. Farraye receives a consulting fee from Arena, BMS, Braintree Labs, Gilead, GI Reviewers, GSK, IBD Educational Group, Iterative Scopes, Janssen, Pfizer, and Sebela. He has ownership interest in Innovation Pharmaceuticals. He lists DSMB for Lilly and Theravance.

Dr. Joseph D. Feuerstein has no financial or proprietary interest in the materials presented herein.

Dr. Sonia Friedman has no financial or proprietary interest in the materials presented herein.

Dr. Kerri Glassner has no financial or proprietary interest in the materials presented herein.

Dr. Idan Goren has no financial or proprietary interest in the materials presented herein.

Kay Greveson has no financial or proprietary interest in the materials presented herein.

Dr. Bilal Hameed has received research grants from Gilead, Intercept, and Pliant.

Dr. Muhammad Bader Hammami has no financial or proprietary interest in the materials presented herein.

Dr. Stephen B. Hanauer is a speaker for AbbVie, American Regent, Bristol Myers Squibb, Janssen, Pfizer, and Takeda. He is a consultant for AbbVie, Allergan, American Regent, Amgen, Arena, Boehringer Ingelheim, Bristol Myers Squibb. Celgene, Celltrion, Genentech, Gilead, GSK, Janssen, Lilly, Merck, Nestle, Novartis, Pfizer, Progenity, Prometheus, Receptos, Salix, Samsung Bioepis, Seres Therapeutics, Takeda, Tigenex, UCB Pharma, and VHsquared. Dr. Hanauer reports clinical research (institution) for AbbVie, Allergan, Amgen, Celgene, Genentech, GSK, Janssen, Lilly, Novartis, Pfizer, Prometheus, Receptos, Takeda, and UCB Pharma. He lists DSMB for Arena and Bristol Myers Squibb.

Dr. Jana G. Hashash has no financial or proprietary interest in the materials presented herein.

Dr. Hans Herfarth has no financial or proprietary interest in the materials presented herein.

Dr. Peter M. Irving has no financial or proprietary interest in the materials presented herein.

Dr. Steven H. Itzkowitz has no financial or proprietary interest in the materials presented herein.

Dr. Sunanda V. Kane is a consultant to Bristol Meyers Squibb, Janssen, Spherix Health, United Healthcare, and TechLab. She is a Section Editor for *UpToDate*.

Dr. Gilaad G. Kaplan has no financial or proprietary interest in the materials presented herein.

Dr. Seymour Katz has no financial or proprietary interest in the materials presented herein.

Dr. Arthur Kavanaugh has no financial or proprietary interest in the materials presented herein.

Dr. Maia Kayal has no financial or proprietary interest in the materials presented herein.

Dr. Laurie Keefer is a consultant to Abbvie, is on the advisory board of Reckitt Health, has equity ownership in Trellus Health, and is on the board of directors for the Rome Foundation.

Dr. *Jami Kinnucan* has no financial or proprietary interest in the materials presented herein.

Dr. *Mark Lazarev* has no financial or proprietary interest in the materials presented herein.

Dr. *Jonathan A. Leighton* provides research for CheckCap and Capsovision and consulting for Zo Diagnostics and Olympus.

Dr. *Irving Levine* has no financial or proprietary interest in the materials presented herein.

Dr. *Alexander N. Levy* has no financial or proprietary interest in the materials presented herein.

Dr. *James D. Lewis*, since 2018, has served as a consultant for Samsung Bioepis, UCB, Bristo-Myers Squibb, Nestle Health Science, Merck, Celgen, Janssen Pharmaceuticals, Bridge Biotherapeutics Inc, Entasis Therapeutics, Abbvie, Pfizer, Gilead, Protagonist Therapeutics, and Arena Pharmaceuticals. He has had research funding from Takeda Pharmaceuticals, Janssen Pharmaceuticals, and Nestle Health Science. He has had educational grant from Takeda Pharmaceuticals.

Dr. *Amy L. Lightner* is a consultant for Takeda.

Dr. *Jimmy K. Limdi* has no financial or proprietary interest in the materials presented herein.

Dr. *Uma Mahadevan* is a consultant for Abbvie, Janssen, Takeda, Pfizer, BMS, Prometheus Biosciences, Lilly, and Gilead.

Dr. *Gil Y. Melmed* is a consultant for Abbvie, Arena, Boehringer-Ingelheim, Bristol-Meyers Squibb/Celgene, Janssen, Medtronic, Samsung Biooepis, Pfizer, Takeda, and Techlab. He receives research support from Pfizer.

Dr. *Oluwakemi Onajin* has no financial or proprietary interest in the materials presented herein.

Dr. *Mark T. Osterman* is a advisory board consultant for AbbVie, Bristol Myers Squibb, Elan, Genentech/Roche, Janssen, Lycera, Merck, Pfizer, Takeda, and UCB. He receives research grant support from UCB.

Dr. *Aoibhlinn O'Toole* has no financial or proprietary interest in the materials presented herein.

Dr. *Baldeep S. Pabla* has no financial or proprietary interest in the materials presented herein.

Dr. *Carolina Palmela* is a consultant for Janssen and Laboratórios Vitória.

Dr. *Remo Panaccione* has no financial or proprietary interest in the materials presented herein.

Dr. *Konstantinos Papamichael* reports personal fees from Mitsubishi Tanabe Pharma (lecture fee), Prometheus Laboratories Inc (consultancy fee), and ProciseDx (scientific advisory board fee).

Dr. *Shabana F. Pasha* has no financial or proprietary interest in the materials presented herein.

Dr. *Shivani A. Patel* has no financial or proprietary interest in the materials presented herein.

Dr. Joel Pekow is a consultant for CVS Caremark and Genetech. He has received grants from Abbvie and Takeda; has been on the advisory boards of Janssen, Takeda, and Pfizer; and has been a consultant to Verastem.

Tamar Pfeffer Gik has served as a consultant in the field of nutrition to Takeda since 2020 and to Strauss-Danone Israel since 2021.

Dr. Ralley Prentice has no financial or proprietary interest in the materials presented herein.

Dr. David T. Rubin has received grant support from Takeda and has served as a consultant for Abbvie, Altrubio, Allergan Inc, Arena Pharmaceuticals, Bellatrix Pharmaceuticals, Boehringer Ingelheim Ltd, Bristol-Myers Squibb, Celgene Corp/Syneos, Connect BioPharma, GalenPharma/Atlantica, Genentech/Roche, Gilead Sciences, InDex Pharmaceuticals, Ironwood Pharmaceuticals, Iterative Scopes, Janssen Pharmaceuticals, Lilly, Materia Prima, Pfizer, Prometheus Biosciences, Reistone, Takeda, and Techlab Inc. He is also co-founder of Cornerstones Health, Inc.

Dr. David B. Sachar has not disclosed any relevant financial relationships.

Dr. Atsushi Sakuraba has no financial or proprietary interest in the materials presented herein.

Dr. Akriti P. Saxena has no financial or proprietary interest in the materials presented herein.

Dr. David A. Schwartz is a consultant for Abbvie, UCB, Janssen, Takeda, Gilead, Pfizer, and Genetech. He reports grant support from UCB and Tract—DSMB member.

Dr. Seth R. Shaffer has no financial or proprietary interest in the materials presented herein.

Dr. Abha G. Singh has no financial or proprietary interest in the materials presented herein.

Dr. Arun Swaminath has no financial or proprietary interest in the materials presented herein.

Dr. Eva Szigethy has not disclosed any relevant financial relationships.

Dr. Norah Terrault has no financial or proprietary interest in the materials presented herein.

Dr. Joana Torres receives advisory board fees from Janssen, Arena Pharmaceuticals, Gilead and Galapagos, and Pfizer.

Dr. Andrew R. Watson has no financial or proprietary interest in the materials presented herein.

Emily Weaver has no financial or proprietary interest in the materials presented herein.

Dr. Roni Weisshof has no financial or proprietary interest in the materials presented herein.

Dr. Rachel W. Winter has no financial or proprietary interest in the materials presented herein.

Dr. Yang (Clare) Wu has no financial or proprietary interest in the materials presented herein.

Dr. Akihiro Yamada receives honoraria for lectures from Takeda, JIMRO, Kyorin, Mochida, and Janssen and payment for educational events from Abbvie and Zeria.

Dr. Toni M. Zahorian has no financial or proprietary interest in the materials presented herein.

INDEX

343

Printed in the United States
by Baker & Taylor Publisher Services